CURING
THE "INCURABLE"

EATING
ALIVE II

Dr. Jonn Matsen, ND

Foreword by Jennifer Beals

Recipes by Irene Hayton & Carol Song
Illustrations by Nelson Dewey

Author of Eating Alive and The Secrets to Great Health

For Fast Results
Go To The
FastTrack Section
Of This Book

Published by Goodwin Books Ltd.
North Vancouver, BC Canada
Toll-free: 1-877-222-9858

Distributed by **Gordon Soules Book
Publishers Ltd.** ● 1359 Ambleside Lane,
West Vancouver, BC, Canada V7T 2Y9
● PMB 620, 1916 Pike Place #12,
Seattle, WA 98101-1097 US
E-mail: books@gordonsoules.com
Web site: http://www.gordonsoules.com
(604) 922 6588 Fax: (604) 688 5442

Revised edition: 2004

Eating Alive II
Published by:
Goodwin Books, Ltd.
156 West 3rd Street
North Vancouver, BC Canada V7M 1E8

Cover Design: Drew Welsh
Technical Editor/Project Manager: Irene Hayton
Editor: Val Wilson

NATIONAL LIBRARY OF CANADA CATALOGUING IN PUBLICATION DATA

Matsen, Jonn, 1949–
    Eating Alive II : Curing the "Incurable"

Includes bibliographical references and index.
ISBN 0-9682853-1-7

    1. Diet in disease.   2. Nutritionally induced diseases—
Popular works.   3. Naturopathy—Popular works.   I. Title.

RM216.M386 2001   615.8'54   C2001-903531-4

I dedicate this book to those who are trying so hard to get well, but who haven't yet found all the missing pieces to their health puzzle.

Notes to the Reader

- It is important that we each assume responsibility for our own actions with regard to our health, well-being, and safety.

- This book is not intended to be a substitute for consulting with your physician and obtaining medical advice and supervision regarding any activity, procedure, or suggestion that might affect your health.

- Neither the author nor the publisher shall be liable or responsible for any loss, injury, or damage allegedly arising from any information or suggestion offered in this book.

Contents

PART I:
FASTTRACK to
THE EATING ALIVE PROGRAM

PART II:
THE FOOD SECTION

PART III:
DETAILS! DETAILS! DETAILS!

PART IV:
HELPFUL RESOURCES

Foreword

By Jennifer Beals

While I've always been physically fit, I haven't always been in great health. In the late 1990s, I was diagnosed with chronic fatigue syndrome and Epstein-Barr virus, which drained my energy for months.

I saw one of the top endocrinologists in New York, who diagnosed me with lupus and thyroiditis, but he was unable to help me. He suggested that I seek the advice of an alternative doctor. In an effort to cure my fatigue, I gave up eating sugar and wheat but was still really tired all the time.

I was in Vancouver, BC, Canada shooting a film, wondering how I was going to regain my energy. I saw Dr. Matsen's first book, *Eating Alive*, on a coffee table in a hotel lobby and started reading it right there. His philosophy that the body is meant to be healthy and can heal itself, once you get the digestive system working properly, really made sense to me. Thankfully his office was close by, in North Vancouver, so I booked an appointment to see him.

I followed his program, which involved changing the way I ate and taking supplements. The results were amazing; three weeks later I was feeling like myself again. I try to avoid sugar, wheat, and caffeine and have even used Dr. Matsen's eating program, along with regular running, to help shed the pounds that I had to put on for the leading role in *A House Divided*.

The results I got from following his program have shown me how important the digestive system is for health and wellness.

Jennifer Beals has been involved in the film industry for the past two decades. The accomplished actress has appeared in more than 30 films, including leading roles in *Flashdance, Devil in a Blue Dress*, and *A House Divided* and has worked with stars such as Gene Hackman, Dustin Hoffman, Faye Dunaway, and Denzel Washington. Jennifer is currently starring in the Showtime Original Series, *The L Word*. She continues to include meditation, healthy eating, and fitness in her lifestyle.

(Excerpted from an article by Jennifer LeClaire in the March 2004 issue of *Better Nutrition* magazine, available at your local health food store or online at www.betternutrition.com)

Acknowledgements

Thanks to Dr. Michael Lyons for opening my eyes to mercury as a missing piece to the health puzzle; and to Pat Connolly and the Price-Pottenger Nutrition Foundation for granting permission for me to use photos from *Nutrition and Physical Degeneration*.

Thanks to Udo Erasmus for the contribution of his article "Fats that Heal and Fats that Kill"; Jennifer Sieberg for her article "Go Organic"; and Dr. Mark Cousins for his help with the written explanation of the ileocecal valve acupressure points.

I'd like to thank the following people for their input:

Gino Gemma and Guy Cramer (hyperbaric oxygen therapy and negative ions); Wayne Obie (mercury) and Pam Floener (DMPS and mercury). Thanks, too, to Andrew Munaweera for providing me with some research articles.

Thanks to Bernie Windham for his tremendous dedication to collecting scientific references on mercury, and for allowing me to use his research in this book.

More thanks: to Val Wilson for her thorough job of editing.

A special thanks to Irene Hayton for her recipes, technical editing, and for all the long hours she spent on every aspect of the book.

Introduction

"…I will prescribe regimen for the good of my patients according to my ability and my judgement and never do harm to anyone. To please no one, will I prescribe a deadly drug nor give advice which may cause his death. If I keep this oath faithfully, may I enjoy my life and practice my art, respected by all men and in all times; but if I swerve from it or violate it, may the reverse be my lot."

Hippocratic Oath

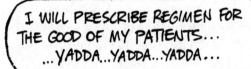

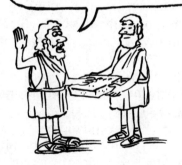

This is the best time to be alive.

If you learn the basics of modern electronics, you can be a millionaire by the time you're 20, and a billionaire by age 40. If you're athletic, you can make more money in a year than your father made in his lifetime.

Even we less-gifted folk have it easier than royalty did a hundred years ago. Just a few of the things we take for granted now—that were only dreams a century ago—are: hot and cold running water; temperature control; the ability to store food safely by refrigeration or freezing, and to quickly cook it with little effort; home access to entertainment, education, news, and sports by turning on the colour TV; instant communication world-wide through telephone, fax, and email; and the ability to travel from continent to continent within a day.

When governments started old-age pensions, the average life expectancy was 65—now it's over 75. Insurance companies recognize that if you're healthy at age 60, you'll likely live to 85. Governments will spend considerable amounts of money every year on your health. The Canadian government spends about $1,600 per person per year on health care; the US government spends about $1,900 per person per year.

Despite this time of affluence and ease we have myriad mysterious chronic health problems for which government-funded health care has few or no answers. Diseases like Alzheimer's, Parkinson's, amyotrophic lateral sclerosis (ALS— also known as Lou Gehrig's disease), cancers, strokes, heart attacks, diabetes, and hiatus hernias are assumed to be more common because the population is living longer.

The younger generation, however, also has a wide range of chronic health problems. Ten percent of young children now have eczema, and asthma and allergies are commonplace among youngsters. One out of 500 children has autism, and diabetes and cancer aren't rare in young children anymore. Dyslexia, hyperactivity, attention deficit disorder, and behavioural problems have made 20 percent of students in some areas learning-disabled.

The age group between young and old has its own rash of health problems such as chronic fatigue; fibromyalgia; rheumatoid arthritis; reflux indigestion; acne; sinusitis; psoriasis; depression; anxiety; cancers; schizophrenia; manic depression; thyroid problems; ankylosing spondylitis; infertility; premenstrual syndrome (PMS); menstrual cramping; prostate enlargement; epilepsy; multiple sclerosis (MS); lupus; Crohn's disease; colitis; and irritable bowel syndrome. Is there anyone that doesn't have a chronic health problem? A recent article in the *Journal of the American Medical Association (JAMA)* stated that 45 percent of Americans have at least one chronic health complaint." [1]

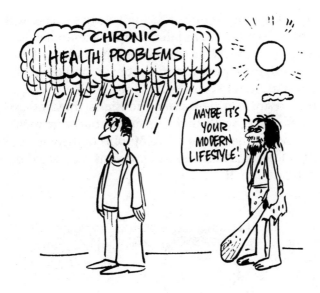

In my first book, *EATING ALIVE: Prevention Thru Good Digestion*, I stated in the Introduction:

"There is an incredible healing power within each of us that knows exactly what and where each of our ailments is, and knows exactly what to do to correct them. That healing power is available to you at little cost and in unlimited quantities. It is, unfortunately, often stifled and dormant."

The incredible healing power within each of us is called **homeostasis**. It is the basic tenet of physiology that your body is a wise, self-adjusting organism capable of monitoring and correcting imbalances, fighting off invaders, and repairing damage. When homeostasis reigns, health is your natural state. Acute disease is your body's gathering of forces to throw off some outside interference, such as a viral infection. When the virus is defeated, the short-lived disease is over, and homeostasis returns your body to its normal, stable functioning. Chronic disease occurs when the body is unable to completely remove the outside influence—or fully correct damage from it—and the full return of homeostasis is thwarted.

Pathology is the study of the failure of homeostasis to return the body to normal physiology. Because physiology (the study of human body function) is one of the first classes in medical school, and pathology is taught later, there is a tendency for medical students to forget about the inherent wisdom of the body to heal itself; they seem to focus more on pathology—otherwise known as *disease*.

When I was in my fourth year at naturopathic medical school in Seattle, Washington, in 1983, my head was bursting with knowledge about all the signs and symptoms of disease, and the multitude of herbs, vitamins, and minerals that could be used to remedy each of the diseases.

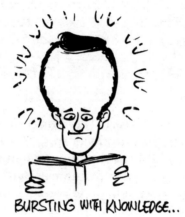

BURSTING WITH KNOWLEDGE...

Then I met Dr. Harold Dick, a gruff, no-nonsense naturopathic physician in Spokane, Washington. He gave little consideration to the joints in an arthritic person or the skin in a psoriatic individual. His key to cure was to get the digestion working so that the improvement in the patients' health would allow their own homeostasis to heal the joints or the skin or whatever disease they had. The focus was on health improvement—rather than disease treatment.

Dr. Dick practised the same way Dr. O. G. Carroll had, 40 years previously, when he reversed Mrs. Dick's arthritis by "jump starting" her digestive system. This technique could be traced from Dr. Dick back to Dr. O. G. Carroll to Dr. Ledoux to Father Sebastian Kneipp, in Central Europe, whom many consider the father of naturopathic practice.

When I began my practice, I modelled it as closely as possible to this time-proven model. Over 17 years in practice, I've seen almost every one of the chronic diseases *disappear*, from young and old, through treatment.

In 1986, I wrote *EATING ALIVE: Prevention Thru Good Digestion* in which I reported the following.

- **Signs and symptoms of chronic disease can only disappear *after* liver function has been fully restored.**
- **Because the liver is the filter of the digestive system, the digestive function must be improved.**
- **And, because the digestive system starts at the mouth, dietary changes are likely to be involved.**

In 1998, I completed my second book, *The Secrets to Great Health*, which went into a lot more detail on liver function and how improving liver function could reverse so many chronic diseases, including breast cancer. In that book, I reiterated the importance of the liver in reversing chronic disease:

"...since the feeling of well-being will only occur after the liver is working properly, it seems obvious that the liver is the junction box from which nearly all symptoms of illness—physical or emotional, and sometimes even mental—must originate."

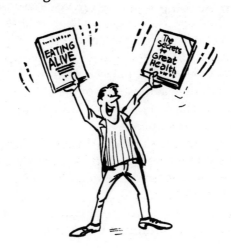

In spite of all the success I was having, I knew something was missing—something I didn't fully understand. I wrote:
"While it's always gratifying to have patients' chronic health problems disappear quickly and effortlessly, there's little to be learned from this. It only reaffirms what I already believe. **There are other patients where the results weren't quick, weren't easy, and weren't complete. Or where the results seemed complete, but the symptoms soon returned.**"

With these patients, it seemed that either the premise of homeostasis—that the body is programmed to be healthy—was wrong, or something was continuing to disrupt their liver function and thus disrupt their ability to heal.

The missing piece to the health puzzle was revealed to me soon after the release of *The Secrets to Great Health*. This new book, *EATING ALIVE II*, will continue on from where *EATING ALIVE* ended. It will also embody the highlights of *The Secrets to Great Health*, and will add the missing piece to show you what you can do to avoid chronic disease—and what you can do to reverse disease, if you already have it. Great health—homeostasis—is still possible, if you can navigate your way through a handful of barriers on your way to health. *EATING ALIVE II* will identify those obstacles and will explain how to overcome them by using THE EATING ALIVE PROGRAM.

Letter from a Patient

Dear Dr. Matsen,

I began following the THE EATING ALIVE PROGRAM about ten months ago. Prior to following the system, I often had sore throats which would turn into an ear infection and a head cold. I was getting sick every couple of months for about a week at a time. My energy level was low to the point it was difficult to function during the day. I had difficulty sleeping at night, headaches, and mood swings.

Within one month of following THE EATING ALIVE PROGRAM, I noticed my energy level had increased. I was able to fill my days with activities. I began to sleep through the night and I haven't been sick or had a sore throat for approximately eight months. My headaches and moodiness have disappeared.

Lydia Burchell-Strand
Burnaby, BC

PART I

FastTrack

to

THE EATING ALIVE PROGRAM

So what is THE EATING ALIVE PROGRAM? And what does *FastTrack* mean?

THE EATING ALIVE PROGRAM includes nutritional and lifestyle guidelines that can help you reverse the symptoms of so-called chronic illnesses.

"EATING ALIVE" refers to that cozy dietary spot found between *EATING TOO BAD* and *EATING TOO WELL.* And, because *healthy eating* isn't enough to prevent or reverse chronic disease, I have created THE EATING ALIVE PROGRAM. It involves:
- Improving diet and digestion.
- Establishing good intestinal flora and eliminating intestinal yeast and bacterial overgrowth.
- Removing/avoiding toxic heavy metals.
- Increasing your intake of oxygen through regular aerobic exercise and laughter.
- Getting enough sleep to allow your body's repair crews to fix the wear-and-tear that your body has endured during the day.
- Learning to relax and respond to stress with positive actions.

1

Your body is meant to be healthy and virtually all chronic health problems can be traced back to a poorly functioning liver. Applying the principles of THE EATING ALIVE PROGRAM allows your liver to work more efficiently so that your body can heal itself.

The *FASTTRACK* section of this book allows you to get started right away. Each *FASTTRACK* previews a Chapter from Part III where the principles of THE EATING ALIVE PROGRAM are explained in greater detail.

Mercury: The Missing Piece

The amalgam in dental fillings is approximately 50 percent mercury; the rest is made up of silver, copper, and tin. Published medical research articles—including autopsy studies, metal allergy tests, chelation research, and clinical studies—show conclusively that mercury vapour continuously leaks from amalgam fillings, and gradually accumulates in the body, especially in the kidneys, brain, and liver.

The leakage of mercury vapour from amalgam fillings is increased by the presence of nearby gold fillings or nickel braces. In the presence of other metals in the mouth, mercury can be subject to galvanic action—the production of electrical currents flowing from one metal to a dissimilar metal—which increases the release of mercury vapours.

Other factors that increase the release of mercury vapours from amalgam fillings are: chewing (especially gum); bruxism (grinding of the teeth); hot foods and drinks; the acidity of foods and beverages; and the brushing, drilling, and polishing of teeth.

Mercury vapour that is swallowed in saliva may react with the hydrochloric acid (HCl) of your stomach, forming **mercuric chloride**. Mercuric chloride can kill off your beneficial intestinal bacteria, allowing the overgrowth of yeast, parasites, and harmful bacteria. Also, when mercury combines with the HCl of the stomach, there is less HCl available for the digestion of food leading to heartburn, bloating, indigestion, and other digestive problems.

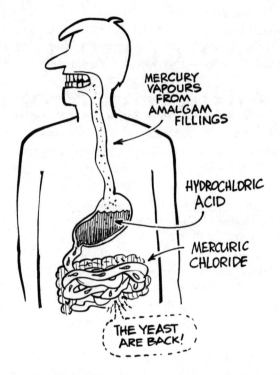

In one research study, a significant percentage of people with degeneration of the basal ganglia of the brain—the part of the brain that is affected by Parkinson's disease—were found to be reactive to mercuric chloride.

The bacteria and yeast in your mouth and intestine can methylate elemental mercury into **methylmercury**. Both methylmercury and mercury vapour that leaks from amalgam fillings can be major contributors to many of the "mysterious" chronic physical, mental, and emotional illnesses—especially those that are neurological or immunological. These illnesses plague industrialized societies today—as they likely have over the last 160 years, since mercury was introduced into dentistry.

Some people who have had relatively low exposure to minor amounts of mercury can have major reactions, due to allergies to mercury. The "Dental Amalgam Patient Information Sheet," put out by the Canadian Dental Association, cites an article from the *Journal of the American Dental Association*. In this article, it is admitted that approximately 3 percent of the general population is likely sensitive (allergic) to mercury. Yet when people with chronic health problems are tested, a much higher percentage is typically seen. Skin-patch testing does not always detect immune reactions to mercury.

Phenylmercury, which is used in root canals to kill bacteria, must be leaking out of the root canals to induce immune reactions, since 14 percent of people tested show reactions to it. **Titanium dioxide** is also a common allergen. Titanium dioxide is used as a white colouring agent in many dental products, including toothpaste, and it is also used in some pain-relief medications.

The removal of mercury-amalgam fillings will spill more mercury into the body, but a dentist who is aware of the adverse health effects of mercury—and who has the right equipment and training—can reduce the spillover of mercury by up to 90 percent.

Replacement of dental amalgams with mercury-free fillings has been shown, in numerous studies of thousands of patients, to give improvement in a wide range of chronic diseases, six to 12 months later.

RECOMMENDATIONS

1. Refuse to allow mercury-amalgam fillings to be placed in your mouth.

2. Avoid phenylmercury in root canals and avoid titanium dioxide, which is found in some dental materials, toothpastes, and pain-relief medications.

3. If you have mercury-amalgam fillings ("silver" amalgams are approximately 50 percent mercury), avoid excessive/unnecessary chewing, especially of gum. Chewing gum or drinking hot liquids can produce 10 to 100 times the normal levels of mercury exposure from amalgams.

4. If you are pregnant or breast-feeding, do not "stir up" mercury—increase your total body burden of mercury—through the removal, addition, or cleaning of mercury-amalgams, and do not attempt chelation of metals. In research studies, exposure of the mother to mercury vapours was found to cause an accumulation of mercury in the fetus. The breast milk of women with seven or more amalgams has been found to have levels of mercury approximately ten times that of the breast milk of amalgam-free women.

5. Have your mercury fillings removed and replaced as you can afford to do so—by a dentist who is properly trained and equipped in the safe removal of amalgams.

6. If you also have gold fillings, have the mercury fillings closest to them replaced first, because galvanic currents between the gold and the mercury increase the release of mercury vapour into your mouth. Nickel in dental appliances (braces, etc.) can also cause increased release of mercury due to galvanic action.

7. Since gold is too soft for fillings, palladium and other metals are added to it to make it harder. In Swedish research studies using MELISA® allergy testing, both gold and palladium have been found to be allergens, although not as commonly as mercury and nickel. Non-metal fillings, such as composites and ceramics, are much safer than metal fillings. Although more expensive than composites, ceramic is harder and less temperature-sensitive.

8. Since metals bind to sulfur in the body, heavy metal toxicity can lead to sulfur deficiency, especially deficiency of the amino acid cysteine. Cysteine as a supplement is considered toxic, so N-acetylcysteine (NAC) is sometimes used. Animal studies, however, have shown that if cysteine binds to mercury, it resembles the structure of the amino acid methionine, and is transported directly into the brain. Using methionine as a sulfur supplement, instead of NAC, should prevent this transfer of mercury into the brain. Methyl-Sulfonyl-Methane (MSM) is also likely to be OK as a sulfur supplement. Because of its high cysteine content, whey protein powder should be used cautiously when "stirring up" mercury through dental work or chelation, until studies show if it is safe to take at that time.

9. Studies show that most people's bodies still contain large amounts of mercury, long after their mercury fillings have been replaced. DMPS or DMSA chelation can remove most of this accumulated mercury, although **great caution needs to be used, because some people's symptoms could become worse if chelation is done inappropriately.**

10. DMPS chelation, followed by a urine test, is the most accurate way to monitor the decrease in mercury levels in the body. DMPS is a sulfur compound that can be given orally in capsule form or mixed in an acidic drink (such as orange juice). Or it can be injected intravenously or intramuscularly. DMPS circulates in the blood and chelates—binds—metals into very stable and non-toxic

molecules that can be excreted primarily by the kidneys. Taking DMPS orally is recommended over intravenous administration.

11. If you are allergic to sulfur or hypersensitive in general, you must inform the person administering the chelation, so that a small trial-dose can be given before a full dose is used.

12. Chelation may also remove minerals, especially zinc, so mineral supplements may need to be taken to replace those lost minerals. Zinc should not be taken within approximately 12 hours of taking a chelation sulfur.

13. Be patient. In mild cases, removing most of the mercury will likely take six months to a year. In most people who've had a major exposure to mercury, it may be a two to three-year project.

14. Elimination of many of the symptoms of metal toxicity can be achieved more quickly by following an appropriate diet, avoiding allergens, and correcting intestinal flora imbalances.

Letter from a Patient

Following a series of surgeries (accompanied by antibiotics) for an incarcerated hernia, I suffered severe digestive problems. I had pain after eating, and constant diarrhea. I lost weight and was constantly exhausted. This lasted over a period of years—in spite of my having consulted two gastroenterologists.

I repeatedly had the usual "invasive procedure" tests; they decided I had "irritable bowel syndrome."

Finally, I went to Dr. Matsen, who found I had a yeast infection and had developed food sensitivities. Thanks to his program, I was much better in six weeks. Now I feel great and have a regained my health.

I only wish I had gone to him sooner.

Natalie V. Rogers
West Vancouver, BC

Vaccines: Unanswered Questions

Vaccines are a highly suspicious factor in a wide range of health problems—including Sudden Infant Death Syndrome (SIDS); attention deficit disorder (ADD); dyslexia; hyperactivity; learning disabilities; autism; asthma; eczema; dermatitis; cerebral palsy; autoimmune arthritis; lupus; Alzheimer's; and others—although more studies are necessary for confirmation.

Mercury in the form of **thimerosal** has been used as a preservative in some vaccines. A recent Italian study of children with dermatitis and eczema found that 42 percent of them were allergic; of all 47 substances tested, thimerosal was by far the greatest allergen. Further studies are necessary to see if thimerosal allergies are related to other diseases.

The two types of vaccines most commonly implicated in lawsuits involving death, brain damage, or autoimmune diseases are pertussis (the P in DPT) and hepatitis B, both of which often contain thimerosal as a preservative.

At least 500 child deaths from pertussis vaccines have been reported over a five-year period in the US, with a billion dollars in damages paid out. Hepatitis B is presently implicated in thousands of lawsuits in France and the US. **No long-term studies on the safety of these or any other vaccines have ever been done**.

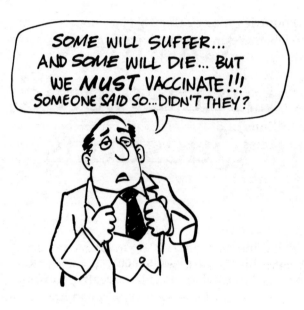

Autopsies done on the brains of people with Alzheimer's have often shown increased levels of mercury and aluminum. Since flu shots commonly contain mercury and aluminum, it is recommended that you avoid flu shots until they are proven to be safe.

RECOMMENDATIONS

1. Vaccines are not mandatory in most countries; you may elect to not have them.

2. In countries where some vaccines are mandatory, such as the US, there are now both medical and religious exemptions.

3. Before receiving a vaccination, ask to see the long-term studies showing its effectiveness and safety. **(Note: in spite of billions of dollars of profit for the pharmaceutical companies that make the vaccines, no studies have been done on long-term side-effects. You're the guinea pig in an experiment where little attention is paid to the guinea pig.)**

4. In spite of the recent bioterrorism fears, absolutely refuse any vaccine that contains the mercury preservative thimerosal. Understand that aluminum, formaldehyde, and monosodium glutamate (MSG)—among other additives—are commonly used in vaccines, as well.

5. Only have vaccinations when in good health, as per the recommendations of the National Vaccine Information Center, which advises *against DPT vaccination if:*
   - the child is ill, which includes having a runny nose, cough, ear infection, diarrhea; if the child has recovered from an illness within one month prior to the DPT; or if the child is currently on antibiotics;
   - the child or a family member has had a severe reaction to a DPT shot;
   - someone in the child's immediate family has a history of convulsions or neurological disease;
   - the child was born prematurely or with low birthweight; or
   - the child has a personal or family history of severe allergies, especially to dairy, or has an allergic disease, such as asthma, dermatitis, hay fever, etc.

6. **If bad reactions occur after a vaccination, avoid having
    any more dosages of that vaccine because reactions can
    worsen with subsequent exposure.**

7. It is also recommended to supplement with extra vitamin
    C before and after the vaccination, because it appears to
    lessen bad reactions.

More information on preventing vaccine injury can be
obtained from *The Consumer's Guide to Childhood Vaccines,*
available from:

National Vaccine Information Center
421–E Church Street
Vienna, VA 22180
(703) 938-DPT3
Fax: (703) 938-5768
www.909shot.com

or in BC, from:

Health Action Network Society (HANS)
#202 – 5262 Rumble Street
Burnaby, BC V5J 2B6
(604) 435-0512
Fax: (604) 435-1561
www.hans.org.

In fact, what a good opportunity to become a member of these
organizations that have devoted so much to protecting your
health interests!

Letter from a Patient

Before starting THE EATING ALIVE PROGRAM, I was labelled a borderline diabetic, with a sugar ratio of 7.0 (7.1 and above is diabetes). I weighed over 200 pounds, was feeling weak, and had no energy.

Since following THE EATING ALIVE PROGRAM, I no longer feel weak and I have lots of energy. My sugar ratio is down to 5.5, and I've lost over 30 pounds. Together with good eating habits and an exercise program, I have been able to maintain my health and fitness over the last two years since finishing THE EATING ALIVE PROGRAM.

Peter J. Galea
North Vancouver, BC

FastTrack for CHAPTER 3

The Liver
Connection

The ability of your body to heal itself depends upon your liver's ability to neutralize toxins arriving from your gut—every minute of every day. Liver detoxification uses a two-step process involving **Phase I enzymes** and **Phase II enzymes**.

Your Phase I enzymes add oxygen to fat-soluble chemicals, called phenols, as the first step in making them water-soluble. Ordinary oxygen molecules have two oxygen atoms (O_2). When one oxygen atom is added to a phenol to make it more water-soluble for your Phase II enzymes, the leftover oxygen becomes a **superoxide radical**. These free radicals can, in turn, create **peroxides**. This production of peroxides is a normal biochemical step; the peroxides should be quickly neutralized by a second set of enzymes—the Phase II enzymes.

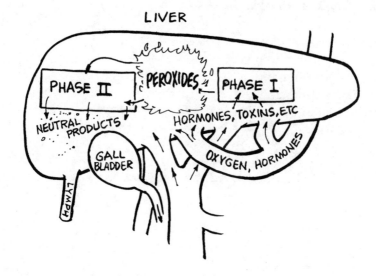

The peroxides can destroy any membrane on contact, if they're not neutralized promptly by your liver.

- If the peroxides spill out of your liver into the bile, they can create digestive and bowel symptoms.
- If they spill into your kidneys, they can cause irritation of your urinary tract or your skin.
- If they spill into your lymph system, they can activate immune and autoimmune reactions.
- If they spill into your bloodstream, they can create heart, brain, and joint irritation, and they can stimulate cancer development.

Peroxides are Bad News when they are not neutralized promptly by your Phase II enzymes.

Glutathione peroxidase is one of the Phase II enzymes; its job is to chop deadly peroxides into harmless water. **Glutathione peroxidase enzyme needs sulfur and selenium to do this and, since mercury binds to sulfur and displaces selenium**, mercury dramatically interferes with your liver's ability to neutralize peroxides. This leaves you vulnerable to virtually any physical, mental, or emotional illness.

You should strictly avoid any dental product, vaccine, or drug that contains mercury. If you have already been exposed (and you probably have been), you will likely be spending some time trying to find ways to eliminate the mercury from your body. Mercury is easy to put in, but very hard to get out. In the meantime, the logical thing to do is **minimize your production of peroxides so that glutathione doesn't have to work so hard**.

RECOMMENDATIONS

1. Reduce your liver's production of peroxides by minimizing your exposure to **tobacco, alcohol,** and **coffee** (even decaffeinated)—all of which increase your liver's production of peroxides. Avoiding tobacco, alcohol, and coffee is *especially* **critical** if you currently have a chronic disease. **Including these things in your diet is** *EATING TOO BAD.*

2. The Phase II enzymes need every known nutrient to neutralize peroxides, so foods that have had their nutrients stripped from them—such as **white sugar, white flour,** and **white salt**—can have devastating effects on your ability to neutralize peroxides. **Including these things in your diet is also** *EATING TOO BAD.*

3. Some foods—such as grapefruit and wheat grass juice—contain nutrients that slow down your Phase I enzymes' production of peroxides. But equally important are the foods and herbs that supply your Phase II enzymes with nutrients they need: pollen (especially rye pollen); green tea; milk thistle herb; whey protein powder or MSM (for sulfur); selenium (200 micrograms per day); cruciferous vegetables (especially broccoli and brussels sprouts); and blue and purple foods such as beets, currants, blueberries, and prunes, which contain **anthocyanidins.**

4. If you have a chronic health problem, supplement with **proanthocyanidins**—such as grape seed extract or pycnogenol—and vitamin C with bioflavonoids. (Vitamin C that is supplemented with bioflavonoids contains the white matter between the skin and the fruit of grapefruit.) If you're not out in the sun regularly, take one capsule of cod or halibut liver oil per day. Following these steps has been proven to *reverse* cancer in some people and therefore, may help *prevent* it in you. Correcting diet is the important first step to *EATING ALIVE!*

Letter from a Patient

Seven years ago, I was diagnosed with irritable bowel syndrome (IBS). For years, I have had unexplained symptoms that were addressed by numerous medical tests—to no avail. It was explained that this was a condition one must learn to live with.

I had been interested in food-combining and diet for many years because I had a suspicion that my symptoms might be related to diet but I could not put my finger on the problem. At a local bookstore, I saw Dr. Matsen's book *Eating Alive: Prevention Thru Good Digestion.* The book was easy to read and explained a lot about food and digestion "in plain English."

At my first appointment a year ago, Dr. Matsen was very optimistic that I would be "as good as new" within six weeks. I viewed that comment with some skepticism, based on my prior experience with doctors.

Dr. Matsen informed me that I was suffering from following a classic "California diet." I thought that my diet of mainly salads, fruit, and low-fat foods was very healthy. He explained that I should eat according to climate—to try soup instead of salad and to have oatmeal for breakfast instead of fruit.

I was put on a regimen of supplements and at the same time, I changed my diet. I have eliminated caffeine, most sugars, dairy products, and fast foods, and I watch my food combinations. I do a lot of cooking and enjoy local, in-season produce immensely.

I only saw Dr. Matsen about four times. A year later, my symptoms are virtually gone—I never thought I'd see the day! I have lost 35 pounds, I am never hungry (cravings are very rare), and my internal organs are remarkably quiet.

Thank you, Dr. Matsen. I encourage everyone to read your books— either to start feeling better or to stay well. It is useful information for everyone.

Patricia Pracher
Vancouver, BC

The Yeast are Back

Your Phase I liver enzymes take fat-soluble chemicals called phenols, and add oxygen to them in the process of making them water-soluble. This **creates peroxides**, which create ill health. In most people with chronic health problems, **the main source of these phenols is yeast living in the intestine**.

Yeast (also known as Candida yeast) are members of the fungus family; they are normal denizens of your intestinal tract. Their job is to turn you into compost when you're dead. Candida yeast are strongly inhibited by acidity, and they are content to hide away in the nooks and crannies of your large intestine—wherever the pH is acceptably alkaline. Your main defence against them is billions of acidophilus bacteria (your good bacteria) that maintain an acid pH in your large intestine (colon), which inhibits yeast growth.

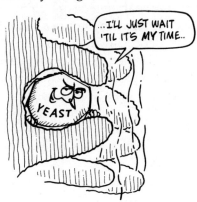

Anything that disrupts the pH of your colon and your good bacteria—such as antibiotics, mercury, antacids, chlorinated water, cortisone, etc.—allows the yeast to begin the composting process while you're still alive. Once they are active, yeast have ways of convincing you that sugar and chocolate are necessary in your diet.

Another way the yeast can become active is when your **ileocecal valve** is weakened. The ileocecal valve is located between your small intestine and your large intestine. This valve is usually kept closed so that the food you've eaten stays in your small intestine long enough to be digested and absorbed fully. It also prevents the good micro-organisms in your large intestine from getting into your small intestine, where their waste products could easily be absorbed. As digestion and absorption are completed in your small intestine, your ileocecal valve opens, and the food passes into your large intestine or colon.

When your ileocecal valve is weakened, the billions of normally "good" bacteria that live in the large intestine get through the ileocecal valve, up into your small intestine— where they're not supposed to be. There, they can become "Bad Guys"—they steal important nutrients like vitamin B_{12} and tryptophan before you have absorbed them, and they can also dump toxins into your liver. Once your good bacteria become bad, yeast soon join the party. The alkaline pH of the small intestine allows the yeast to multiply vigorously.

Your ileocecal valve can become weak when your calcium levels are low for more than five days—calcium helps to strengthen this valve. Increasing your calcium intake doesn't necessarily solve the ileocecal valve problem, because the solution depends on whether the calcium is being *absorbed* by your body. **Vitamin D** is required for calcium absorption: it stimulates your intestinal cells to make a calcium-binding protein that dramatically increases your absorption of calcium. Vitamin D is made by your skin when exposed to the ultraviolet (UV) rays of the sun, and then it is stored in an inactive form in your liver.

When vitamin D is released from liver storage, your liver converts it into a weak form of vitamin D, which then activates calcium absorption to a small degree. This might be sufficient activation if you were out in the sun regularly, when your skin can make a lot of vitamin D. Your kidneys convert this weak form of vitamin D into a much stronger form that can improve calcium absorption up to 1,000 times. This strong activation of vitamin D is especially crucial for wintertime when there is little sun around to make vitamin D directly through the skin.

Your kidneys are in charge of regulating calcium levels by altering the activation of vitamin D with the changes in the seasons. Because the kidneys can't see outside to know what the weather is like, they monitor the ions in the foods and the beverages you're consuming. The sodium/potassium ion ratio tells the kidneys what to do with regard to the activation of vitamin D.

Your blood contains 3 percent sodium, a percentage similar to that found in the ocean and in animals. Your kidneys maintain a 50/50 ratio of sodium and potassium at all times. Excess sodium in the diet is eliminated through the kidneys, giving a warming effect to your body and making you more active, while an excess of potassium has a cooling effect, which slows you down.

All plants contain potassium; generally, the more sun they're exposed to, the more potassium they contain. Eat a banana, which has lots of potassium, and your kidneys will think that you're in Hawaii, and that your skin must be roasting in the sun—making vitamin D—so they stop activating vitamin D. If you're not actually out in the sun, you could quickly lose your calcium absorption—and within five days, your ileocecal valve could be weak enough to allow your billions of good bacteria to stampede into your small intestine, where they could become Bad Guys.

A vegetarian animal on a high-potassium diet needs access to salt, while a carnivorous animal gets its salt from the 3 percent sodium found in the vegetarian animal that it eats. In the winter, an Inuit would be on a high-sodium animal-protein diet, which would tell the kidneys that the weather is not sunny, so his kidneys would activate the vitamin D much more vigorously.

If your skin is going brown from the sun, you can eat a slight excess of potassium; otherwise you should eat a slight excess of sodium. This is the basis of the concept in Asian medicine of "yin and yang"—warming and cooling. Even though most Asians don't have high-calcium dairy products in their traditional diets, they generally have much lower incidences of dental cavities and osteoporosis than do Westerners who use dairy—and who also eat a lot of fresh fruit, juices, and salads, even in winter.

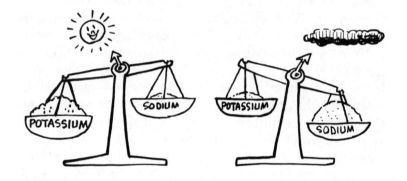

The ileocecal valve problem is commonly seen in **PEOPLE WHO *EAT TOO WELL*!** That is, they consume too many foods and drinks high in potassium, and don't consume enough sodium in the form of animal protein or salt. This confuses the kidneys into assuming they are in the hot sun of mid-summer, so they deactivate vitamin D.

While the kidneys' activation of vitamin D is crucial to getting calcium from the gut to the blood, it is **vitamin K** that delivers calcium from the blood into the bone. Vitamin K also prevents calcium from sticking in the arteries—thereby reducing the risk of heart disease and stroke. Vitamin K is found in leafy greens; cooking them slightly and salting them will help prevent ileocecal valve problems when you're not actually out in the sun.

RECOMMENDATIONS

1. Vitamin D is crucial for the absorption of calcium. If you're out in the sunshine and your skin is exposed to the UV rays of the sun, it will make vitamin D. If you're unable to get regular sun exposure, take vitamin D as a supplement—one capsule of halibut or cod liver oil per day. These sources of vitamin D seem to be more active than the irradiated yeast used in vegetarian vitamin D supplements.

2. Vitamin D is relatively passive until it's activated by your kidneys, which change the activation of vitamin D as the weather changes. Sodium in the diet tells the kidneys it's *not* sunny, so they activate vitamin D—while potassium tells the kidneys it *is* sunny, so they don't activate vitamin D. So, eat according to the climate in which you are living.

3. If you eat animal products, you get adequate sodium; if you eat vegetable products, you need to add salt. Unrefined sea salt carries myriad trace minerals that buffer the potential side-effects of pure sodium chloride. Salt, however, including most sea salts, has had these important trace minerals stripped off and sold to the industrial mineral market. The salt I recommend is Celtic Sea Salt® from Brittany in France—it still contains its key trace minerals. Having these minerals in your diet can be critical to your health because fertilization of the soil with nitrogen, phosphorus, and potassium has depleted trace minerals from heavily farmed soils. Organic gardeners are attempting to correct these deficiencies by adding rock powder to the soil. Celtic Sea Salt® can be purchased from:
   The Grain and Salt Society, Canada
   17 Matilda Street
   Tara, Ontario N0H 2N0
   1-888-725-8386 or (519) 934-9948
   Fax: (519) 934-9908

4. While activated vitamin D will transport calcium from your gut into the blood, it's vitamin K that puts it into your bones and keeps it out of your arteries. Eat leafy green vegetables regularly for their vitamin K. Eat salads when you're out in the warm sun, and steamed greens—with a little sea salt—the rest of the year.

5. Eat foods containing acidophilus bacteria—such as fresh yogurt—to inhibit yeast. Or take acidophilus capsules. I recommend 1 acidophilus capsule two times per day on an empty stomach: in the morning upon rising (then try to wait at least 20 minutes before eating) and at night before bed. Use garlic, oregano, basil, rosemary, thyme, savoury, turmeric, curcumin, etc., for their anti-yeast and anti-inflammatory properties.

6. Make sure that you get enough sleep to allow your body's repair crews—such as growth hormone and thymus hormones—to fix the wear-and-tear that your body has endured during the day, so you are rested, repaired, recharged, and ready for another busy day.

Letter from a Patient

Since going to see Dr. Matsen 15 years ago, I have rediscovered my natural energy. All over again!

I had been devastated with dreadful stomach pains, awful abdominal gas, a feeling of exhaustion, and to some extent, was depressed about the way I was feeling.

Within three weeks, I began to notice a big change. I bought the book *Eating Alive* and followed the instructions given at the time of my visit to see Dr. Matsen. I then bought THE Book for my family members, to share the eating techniques I had learned.

I seem to get into eating difficulties cyclically. I either rush the spring into summer by eating off-season fruit, or in the fall, I eat fresh, raw vegetables—even as the days grow short and dark!

I am currently on a detox program that Dr. Matsen has recommended. The results are as before—the recovery is quick, and my energy returns fully.

I am very pleased to have this opportunity to thank Dr. Matsen for his patient care, and for the pleasant experience it is to visit the office. The staff are just great, assisting in every way possible!

Sincerely,
Mary A. (Pat) Ferguson
North Vancouver, BC

Oxygen: Nature's Best Cure

Oxygen is the most important nutrient to your health. And it's still free! Approximately 90 percent of the oxygen you breathe is used to give you bountiful energy in the form of adenosine triphosphate (ATP). The other 10 percent plays a key role in liver detoxification, and is an important source of ammunition for your immune system.

Oxygen is moved into your body by the process of breathing. The deeper you inhale, the more oxygen you take in. Numerous studies have shown that people who exercise regularly outlive those who are sedentary, and they are also more immune to many of the degenerative diseases of modern society.

Breathing is also the "pump" for your liver. When your diaphragm and abdominal muscles are working together during deep breathing, they "pump" your liver and play an important part in its functioning. Stress and worry can dramatically decrease breathing. When we are stressed or worried, deep abdominal breathing disappears and breathing moves to the upper chest in the form of shallow breaths. Exercise can help to decrease stress and worry.

Hyperbaric Oxygen Therapy (HBOT)—breathing oxygen under pressure in a hyperbaric chamber—can increase the body's absorption of oxygen. HBOT can therefore help in the healing of problems that involve oxygen deficiency—such as carbon monoxide poisoning, strokes, heart attacks, and some stubborn infections.

RECOMMENDATIONS

1. Get up and get moving. Engage in aerobic exercise on a regular basis—brisk walking, jogging, cycling, swimming, for example. Not only does aerobic exercise increase your oxygen intake and act as a pump for the liver, but it also burns fat, tones muscles, improves the cardiovascular system, speeds up lymph drainage, and decreases stress by releasing endorphins (the feel-good hormones). Keep in mind that optimistic athletes tend to get better faster than sedentary worriers.

   If you are unable to do aerobic activities on a regular basis, due to physical impediments, then do something lighter, like Tai Chi or yoga.

2. If you're unable to do even light exercise, develop a good sense of humour because laughter also increases breathing and liver function.

3. If you're unable to laugh due to ill health, consider hyperbaric oxygen therapy, which can increase your oxygen intake 14-fold.

Letter from a Patient

In late October 2000, I started having diarrhea frequently. There was mucous, then blood, in my stool. I also had gas and bloating. I visited my GP [general medical practitioner], which started a long process of stool samples, antibiotics, and referrals to a surgeon and a gastroenterologist. I was put on medication and had a sigmoidoscopy.

The conclusion was ulcerative colitis. I was to continue with the medication and if my condition got worse, I was supposed to go back to the gastroenterologist.

Thank goodness my mom had a friend who recommended I see Dr. Matsen. He had a very definite plan of action and expected me to feel much better within six weeks! WOW! With some healthy changes to my diet and the addition of supplements, my symptoms quickly disappeared.

I am so impressed and grateful.

Michele Heit
North Vancouver, BC

Negative Ions: Positively Good

Fresh air contains small amounts of positive and negative ions that are crucial to our utilization of oxygen, and that affect various hormones, such as serotonin.

There are ebbs and flows of ion levels, with the daily rising and setting of the sun and the monthly movements of the moon. Fluctuations also occur with the movements of weather fronts and winds, and the presence of water and plants.

Geographical areas that have naturally high levels of negative ions—such as mountains, waterfalls, and the seashore—are places that people like to go to rest and recover from stress. A decrease in negative ions and an increase in positive ions has profound ill effects on many people. Areas with drying winds are known to be unpleasant because of the lack of negative ions and the increase in positive ions.

Much of the man-made air in sealed buildings, cars, airplanes, and cruiseships is stripped of negative ions, due to the metal ducting of the air conditioning and heating systems. This can increase physical, mental, and emotional stress to the occupants, and can increase susceptibility to infections.

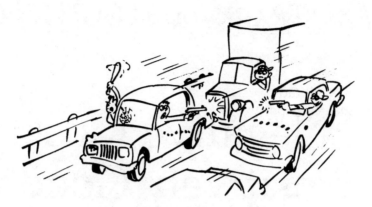

ANOTHER LOW NEGATIVE ION DAY
ON THE CALIFORNIA FREEWAY...

Numerous studies with negative ion generators have shown that people function better with an excess of negative ions. Mental function is sharper; people are more amiable, and are physically much more resistant to illness.

Russian studies have shown that the stamina, quickness, and mental sharpness of athletes increased when training while exposed to negative ions from negative ion generators.

RECOMMENDATIONS

1. Go for regular walks or runs outdoors in the fresh air—
   especially along creeks, rivers, beaches, waterfalls, and in
   high altitudes with natural vegetation. You will get your
   greatest exposure to negative ions in these areas.

2. If you are regularly confined in an enclosed artificial
   atmosphere—such as home, office, car, airplane,
   cruiseship, bus—try putting a negative ion generator
   in that area. Or you can buy a much cheaper portable
   negative ion generator that you can wear on your clothing,
   near your face. See www.hyperstealth.com or call
   (604) 408-3600.

Letter from a Patient

Dear Dr. Matsen:

It is just over six months since I started treatment at your clinic. I already feel younger and more energetic. I no longer suffer from the stabbing pain, bloating, and headaches that had lasted for almost 30 years.

I was diagnosed several times over the past 30 years—by medical specialists—as having "Irritable Bowel Syndrome." I was told there was no cure, and that I would simply "have to learn to live with it."

Thank you for changing my life.

Sincerely,
Mary Walsh
Burnaby, BC

Putting It All Together

The last 50 years have brought affluence and wealth to many—but they have also brought increased exposure to heavy metals, antibiotics, vaccines, anti-inflammatories, anaesthetics, x-rays, pesticides, herbicides, solvents, dioxins, automobile exhaust, processed foods, and man-made air.

Survival of the fittest is as relevant today as it was with our ancestors, but the daily physical struggle to eke out a niche in nature is less relevant. Today, survival is more related to the ability of your liver's detoxification enzymes to process the countless chemicals to which it is exposed on a daily basis. In a study done by the Environmental Protection Agency, 100 percent of the North American population sampled has been shown to have accumulated four solvents and one dioxin in their bodies; over 90 percent of the population has accumulated another nine chemicals—four more solvents, one furan, three more dioxins, and DDE (a breakdown product of DDT). This goes to show the tremendous amount of exposure we have all had.

All these man-made chemicals—and any phenols originating from your intestinal flora—must be processed by your Phase I liver enzymes. During this process, dangerous peroxides will be formed. The production of peroxides is greatly increased by the intake of three physically or socially addictive drugs: tobacco,

alcohol, and coffee. The whole future of your health and
survival depends upon one enzyme's ability to chop those
deadly peroxides into harmless water. This key enzyme needs
nutrients that are not supplied by modern processed foods and
drinks. This same key enzyme is strongly inhibited by heavy
metals, such as the mercury commonly found in dental
amalgam fillings and used as a preservative in vaccines—both
of which are widely used in industrialized societies.

It is evident from the number of chronic diseases seen in all
age groups, that a large percentage of people are already
suffering from their liver's failure to neutralize their exposure
to the onslaught of metals and chemicals. At least 45 percent of
Americans have a chronic health problem.

The regulation of the chemical, pharmaceutical, dental,
medical, and food industries has been entrusted by us to the
"health" departments of our governments. It is obvious that
they have failed miserably in their job of protecting public
health—with the possible exception of Sweden. This failure is
partly due to lobby groups that overly influence political
decisions, which then override the researchers—although much
of the research has already been hijacked by corporate interests.

Except for the most severe genetic disorders, you are
programmed to be healthy, given the right conditions.
Researchers appear to be overlooking these conditions in their
desire to begin resplicing our DNA—now that they have
managed to gain patents on much of it. It would seem that the
elimination of mercury, chemicals, and processed foods would
go a long way toward avoiding the need to tinker with our
DNA, as the researchers seem to be intent on doing in the near
future.

As a member of a profession that has always focused on
building health, rather than *treating disease*, the impression I'm
left with is this: if you're waiting for the government to deliver
you good health, you're likely going to have a long, lonely, and
disappointing wait because our tax dollars have been mainly
shunted into pharmaceutical medicine.

My intention in writing this book is to help guide that
segment of the population that wants to be in charge of its

health by eating the right foods, minimizing exposure to heavy metals and chemicals, getting more exercise, taking the right supplements, getting adequate sleep, and beginning the restoration of their intestinal flora and liver from the effects of whatever damage has been done by chemicals and metals. Be patient and be persistent. You're on the first step to taking control of your health.

The diagram on the next page shows that a number of factors can cause the liver to create peroxides. Some factors come under the category of *EATING TOO BAD*, some from *EATING TOO WELL*, while others have been acquired through dental and medical treatments. The more of one factor you're exposed to, the less leeway you'll have with the others. This is particularly true of mercury exposure because it can so profoundly affect your liver's ability to neutralize peroxides.

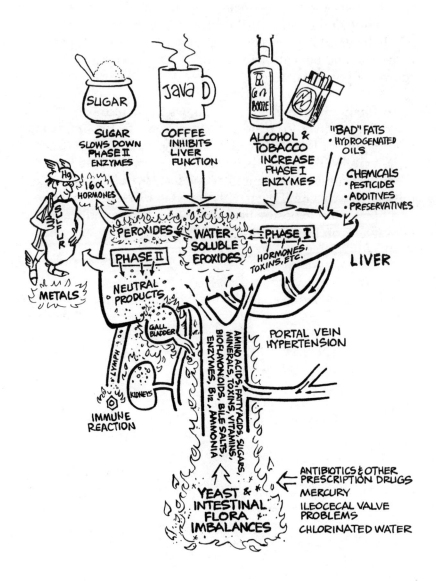

SIGNS AND SYMPTOMS

Let's take a closer look at some of the symptoms that might be manifested by "disrupted" intestinal flora, and by peroxides that are made in the liver, but not fully neutralized.

INTESTINAL FLORA IMBALANCES—Digestive and bowel problems

Your intestine is sterile when you're born, but it soon picks up a collection of hundreds of different species of bacteria and several species of fungi, dominated by Candida yeast. This motley crew of bacteria and fungi proliferate in the billions in the large intestine, and generally establish their own equilibrium. Lactobacilli, especially *Lactobacillus acidophilus* (acid-lovers), keep the large intestine acidic, which inhibits the fungus from growing, until you and your acidophilus die—at which time the fungus will recycle you into compost. Anything that knocks down your acidophilus prematurely, such as antibiotics and mercury, allows the fungi to grow prematurely—especially if you have a diet high in sugar. The yeast and other fungi create hordes of fatty toxins called phenols that must be neutralized by the liver. Weakness of the ileocecal valve due to poor calcium absorption can allow bacteria and yeast into the small intestine, where the alkaline conditions allow the yeast to proliferate.

- The most common symptoms of yeast overgrowth are gas, bloating, and cravings for sugar and chocolate.
- Frustration is the emotion most applicable to ileocecal valve problems.
- Other symptoms include bad breath and irregular bowel movements.

LIVER—Liver and blood problems

If the peroxides made by your Phase I liver enzymes are not quickly neutralized by your Phase II enzymes, the following conditions may result.

- Fatty liver
- Cirrhosis of the liver
- Susceptibility to hepatitis
- High cholesterol
- Type II diabetes
- Hypoglycemia

METALS—Liver, kidney, nerve, and immune problems

- Metals in the body, especially mercury, bind to sulfur, thereby interfering with the function of many sulfur-containing enzymes—notably glutathione transferase and glutathione peroxidase. They are the two critical Phase II enzymes in your liver that neutralize peroxides. When mercury binds to the sulfur of these enzymes, peroxides may spill out of the liver into the bile, kidneys, and lymph, and push hormones into the C-16 pathway, which creates "bad" hormones (see 16α HORMONES).

- Metals can directly cause neurological problems, such as memory and concentration problems, behavioural and learning disorders, spasticity, Parkinson's Disease, MS, Alzheimer Disease, ALS (Lou Gehrig's disease), schizophrenia, and autism.

- Metals can create immunological problems— especially autoimmune reactions such as arthritis and fibromyalgia—in addition to causing decreased functioning of the immune system (see IMMUNE REACTIONS).

- Metals—especially mercury—can come from "silver" amalgam fillings. Mercury and aluminum are also used in vaccines and flu shots. Even if you were exposed to metals a long time ago, they can still be present in your body today, although some people seem to have the ability to gradually eliminate metals.

GALLBLADDER—Digestive and bowel problems

When peroxides spill out of the liver into the bile, they create toxic bile symptoms, which include the following.

- Acid reflux; heartburn; pain under or below the sternum; pain in the centre of the chest; shortness of breath; heaviness after eating—especially spicy or fatty foods; fatigue or dizziness after eating; hiatus hernia; nausea; vomiting; pain under the right rib cage; gallstones; gas; bloating; cramping; diarrhea/ constipation; pain between the shoulder blades; fatigue that's worse in the morning but that lessens later in the day; fluid retention that's worse in the morning and that lessens later in the day.
- Nightmares, bad dreams, waking between 1 a.m. and 3 a.m.
- Eye sensitivity or blurring; migraines; neck pain that's worse in the morning and less painful later in the day.
- Weakened connective tissue leading to hernias, sprains, varicose veins, bruising, prolapses, and joint dislocation.
- Melancholia, moodiness, depression, anger, irritability, and indecisiveness.

KIDNEY—Urinary tract and bladder problems

When peroxides spill from the liver into the blood, the kidneys are forced to filter them. However, the kidneys are dependent on the liver for glutathione to neutralize the peroxides. If glutathione does not neutralize the peroxides, these symptoms can result.

- Frequent urination; irritation on urination; chronic bladder infections; urethra spasm; high blood pressure; low back pain; neck pain that feels better in the morning and worse later in the day; fluid retention that's less in the morning and worse at the end of the day.
- Skin problems

- Fearfulness/anxiety
- Decreased sex drive

IMMUNE REACTIONS—Overactive and underactive immune system problems

When the liver spills peroxides and proteins into the lymph, the immune system attacks them as if they were dangerous invaders. The immune reactions can create the following.

- Congestion and swelling in the lymph glands, which can make the person more susceptible to sore throats, ear infections, bronchitis, sinusitis, and rhinitis.
- Allergies, asthma, eczema, dermatitis, hives, achy joints.
- Autoimmune diseases such as lupus; scleroderma; sarcoidosis; type I diabetes; psoriasis; atherosclerosis; MS; colitis; Crohn's disease; fibromyalgia; rheumatoid arthritis, etc.
- Severe fatigue.

16α HORMONES—Organ irritation

When the liver has a build-up of peroxides, they may interfere with the breakdown of steroid hormones. Because women also have testosterone (6 percent of the amount that men have) and men also have estrogens (20 percent of the amount that women have), poor liver function can wreak havoc with the hormones in both sexes.

The ideal way for your liver to break down estrogens is through what's known as the C-2 pathway, in which the end-products are mild hormones. The alternative breakdown pathway—which is more commonly used when there is a build-up of peroxides in the liver—is known as the C-16 pathway. This pathway breaks down estrogens into products such as 16α-hydroxyestrone, which can aggravate the reproductive organs.

The C-16 pathway creates nasty hormones that can:
- cause irregular periods, menstrual cramping, PMS, fibroids, ovarian cysts, fibrocystic breast disease, endometriosis, and unexplained infertility;
- cause breast cancer, cervical cancer, and ovarian cancer;
- contribute to prostate enlargement and prostate cancer;
- contribute to lung cancer, colon cancer, and lupus; and
- cause hair loss.

DNA—Mutations

If your Phase II enzymes don't neutralize the peroxides and epoxides that are made by your Phase I enzymes, some of these toxic epoxides can bind to and damage your DNA. This can lead to mutations that can cause benign tumours and eventually, cancer. The peroxides can damage p53, the gene that controls the replication rate of your DNA. Without p53's supervision, mutated DNA can grow rapidly, creating benign tumours or cancer.

PORTAL VEIN

When your liver's detoxification enzymes can't keep up with incoming toxins, that can lead to the closing of your liver's inlet valves, which creates back-pressure on the portal vein itself—called portal vein hypertension. This can cause problems anywhere in the digestive system, such as:
- "bay window" belly;
- swelling of the hemorrhoidal veins, proctitis, fissures, fistulas, etc.; and
- swelling of the esophageal vein, colitis, diverticulosis, Crohn's disease, gastritis, and ulcers.

The First
Two Weeks

You can see from the preceding information that virtually any health problem can occur when the liver is overwhelmed with peroxides. Since there is no alarm system installed in your liver to tell you when you are producing peroxides, each and every one of your systems acts as a peripheral alarm, to let you know you're in "peroxide trouble."

In 1983, I had the good fortune to sit in with an old naturopathic doctor who knew implicitly that to help a person become healthy, you had to get his or her liver working better. To accomplish that, you had to improve the person's digestion, starting with the diet and then working from the mouth down the digestive system, until the liver regained its function.

Applying this basic insight, I began my practice, and soon found that 70 percent or more of my patients achieved dramatic results within several months. However, I was stumped as to why 20 to 30 percent of the patients struggled for improvement—even though they claimed to be following my treatment program.

In retrospect, I can see now that for those patients, the main detriment to their liver function was the presence of metals— mainly mercury—in their bodies. Removing all the other factors wasn't enough to help them regain their health. They still had a long and expensive journey ahead to gain improvement.

Yet most people with high levels of mercury, including myself, were able to regain a sense of well-being simply by following a healthy diet and improving their intestinal flora and liver function. I still can't predict who will respond to the dietary/digestion adjustments. But because removing metals from the body is a relatively slow and expensive process—compared to improving diet and digestion—I still prefer to remove the metals last.

After several years in practice, I wrote *EATING ALIVE: Prevention Thru Good Digestion* in 1987. I quote from *EATING ALIVE*:

"There is no doubt that a person with a strong genetic constitution, healthy intestinal flora (not ravaged by Western medicine), and a digestion free from the worries and troubles of life, can eat and drink with abandon for a considerable period of time. However, the prevalence of chronic disease (physical, mental, and emotional) in our society indicates that eventually, there are limits."

Avoiding coffee, alcohol, tobacco, white sugar, and white flour are obvious goals to set. At the same time, it's important to be careful not to go too far in the other direction—you can weaken your ileocecal valve by eating *too many* fruits and salads, as most diet and weight-loss books would recommend. I quote again:

"The confusion over diet is mainly because changing diet by itself doesn't improve digestion, so a person remains highly sensitive to many different foods."

"If a person can increase digestive vitality, the dietary range can also be increased."

Since it's going to take six to eight weeks to regain your proper intestinal flora, and one to three years to strip accumulated metals from your body, I'll give a few quick tips that may help you to at least obtain some fairly quick improvement in your symptoms within a week or so.

TWO QUICK WAYS TO TUNE UP THE KIDNEYS

If you have eaten a diet high in regular table salt and you're retaining fluid, and perhaps have high blood pressure, your kidneys may be swamped from excess sodium and may be deficient in potassium. This can be rectified by drinking a **potassium broth** made by thoroughly cooking potato skins, carrots, celery, and perhaps some other vegetables in a pot of water, and then straining the broth. You can drink this broth liberally throughout the day and, within a week or so, excess salt and fluid retention should be decreased or eliminated. The celery also helps loosen stiff and achy joints, and can be used in juice form. This broth should not be consumed by those with kidney damage, because too much potassium could interfere with heart function.

If you have bloating and fluid retention but have been "health-conscious"—reading health books, following weight-loss programs, undergoing colon irrigation, fasting, or if you are a vegetarian who has intentionally avoided salt—you probably have the opposite kidney problem: low sodium, with an associated weakened ileocecal valve, especially if you have low blood pressure.

The two main sources of sodium are **animal protein** and **salt**. Adding Celtic Sea Salt® to the diet is imperative for those eating vegetable foods. In several cases, the blood pressure of my patients was so low from a strict vegetarian diet (80 over 50) that I asked them to mix a half-teaspoon of Celtic Sea Salt® in a glass of warm water and drink it several times a day. Obviously this should not be done if you have high blood pressure because, while sodium is not the cause of high blood pressure, it can worsen this condition once you have it.

ILEOCECAL VALVE TIP

While the aforementioned quick tips should help give your kidneys a little improvement, it might be several weeks before you will be ready to tackle killing off the yeast in your intestine. Since most of my patients have bacteria and yeast in the *small intestine*, rather than in the *large intestine*, it's imperative to close the ileocecal valve before trying to kill the yeast. The reason is that yeast are quite toxic when they die off, thereby putting a heavier load on the liver's detoxification enzymes. If constipation is present, this load will be worsened dramatically.

If the ileocecal valve remains open while you are taking a yeast-killer, more bacteria and yeast from the large intestine will move into the small intestine—virtually as fast as you kill them off. The net effect over a period of time can be to gradually jam up your liver with peroxides made by the dying yeast. Normally I check the patient's ileocecal valve before advising the use of a yeast-killer.

I've included a few acupressure exercises you can do to help your ileocecal valve function better. Years ago, I used to routinely give similar exercises to my patients, before I understood that calcium absorption via the kidneys' sodium/ potassium levels was the key to getting the valve working.

ACUPRESSURE POINTS FOR BALANCING THE ILEOCECAL VALVE

Rub each of the following points, two or three times per day. You do not have to rub them hard and inflict pain—just apply enough pressure to stimulate them.

1. Place your hands halfway between your navel and the prominent hip bone on each side of the body—your little fingers should be at the inside edge of the hip bone. Your right hand is over the ileocecal valve and your left hand is over the Houston valve. Now rub the fingers of each hand up and down over these areas for 20 to 30 seconds. The areas you should rub are approximately six inches in length.

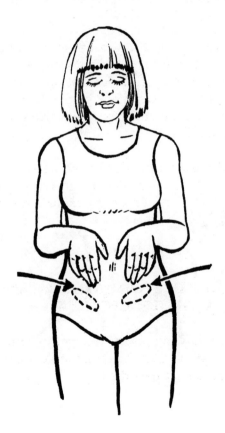

2. The next two points are located at the top of the neck where it meets the skull. With each hand, follow the edge of the bottom of the skull; start at the bones behind the bottom of the ears, and move your fingers toward the middle of the back of the head. The acupressure points are located about one-third of the way to the middle, where you will feel an indentation, groove, or notch that goes up toward the top of the head for about half an inch. These are gallbladder points; they may feel very tender if you have toxic bile. Stimulate them for 20 to 30 seconds.

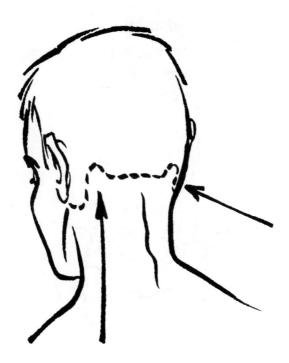

3. To locate the next two points, cross your arms so that the
    fingers of each hand are touching the upper arm—halfway
    between the elbow and the shoulder—on the opposite side
    of the body. The acupressure points are located between
    the biceps muscle (the one at the front of the arm that
    people flex to show how strong they are) and the triceps
    muscle (the muscle at the back of the arm). These are
    kidney points. Now rub the fingers of each hand up and
    down over these areas for 20 to 30 seconds. The areas you
    should rub are approximately six inches in length.

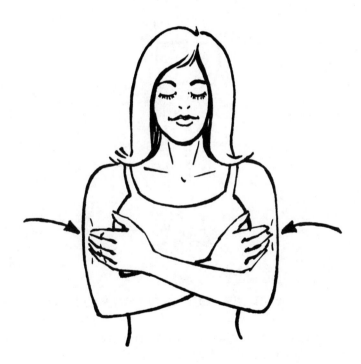

4. Rubbing these last two points is optional. Stand straight and allow your arms to hang comfortably by your sides. The points are located where your middle fingers meet the outside of your thighs. These are gallbladder points; they may feel very tender if you have toxic bile. Rub for 20 to 30 seconds.

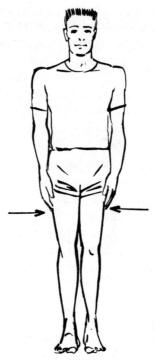

A QUICK DIGESTION AND LIVER BOOSTER

One way that you can quickly speed up your digestion is by following basic **food-combining**—which is actually the opposite of the way it sounds. Food-combining involves the *separation* of foods. Proteins (flesh proteins, at least, such as fish, poultry, and red meat) need hydrochloric acid to be digested, while starches (grains, legumes, beans, and starchy vegetables such as potatoes and corn) need alkaline digestive juices; thus, when they are eaten at the same meal, these foods inhibit each other's digestion. This may not be important when the digestive system is at its peak, but when the digestion is weakened due to stress and/or peroxide-laden bile—which inhibits the production of digestive juices—then the combination of animal protein and starch may be too much of a burden on the system, resulting in fatigue after eating, and digestive "heaviness."

Eating **protein** and **non-starchy vegetables**, while excluding starches, will often quickly improve the digestion; energy levels will usually rise. Since starch is sugar, and surplus sugar is stored as fat, weight loss often accompanies this approach to eating. The decreased intake of sugar will sometimes give symptoms of low blood sugar, which can be rectified by drinking **unsweetened Concord grape juice**, as needed. The anti-peroxide bioflavonoids of the grape juice will also help inhibit peroxides in the liver. If ileocecal valve problems are suspected, do not drink the grape juice. Other things that might be used in place of Concord grape juice are **blueberry juice, blue elderberry juice, black currant juice**, and **beet juice**.

Beets should be eaten daily in the diet, as part of one of your meals. Sliced pickled beets are commonly used in sandwiches and hamburgers in countries such as Australia.

Unsweetened cranberry juice can also be used. Like blueberries, cranberries have bioflavonoids that make it difficult for bacteria to cling to the walls of the urinary tract. Read labels carefully, because cranberry drink and cranberry cocktail can be loaded with added sugar. Diabetics should avoid using such drinks, even the unsweetened ones, unless they are carefully monitoring their blood-sugar levels.

Having animal protein, non-starchy vegetables, and Concord grape juice at the last meal of the day is especially beneficial, because digestion tends to weaken as the day goes on. This combination can be repeated as needed. The fats in poultry and fish are easier to digest than those in red meat. The high potassium in the grape juice means that sodium in the form of sea salt must be added into the diet somewhere, to avoid problems with the ileocecal valve. Also, if a person loses too much weight, he or she should add starches back into the diet, as needed.

If there is cramping in the digestive system, drinking **fennel seed tea** will usually relieve it.

A QUICK GALLBLADDER TONIC

Since the majority of digestive symptoms come from peroxide-laden bile, those with gallbladder symptoms should consider having a **lemon drink** in the morning, because lemon stimulates the flushing of the bile from the gallbladder. Ten to 20 minutes before breakfast, having approximately 3 teaspoons of lemon juice in warm water, perhaps with **ginger**, will give the gallbladder a little tune-up after about a week. Those with acid reflux may find the lemon too irritating; these individuals might do better just having ginger in warm water.

The lemon drink can be repeated as needed. Also, because lemon is high in potassium, an equal amount of sea salt must be added into the diet somewhere, to maintain the calcium levels of the ileocecal valve.

WEAKEN THE YEAST

Throughout the first few weeks, you should be taking **acidophilus**, in the form of yogurt or capsules, to inhibit any yeast in the intestine. Acidophilus isn't known as a yeast-killer but it can slow the yeast down a little—which is all you want at the beginning, anyway. You can also weaken the yeast if you stop feeding them refined carbohydrates. Before you consider killing off the yeast and bacteria, render the yeast a little weaker and make your liver a little stronger.

SUPPORT THE LIVER

Now that I understand the ramifications of the tremendous quantities of mercury found in myself and many of my patients, I use far more supplementation than in the past. In my practice, I use several different remedies that consist of a combination of ingredients to reduce liver peroxides, but you can also make your own—although it might be more expensive.

The main liver enzyme you need to support is glutathione peroxidase, which requires two key ingredients: **selenium** and the amino acid **cysteine**—which contains sulfur. Many soils in which we grow food are selenium-deficient, but selenium can be readily supplemented at 200 micrograms per day at little expense and with no side-effects. This dose has been documented to reduce your chances of getting many cancers, by about 50 percent.

While any animal protein will have cysteine, the food that is highest in cysteine is whey protein powder—long considered a useless leftover from cheese-making after the curds have been extracted from milk. Now it is known as one of the medicinal parts of dairy, if it is micro-filtered and not heated—so that the precious enzymes and sulfur are not destroyed. One of the side-effects of whey is weight gain, due to muscle-mass increase. Whey is much less allergenic than milk, but some people still have trouble taking it. Taking 1 to 2 tablespoons, one or two times per day, is adequate when using the other synergistic liver supplements. **Do not take whey or any other cysteine while mercury is in the blood—for example, after dental work or chelation—because the mercury may bind to cysteine, and be transported into the brain.**

Another form of sulfur to which few are allergic is **Methyl-Sulfonyl-Methane (MSM)**, which helps strengthen membranes throughout the body.

The herb **milk thistle** is known for its ability to activate glutathione peroxidase, after it has been taken regularly for about three days.

It's also important to take **vitamin C with bioflavonoids**, to help neutralize peroxides and also to help strengthen connective tissue. Some brands use bioflavonoids from grapefruit—not the fruit or the skin, but the white matter found between them. These grapefruit bioflavonoids are believed to be the best at dissolving plaque out of the arteries—the way lemon in dishwashing liquids cuts grease on a plate. Grapefruit bioflavonoids also have the ability to decrease the Phase I enzymes that make peroxides. For an adult with a chronic health problem, a minimum dose of vitamin C (usually a *buffered* C) with bioflavonoids is 500 milligrams, three times per day. Linus Pauling found that vitamin C only lasts up to four hours in the body, so he recommended taking it up to six times per day.

Rounding off a liver remedy should be a **multivitamin/mineral supplement** including **the B vitamins** and **zinc**, and perhaps desiccated liver, as well.

During the first week, there will be some ups and downs as you go through withdrawals from addictive substances, and as your liver starts to flush out some of the accumulated toxins. It's important to keep your bowels working well—toxins from the bile should be expelled promptly. Getting regular exercise and drinking plenty of spring or filtered water can help; so can **psyllium** or **flax seed powder**.

If you're doing things right, after five to ten days, your ileocecal valve should be closed due to improved calcium absorption, and the flood of bacteria and yeast from your large intestine into your small intestine should be over. Also, your liver should be functioning a little better. As your liver improves, your energy should increase, digestive symptoms should decrease, sleep should deepen, and moods should brighten—although the biggest improvement is yet to come.

The illustration below shows the things that are GOOD for the liver.

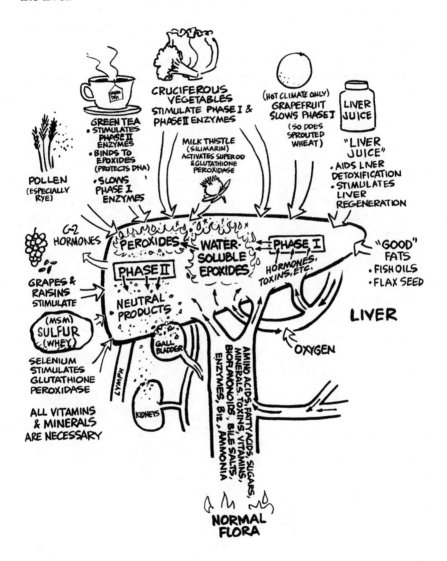

The Next Four Weeks

There comes a point where you may hit a plateau, between one to two weeks into the program. Some energy and digestive symptoms might have improved, but immune reactions and hormonal problems won't have shown any improvement at all. Continue supporting the liver as you move on to kill the yeast.

My favourite yeast remedy is Latero-Flora™—*Bacillus laterosporus*—a famed fungus and bacteria "assassin" discovered in the soil of Iceland. Latero-Flora comes in a dried powder form; the bacteria are dormant and become active when moisture is added, so it's best to store the container in a dry cupboard rather than the fridge. Although the dosage recommended on the bottle is 1 teaspoon per morning, I recommend a *lower* dosage, based on the amount of metals suspected to have accumulated in the person.

If metals such as mercury bind to the key detoxification enzymes of the body, it only makes sense to detoxify at a slower pace, to avoid aggravation. For most adults, I suggest ⅛ to ½ teaspoon every *third* morning (for children, ⅛ teaspoon every *third* morning).

It's usually not necessary to increase it more than that because, by the time one month has passed, the bacteria and yeast have usually been eliminated from the intestine.

I found that, for many patients, after they stopped taking Latero-Flora™, the yeast came back quite quickly. Now I suggest that my patients keep taking it several times a week, indefinitely, especially if they have mercury fillings.

On the days when you take the Latero-Flora™ in the morning, you can skip the morning dose of acidophilus, but you can continue to take acidophilus at night.

Other yeast-killers—such as wild oregano, caprylic acid, and even garlic, as is used in herbal heart remedies—can kill yeast most of the time, but not always. A yeast-killer I sometimes recommend, if the person has advanced skin fungus, is grapefruit seed extract. In the health food store, it is called Nutribiotic®. The stronger version, Citricidal®, is sold by health practitioners. I've even used it successfully in the Citricidal Plus® form (it has two extra herbs: echinacea and *artemesia annua*), to help fight the antibiotic-resistant bacteria *Enterococci*. The dose was 1 capsule, three times per day, although the biggest improvement in one client didn't occur until after the yeast was cleared out of her intestine with Latero-Flora™.

Olive leaf extract can be used to kill mycoplasma—another yeast-like Bad Guy—that is sometimes seen in fibromyalgia and rheumatoid arthritis. I suggest that you go slowly, taking 1 capsule, one to four times a day, increasing gradually.

When patients first come to my office, it's not unusual for them to have ten or 12 different complaints. After the first two weeks, a few of these symptoms are usually reduced slightly, but the rest are the same. By the time they've been through four weeks of the yeast-killer, most of their symptoms are usually either gone or greatly reduced. Typically, the symptoms that aren't completely better yet are immunological, neurological, and/or hormonal.

Sometimes it just takes a little more time for these symptoms to fade away; sometimes they still don't get better. Every one of my patients who has been slow to respond to my treatment program, and who has subsequently had a "DMPS chelation challenge," has shown the presence of incredible amounts of mercury in his or her system. Some of these patients have now completed one to two years of chelation; they have removed much of the mercury from their systems, and they are showing improvement. I haven't yet found the end of the "mercury trail" but so far, it seems to explain the stubbornness of the health difficulties that many patients are experiencing.

As I finish off our little journey, I repeat my earlier warnings: **Don't let anyone—doctor, nurse, or dentist—put mercury into your body through vaccines or amalgam fillings, because it can take a very long time to remove mercury from your body.**

The Nutritional Steps of THE EATING ALIVE PROGRAM

The Nutritional Steps of THE EATING ALIVE PROGRAM consist of both dietary guidelines and nutritional supplements, to achieve the following results.

- Replenish your body with the nutrients it needs. This is especially important to improve the functioning of your digestive system, particularly your liver.
- Repair your ileocecal valve.
- Restore your good intestinal flora.

Part II of this book contains Menu Suggestions and many delicious, easy-to-make recipes to help you follow these nutritional steps. Part II also contains information about the importance of consuming healthy fats and oils, and the benefits of organic foods.

REPLENISH

Your liver has hundreds of jobs to do, so it's important that it functions effectively. Some of its jobs include the following.

- Neutralize toxins
- Deactivate hormones
- Activate vitamin D
- Make bile salts
- Oxidize fats for energy
- Store iron and vitamins A, D, and B_{12}
- Change sugars and amino acids into fats such as triglycerides
- Remove ammonia by the formation of urea
- Produce amino acids and plasma proteins
- Make CoQ_{10} and other nutrients crucial to your health
- And many, many more.

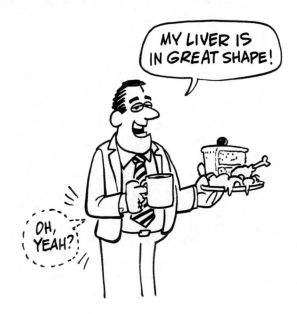

Healthy eating includes proteins, fats, and carbohydrates—all of which are required by your body to obtain the nutrients it needs. Use the **Food Chart** on pages 78 and 79 as a guideline for choosing what to eat (see also the Menu Suggestions in Part II). The Food Chart is divided into three columns.

Left Column
The left column contains *warming* foods and consists of proteins and fats, which are usually found together in foods.

Animal proteins already have the proper sodium/potassium balance so they don't need to be salted. The best choices of protein include: fish; skinless chicken and turkey breast; venison; ostrich; eggs (poached or soft-boiled); and whey protein powder (choose unsweetened varieties). Soy products such as tofu, tempeh, soybeans, and soy protein powder are healthy sources of protein but should be eaten in moderation. Compared to the other proteins listed, eggs and cheese have a higher fat content in proportion to protein. Whenever possible, choose egg whites, rather than whole eggs, and reduced-fat cheeses. Low-fat milk and plain yogurt are mixed protein-carbohydrate choices.

Certain fats are vital to a well-balanced, healthy diet because they provide **essential fatty acids (EFAs)—omega 3 (O-3)** and **omega 6 (O-6) fatty acids**—those that your body cannot synthesize itself.
The recommended choices for the fat portion of your diet include: Udo's Choice Ultimate Oil Blend® (a combination of O-3 and O-6); hemp oil (O-3 and O-6); pumpkin seeds and pumpkin seed butter (O-3 and O-6); flax seed oil and flax seeds (O-3: the seeds should be ground—to release the oil—and be eaten immediately after doing so); tahini (sesame seed paste) and sesame oil (O-6); almonds and smooth almond butter (O-6); extra virgin olive oil (no EFAs but suitable for cooking); and sunflower and safflower oils (O-6).
Choose oils that are unrefined, minimally processed, and expeller pressed. These oils should be stored in dark containers that won't allow light in and that have an expiry date on the bottle. They can be found in health food stores; they are more expensive than the processed oils found on the grocery store shelves, but they are worth the extra cost. Most oils (except

olive oil and ghee) should be kept in the fridge. (For more information on healthy fats and oils, please see the article by Udo Erasmus in Part II.)

One of the best sources of healthy fat is fish, which contains two O-3 fatty acids called DHA (docosahexaenoic acid) and EPA (eicosapentaenoic acid). DHA is used in the nervous system as a building block—for brain cells, for example. EPA has broad-acting anti-inflammatory properties. The oilier fish have the most EPA. Ideal choices include wild salmon, albacore tuna, sardines, herring, and mackerel.

Right Column
The right column contains fruits (carbohydrates) that are *cooling* foods—those that are naturally high in potassium and/or sugar.

Centre Column
All the foods in the centre column are carbohydrates; they include non-starchy vegetables and starchy carbohydrates—grains, legumes (beans, peas, lentils, peanuts), and starchy vegetables such as potatoes and corn. These foods should be salted with Celtic sea salt before being eaten; they're high in potassium, but when you add sea salt to them, the sodium in the sea salt combines with the potassium of the plants to make them *neutral*—neither warming or cooling.

Vegetables should be lightly steamed or stir-fried as often as possible, especially during cooler weather; this makes them easier to digest and helps avoid irritating a sensitive ileocecal valve. Cruciferous vegetables are those that belong to the cabbage family; they have anti-cancer properties and should be eaten several times a week.

You'll notice on the Food Chart that the starchy carbohydrates, fruits, and dairy products have two letter values beside them—for example, L/L. The first letter represents the **Glycemic Index** or **GI** of that particular food. A low value (L) denotes a GI of 55 or less; a medium value (M) means a GI of 56 to 69 inclusive; and a high value (H) denotes a GI of 70 or more. The second letter represents the **Glycemic Load** or **GL** rating of that particular food. A low value (L) denotes a GL of 10 or less; a medium value (M) means a GL of 11 to 19 inclusive; and a high value (H) denotes a GI of 20 or more. A few of the foods have ranges for one or both of these ratings, for example L to H. Read further for a more detailed explanation of GI and GL.

Value	Glycemic Index (GI)	Glycemic Load (GL)
Low (L)	55 or less	10 or less
Medium (M)	56 to 69	11 to 19
High (H)	70 or more	20 or more

The Glycemic Index or GI is a rating system that indicates how different carbohydrates affect the rise in blood sugar (glucose) levels. Carbohydrates are made up of sugars that are bound together. The digestive process breaks these bonds and the simple sugars then enter the bloodstream, affecting blood sugar levels and insulin production. Insulin is a hormone that is secreted by the pancreas in response to an increase in blood sugar levels shortly after meals. Insulin helps to regulate blood sugar levels.

Generally speaking, the more processed a food is, the higher its GI value. For example, fruit juices have higher GIs than their whole fruit counterparts, and flours (and foods made from them) have higher GIs than the whole grains from which they're ground.

Foods that have a low GI enter the bloodstream slowly, cause a slow, moderate rise in blood sugar, and therefore a moderate insulin response. Foods that have a high GI enter the bloodstream quickly, cause a quick, sharp rise in blood sugar, and a corresponding sharp rise in insulin.

Excessive amounts of insulin in the bloodstream have the following effects.
- Insulin lowers blood sugar levels by promoting the uptake of glucose into most of your body's cells, especially the muscles, liver, and fat cells. *Excess*

insulin causes *rapid* absorption of glucose. As a result, blood sugar quickly falls below a critical level and your body calls out for more glucose, which the brain requires in order to function. Thus, you experience carbohydrate cravings and blood sugar swings.

- Insulin increases the use of glucose by most of your body's cells, which automatically *decreases* the use of fat as an energy source.
- Insulin causes excess glucose in the liver to be converted into fats, which are then transported to fat cells to be stored.
- Insulin inhibits the action of lipase, the enzyme responsible for breaking down fat molecules.

In the GI rating system, glucose is assigned a GI of 100 and other foods are assigned GI numbers in comparison to it. In *The Secrets to Great Health* and in the first printing of this book, as well as in my clinical practice, we had only ever included the GI of carbohydrate-containing foods (GL values were not included). The values that were used were based on information contained in "International Tables of Glycemic Index" published in 1995 in the *American Journal of Clinical Nutrition*. We used the white bread index in which white bread was assigned a GI of 100. We've now chosen to switch to the glucose index in which glucose has a value of 100 so as to be less confusing to my patients and to readers, since most other publications use this method.

Another change that we've made is to assign more general ratings of Low, Medium, and High rather than actual numerical values, as we did in the past. We've chosen this method to make it easier to understand because for some foods, there's a wide variation of numerical values.

One of the drawbacks of using only the GI is that it can be misleading because GI tests aren't based on typical portion sizes of foods. Instead, researchers use a standard measure of 50 grams of carbohydrate of the foods that they are testing; therefore, portion sizes vary depending on the amount of available carbohydrate in the particular food. For example, a carrot contains only 4 to 6 grams of available carbohydrate so you'd need to eat about 10 carrots to consume 50 grams of carbohydrate—and nobody eats that many carrots at one meal! We found that many patients were avoiding carrots and other nutritious high-GI foods, such as beets and squash, because of their higher GI values. This is where the Glycemic Load or GL proves more useful.

GL is a relatively new tool that takes into account the GI as well as the amount of carbohydrate in a typical portion size of a given food. The GL is calculated by dividing the GI numerical value of that food by 100 and then multiplying by the grams of carbohydrate that a typical serving contains. As an example, in some studies, carrots have a *high* GI rating of 92. One medium carrot only has about 6 grams of available carbohydrate, so the GL would be 92 divided by 100 then multiplied by 6, giving a *low* GL rating of approximately 5. In contrast, white rice has a *low* GI of 51. A one-cup serving has 42 grams of available carbohydrate, so the GL would be 51 divided by 100 then multiplied by 42, giving a *high* GL rating of approximately 21.

Highly processed foods, starchy high-GI foods like white bread and white rice, and foods and beverages that contain a lot of sugar—such as cakes, cookies, candy, and soft drinks—generally have high GL values. These are lacking in nutrients and are not recommended foods of The Eating Alive Program.

No GI/GL values are available for some of the grains such as spelt, amaranth, kamut, quinoa, and oat groats, but when cooked in their whole form, the glycemic values would generally be assumed to be in the low to medium range. 'Whole form' means the whole grain itself, not the flours or flakes made from them. (As an example, because they are more processed, rolled oats would have higher glycemic values than old-fashioned, large flake oats and oat groats would have even lower values.)

Non-starchy vegetables have no glycemic values because they contain either no carbohydrate or too small an amount of available carbohydrate for glycemic testing to be feasible. This may also explain why there are no GI/GL values for lemons, limes, nuts, avocadoes, and most of the berries, so we assume these values to be in the low range.

The best choices for carbohydrates are those that have low to medium or no GL ratings, as outlined below. These foods help to keep blood sugar levels stable and provide vitamins, minerals, phytonutrients, and fibre.

As a general guideline, fill half your plate with cruciferous and/or other non-starchy vegetables, particularly leafy greens. Feel free to load up on these foods at snacks as well as for meals.

One quarter of your plate can be filled with a serving of starchy carbohydrates that have low to medium GL values (a ½ cup serving is approximately equal to the size of a small clenched fist). They include the following:

- Lentils, chickpeas, and most beans—these also contain protein (½ cup)
- Oatmeal (slow-cooking type only, ⅓ to ½ cup)
- Whole grains such as oat groats, brown rice, barley, rye and wheat kernels, buckwheat, kamut, spelt, quinoa, and amaranth (⅓ to ½ cup)
- Whole-grain rye bread and other whole-grain breads (1 slice)
- Whole-grain pastas, and beanthread or mung bean noodles (½ cup)
- Starchy vegetables, such as corn, new potatoes, squash, carrots, beets, and sweet potatoes (½ cup).

Looking at the Food Chart, you'll notice that most of these foods have low GL values. Those that have medium GL values are still nutritious—just don't eat large quantities of them. The same goes for those foods that have medium or high GI values, but low GL values, such as carrots and beets. Carrots, squash, and sweet potatoes are foods that you want to include in your diet because they're good sources of vitamin A and other nutrients; beets are an excellent source of anthocyanidins. So go ahead and eat them, just have them in moderate amounts along with other vegetables and some lean protein and/or healthy fat. Eating protein and fat with carbohydrates tends to slow down their rate of entry into the bloodstream, thus lowering their glycemic effect.

The remaining quarter of your plate can be filled with a serving of healthy protein (see Food Chart and page 69 for recommended choices). An average serving of animal protein, about 3 to 4 ounces, is approximately the same size as the palm of a woman's hand or a deck of cards. Nuts, seeds, low-fat milk and yogurt, and legumes (beans, peas, lentils) also contain some protein.

Most fruits (excluding fruit juices, bananas, raisins, dried dates, and dried figs) also have low GL values. Fruits can be eaten for snacks, either by themselves or—for those whose digestive system can handle it—with low-fat plain yogurt, nut butters, or seed butters. A typical serving size is about ½ cup or a small piece of fruit. **Choose fruit that's "in season" for the climate in which you live** and limit consumption to a maximum of one serving per day. Do not eat fruit with animal protein.

For those who'd like to lose weight, choose the majority of your carbohydrates from those that have no GI/GL values (such as cruciferous and other non-starchy vegetables) and those with low GL values. And remember that regular aerobic and strength-training exercises are also an important part of any weight-loss program.

In order to keep blood sugar levels stable, try to include some protein, carbohydrate, and fat at each meal and remember to have snacks. The amount of food needed on a daily basis will vary from person to person depending upon one's size, activity level, and metabolism. Those with larger body frames and/or who are more active will require more protein than those who are smaller and/or more sedentary. Those who are very active will need to consume larger quantities of healthy carbohydrates. Glucose is stored in your body as glycogen. If intense muscle activity occurs—such as when you engage in heavy exercise for an hour or longer—you may deplete your glycogen stores. A high-carbohydrate diet will help to renew depleted glycogen within two days, while a high-protein, low-carbohydrate diet might take five days or longer to do so.

One of the problems with using glycemic values is that they don't take into consideration the nutritive value of a particular food. For example, a small serving of low-fat ice cream has a low value for both GI and GL but it's hardly nutritious; it's usually loaded with sugar or sugar substitutes and provides little in the way of vitamins, minerals, antioxidants, and fibre. The GI/GL values are not the only criteria that you should use when choosing what to eat; instead, use them in conjunction with the other principles of THE EATING ALIVE PROGRAM. Remember to eat according to the climate in which you live; avoid foods to which you may be sensitive; watch your portion sizes; and eat balanced meals composed of the recommended carbohydrates, lean protein, and healthy fats.

The important thing to remember is to listen to your body; when you replace processed foods with nutritious, whole foods and improve your health, it becomes clearer as to what is good and bad for you.

For more information on GI and GL values, see the "Revised International Table of Glycemic Index and Glycemic Load Values-2002" at http://diabetes.about.com/library/mendosagi/ngilists.htm

Food Chart

FOOD CHART

• WARMING

PROTEIN

Recommended
All or most of the time

wild salmon, sardines, mackerel
albacore tuna, herring
halibut, trout
cod, bass, sole
venison
ostrich
chicken breast (free run)
turkey breast (free run)
eggs (poached or soft-boiled)
whey protein powder

In Moderation

tofu, tempeh, miso
shellfish, anchovies
lamb
reduced-fat cottage cheese
reduced-fat cheese
quark
veal
beef (lean cuts)
duck
pork
calf liver

PROTEIN/CARBOHYDRATE

goat's milk or yogurt	(not avail.)
low fat milk or yogurt	L/L
soy milk or yogurt	L/L

• NEUTRAL (if salted with sea salt)

CARBOHYDRATES
Lightly cook: steam or stir-fry.

Cruciferous Vegetables

broccoli; cauliflower
brussels sprouts; cabbage
broccoli rabe (rapini)
collard greens; kale; bok choy
mustard greens; watercress
kohlrabi; radishes
turnips/rutabagas

Other Vegetables

swiss chard; spinach; romaine
green and red leaf lettuces
arugula; radicchio; chicory
beet greens; nettle
endive; dandelion greens
sea vegetables
garlic; onion; leek; chive
shallot; scallion (green onion)
artichoke; asparagus
celery; jicama
green and wax beans
eggplant; okra; sweet peppers
tomatoes; cucumber
zucchini, yellow squash
snow peas; mushrooms
fresh herbs
sprouts

• COOLING

FRUITS (CARBOHYDRATES)
Limit the amount of fruit you eat.
Select fruits that are in season for the climate in which you live.

With GI/GL values

lemons; limes	
raspberries; blueberries	
blackberries; cranberries	
strawberries	L/L
cherries	L/L
plums; prunes	L/L
grapefruit	L/L
peaches	L/L
pears	L/L
apples	L/L
grapes: red and green	L/L
oranges	L/L
kiwi fruit	L/L
mangoes	L/L
apricots, dried	L/L
fresh	M/L
bananas	L/M
pineapple; papaya	M/L
cantaloupe	M/L
watermelon	H/L
raisins	M/H

FATS

avocado (guacamole)
olives

FATS

Recommended (unrefined oils)
Udo's Choice Ultimate Oil Blend®
hemp oil
pumpkin seeds, pumpkin seed butter
flax seeds, flax seed oil
sesame oil, tahini
almonds, almond butter
olive oil
sunflower, safflower oils

In Moderation
butter, ghee
coconut butter
walnuts
brazil nuts (1 per day)
other nut & seed butters

Use Sparingly
mayonnaise
cream cheese, sour cream

OTHER
ginger

• BEVERAGES
water
dandelion or herbal coffees
herbal tea
green tea
vegetable or chicken broth
ginger tea

STARCHY CARBOHYDRATES

	GI/GL
green peas; peanuts	L/L
lentils; chickpeas	L/L
beans: soy; kidney; black; lima	L/L
beans: pinto; romano; mung	L/L
navy beans; black eye beans	L/M
broad beans	H/L
barley, bulgur	L/M
wheat, whole kernels	L/M
rye kernels; buckwheat	L/M
brown rice; wild rice	L to M/M
white rice; couscous	M/H
porridge: thick oat flakes	L/M
rolled oats	M/M
sweet corn	L to M/M
new potato	L/M
sweet potato	M/M
baked potato; millet	H/H
beets	M/L
carrots; pumpkin	H/L
parsnips	H/M

Breads:

	GI/GL
pumpernickel (rye kernel)	L/L
sourdough or wholemeal rye	L/L
barley kernel; oat bran	L/L
buckwheat; whole wheat	L/L
spelt multigrain; wheat tortilla	L/L
cracked wheat; corn tortilla	L/M
barley flour	L to M/L to M
white spelt wheat	H/M
gluten-free multigrain	H/L

Pasta/Noodles:

	GI/GL
beanthread/mung bean noodles	L/M
wholemeal spaghetti	L/M
white flour pastas/noodles	L-M/M-H
rice noodles/pasta	M-H/M-H
corn pasta	H/H

No GI/GL values are available for the following grains: spelt, amaranth, kamut, quinoa, and oat groats, but when cooked in their whole form and eaten with some protein and/or fat, the glycemic values would generally be in the low to medium range.

Value	Glycemic Index (GI)	Glycemic Load (GL)
Low (L)	55 or less	10 or less
Medium (M)	56 to 69	11 to 19
High (H)	70+	20+

Remember that a balanced diet includes proteins, carbohydrates, and fats.

If you want to lose weight, choose carbohydrates with no GI/GL values (cruciferous and other non-starchy vegetables) and those with GL values of L.

- **Beverages**

  Water is the preferred beverage of The Eating Alive Program. Water is one of the most important substances in our bodies, making up more than half our body weight. It is vital to many processes in the body, including circulation, digestion, absorption of nutrients, removal of wastes, and maintenance of a constant body temperature. Water is involved in many of the chemical processes that take place in each of our cells. Drink plenty of spring or filtered water to make up for the amount that you lose through perspiration and excretion, and to help with detoxification.

  Substitute **herbal coffees and teas** for regular coffee and tea. **Green tea** is also a good choice. Although it does contain some caffeine (approximately 3 percent), the anti-cancer properties of green tea far outweigh the detriments of this small amount of caffeine, which can be tolerated by most people. Green tea contains bioflavonoids, which stimulate the antioxidant activity of liver enzymes such as glutathione peroxidase and catalase. These bioflavonoids can also bind and neutralize toxic epoxides, and they inhibit the formation of toxic nitrosamines, which are carcinogenic compounds. Green tea also helps digest fatty foods.

  If you consume them regularly, wean yourself off caffeine-containing products (coffee, black tea, colas, chocolate) *slowly*, over a period of 1 to 2 weeks, rather than quitting "cold turkey." This will help ease the side-effects of withdrawal, such as headaches and fatigue.

- To regain liver and stomach function, **avoid white sugar, coffee, black tea, chocolate, alcohol, and pop.** Besides having no nutritional value, these substances make extra work for your liver. **Also avoid anything to which you know you have sensitivities.**

- **To help your intestine, avoid eating refined foods** (such as white rice, white flour, white pasta) **as much as possible.** Use whole-grain rice, pasta, and flours instead (such as brown rice, whole-wheat, corn, kamut, or spelt pasta and rye, whole-wheat, spelt, kamut, barley, or oat flour) unless you have a *very sensitive* ileocecal valve.

- **Avoid processed foods as much as possible.** They are low in nutrients and they usually contain sugar, hydrogenated fats, and/or additives.

- **Choose organic foods as often as possible** to reduce the amount of chemicals that your liver has to deal with. For more information about the benefits of organic foods, see the article "Go Organic" in Part II.

- **Try to include some protein, carbohydrates, and fat at each meal,** to keep your blood sugar levels stable. An average serving of protein is 2 to 4 ounces. As a guideline, a 3 to 4 ounce serving is about the same size as the palm of your hand or a deck of cards. If you're eating high-GL foods, do so in moderation. If you're not eating a protein-rich food, choose low GI/GL carbohydrates. Be sure to include plenty of vegetables at lunch and dinner (for snacks, too). By stabilizing your blood sugar levels through diet, the liver and pancreas do not have to work as hard; this results in surplus energy. The amount of food required on a daily basis will vary from person to person, depending upon one's size, activity level, metabolism, etc.

- **Do not mix sweets with proteins.** (Sweets include fruits, fruit juices, sugars, and desserts.) Proteins require hydrochloric acid (HCl) for digestion in the

stomach. Carbohydrates can inhibit HCl production—
the sweeter the carbohydrate, the greater the
inhibition of HCl. Combining sweets and proteins
results in a slower rate of digestion, allowing yeast
and bacteria more time to create toxins. *If* you are
going to have sweets, wait three to five hours after a
protein-containing meal.

- **It's very important to keep your bowels working
  well to eliminate toxins.** If you're exercising
  regularly, drinking enough water, and eating plenty of
  whole grains and vegetables, but find that you're
  constipated, try taking flax seed powder and/or
  psyllium powder.

These nutritional supplements have proven useful during
detoxification.
- Milk thistle
- Selenium
- MSM or whey protein powder
- Vitamin C with bioflavonoids—choose a buffered
  vitamin C
- Multivitamin/mineral supplement—choose one that
  contains the B vitamins and zinc
- Acidophilus (see REPAIR Section below)
- Proanthocyanidins—such as grape seed extract or
  pycnogenol—for those with chronic health problems

REPAIR

The majority of my patients have an ileocecal valve problem.
This valve can become weak when your calcium levels are low
for more than five days; it must be repaired before you can start
killing any of the yeast in your system.

Repair your weakened ileocecal valve by strengthening it—
you can do this by eating according to the climate in which you
live. This means you should eat fruit that grows in your area.
Fruit can be eaten raw *when it is in season* and if you're getting

some exposure to the sun. During cooler weather, fruit should be cooked: for example, add berries, pears, apples, or raisins to your hot cereal while it's cooking; bake apples or pears; use unsweetened applesauce. Fruit should only be eaten if you *do not* have an overgrowth of yeast in your intestine, and even then, in moderation only.

Be sure to eat several servings of vegetables each day. Vegetables may be eaten raw, in moderation, when they are "in season" in the area where you live, and if you're getting some exposure to the sun. During cooler weather, vegetables should be lightly cooked (steamed or stir-fried) and salted with sea salt.

Your kidneys are responsible for maintaining the proper balance of minerals (such as sodium, potassium, and calcium) and for helping to adjust your body temperature according to the climate in which you're living. The kidneys control the absorption of calcium by activating, or not activating, vitamin D—they can increase the absorption of calcium 1000-fold, depending on the weather. The skin makes vitamin D from the ultraviolet rays of the sun. If the skin is making lots of vitamin D in hot, sunny weather, the kidneys don't need to activate vitamin D. If there's *no sun*, then the kidneys should activate vitamin D.

Your kidneys determine what the weather is like outside, based on the foods you eat. They adjust the minerals levels and body temperature accordingly. During cold weather, when you eat foods that are high in potassium and/or sugar (such as fruits and salads), the high potassium and sugar levels alert your kidneys that you must be out in the hot sun (because these foods grow in hot climates), and that your skin must be making lots of vitamin D from the sun. Therefore, your kidneys don't activate the strong form of vitamin D, and calcium is not absorbed. This results in low calcium levels, forcing the body to take calcium from other sources, such as the bones, teeth, and membranes, thus weakening these structures. Weakened membranes (such as those of the sinuses, nose, throat, bladder, nerves, intestine, ileocecal valve) then become more sensitive.

Even in hot weather, too many cooling foods (those high in potassium and/or sugar) can create problems, because your kidneys need equal amounts of sodium and potassium to work properly. A warming diet should immediately be resumed when warm/hot weather suddenly turns cold.

By eating according to the climate in which you live, you enable your kidneys to activate the strong form of vitamin D when it's needed, and your calcium absorption will improve. In a week or so, your calcium levels should be up enough to repair your weakened ileocecal valve.

Eat leafy green vegetables regularly to get vitamin K, which delivers calcium from the blood into the bones. Eat salads if you're out in the sun—if you're not out in the sun daily, switch to steamed greens with a little sea salt added.

Once the ileocecal valve is weakened, it becomes sensitive to spicy foods and coarse, scratchy fibres. **If you have a sensitive ileocecal valve, you should avoid spicy foods for approximately three to six weeks; you should also reduce the amount of coarse, scratchy fibre that you eat,** such as raw fruit, raw vegetables (including lettuce), popcorn, rice cakes, tortilla chips, crackers, granola, dry cold cereal, bran muffins, and nuts (smooth nut and seed butters are OK). Those with a *very sensitive* ileocecal valve may need to avoid whole-grain cereals and rice, as well, until the ileocecal valve becomes stronger.

RESTORE

As I mentioned before, there are two ways that a yeast overgrowth can occur. One way is when the pH of your colon and your good bacteria are disrupted by antibiotics, mercury, antacids, chlorinated water, cortisone, and so on. The other way is when your ileocecal valve is weakened due to low calcium levels.

So you need to restore your good intestinal flora and get rid of the yeast and other "Bad Guys." This is a two-part process. During the first two weeks, your goal is to weaken the yeast while you're strengthening the liver and the ileocecal valve. During the next four weeks—once your liver is replenished enough to handle the yeast die-off, and your ileocecal valve is repaired—your goal is to kill off the yeast and other "Bad Guys," while continuing to support the liver.

To weaken the yeast, you need to do the following.

- Stop feeding them what they like—refined carbohydrates such as white sugar and white flour.
- Eat foods containing acidophilus bacteria—such as fresh yogurt—or take acidophilus capsules. Acidophilus bacteria help to inhibit the yeast by direct competition, and by creating an acid pH, which yeast don't like. I recommend 1 acidophilus capsule two times per day on an empty stomach: in the morning upon rising (then try to wait at least 20 minutes before eating), and at night before bed.
- Use garlic, oregano, basil, rosemary, thyme, savoury, turmeric, curcumin, etc., for their anti-yeast and anti-inflammatory properties.

The following nutritional supplements may help satisfy/reduce your cravings for sugar.

- **Stevia**. This plant grows in South America. Stevia is 200 to 300 times sweeter than sugar and has a slight licorice taste. It doesn't feed yeast and other "Bad Guys," doesn't cause an increase in blood sugar levels, and doesn't promote tooth decay. You can buy stevia in a powder form and use it in place of sugar. (See Part II for more information on stevia.)
- **Minbal**™ by Nutri-West. It helps reduce sugar cravings. If Minbal™ is not available in your area, you could use chromium, but it is slower-acting.

Nutritional supplements that are helpful for killing yeast.

- **Latero-Flora™**
- See THE NEXT FOUR WEEKS section for suggestions for more specific problems.

OTHER HELPFUL GUIDELINES

- **Chew your food well**. A large part of the digestive process takes place in your mouth. Enzymes that digest carbohydrates are secreted in your saliva; the process of chewing will break down protein foods into smaller pieces before they reach your stomach. This makes less work for the rest of your digestive system.

- It's important that you **eat breakfast every morning,** to provide energy and avoid drops in blood sugar levels. If you don't eat breakfast because you don't have time in the morning, make it a point to get up a little earlier to allow yourself time to sit and eat. If eggs or oatmeal are too heavy for you first thing in the morning, try having a lighter breakfast such as plain yogurt, toast with nut or seed butter, or a blender protein drink.

- **Most people shouldn't go without eating for more than three to four hours.** Include snacks to help regulate your blood sugar levels.

- Keep in mind that **there's no magic pill available for improving your health.** Achieving great health requires lifestyle changes, and for most people, the first place to start is with their diet.

- **Make changes gradually**, if necessary—especially if your current eating habits differ considerably from the recommendations outlined here.

- **Be realistic**. Don't allow yourself to become stressed-out if you can't follow these dietary guidelines 100 percent of the time; stress is just as bad for your liver as poor dietary choices. Even if you follow the dietary guidelines only 70 to 80 percent of the time, you will still achieve some positive results.

- **The nutritional guidelines of** THE EATING ALIVE
  PROGRAM **are ones you will need to follow forever,
  not just for the short term—if you want to maintain
  great health**. This doesn't mean you can't *ever*
  consume things that aren't included in this eating
  plan, such as sugar, coffee, and alcohol. Just don't go
  overboard; make them "once-in-awhile" indulgences,
  if you are so inclined. Remember that *moderation is the
  key*, as with anything in life. Of course, the more
  serious your health problem, the less leeway you'll
  have when it comes to indulging.

- **Keep a positive attitude**. Try not to look at these
  dietary changes as deprivation of the things you like
  to eat and drink. Instead, see this as an opportunity to
  introduce new foods and beverages into your life.
  - ❑ If you're sensitive to dairy products, try soy milk or rice
    milk, and soy or rice cheeses as alternatives.
  - ❑ Substitute coffee with green tea and/or herbal coffees
    (Bambu®, Caf-Lib™, or dandelion varieties). Or check
    out the wide variety of herbal teas available in your
    grocery store. You may have to try several before you
    find one you like.
  - ❑ If you eat a lot of red meat, gradually replace it with
    fish, chicken, or turkey. Use ground chicken or turkey
    instead of ground beef.
  - ❑ Increase your consumption of fish. There are probably a
    lot of varieties you haven't even tried yet.
  - ❑ Experiment with the wide variety of beans and
    legumes, as well.
  - ❑ If you're sensitive to the grains that you typically eat,
    such as wheat or corn, try some alternate grains, such as
    spelt, quinoa, kamut, buckwheat, and amaranth.
  - ❑ Replace sugary cereals with cooked oatmeal or other
    types of cereal flakes that you cook, such as barley,
    buckwheat, rye, spelt, or kamut flakes.
  - ❑ If a wheat sensitivity limits your choice of pastas, try
    spelt or kamut pastas.

❑ Try vegetables that you've never eaten before. Check out daikon radish, eggplant, fennel, sea vegetables, jicama, kohlrabi, and the wide variety of greens such as kale, spinach, swiss chard, collard greens, mustard greens, watercress, rapini, beet greens, sui choy, and bok choy.

- **Be patient**; your liver didn't become overloaded overnight, so don't expect immediate results. It's not uncommon to feel worse before you feel better, especially if your body has been waiting a long time to be detoxified.

- **Listen to your body.** Note how you feel after eating; results are not always immediate. As you become healthier, you'll lose your cravings for things like sugar, coffee, and junk food and you'll want to eat healthy foods instead.

- Many people wonder how they'll get the vitamins their body needs if they don't eat a lot of fruit. Vegetables also contain vitamins—as well as other important nutrients—so **be sure to eat several servings of vegetables per day.** For example, broccoli, brussels sprouts, cabbage, cauliflower, red peppers, leaf lettuce, sweet potatoes, and tomatoes are all good sources of vitamin C; and asparagus, broccoli, carrots, pumpkin, squash, sweet potatoes, and green, leafy vegetables such as kale, leaf lettuce, spinach, and swiss chard are all good sources of vitamin A. (Fish liver oil and eggs are also good sources of vitamin A.)

- **To speed up lymph drainage, rub your chest and legs daily with a shower brush or loofah sponge.** Your lymphatic system is designed to drain excess fluid from your cells and take it back into the circulatory system. Fifty percent of your lymphatic system originates in your liver, 25 percent comes from your intestine, and 25 percent comes from the rest of your body. As lymph travels through the lymph vessels, it flows through lymph nodes, which act as defence stations, guarding against invading bacteria and other foreign materials.

Letter from a Patient

Dear Dr. Matsen

All our family of six came in for consultations with you in 1990. At the time, we were concerned about one of our family members who had asthma and numerous bouts of bronchitis.

Dr. Matsen, you opened up the whole new world of Naturopathic medicine for us. Thank you! We followed your program carefully and read your first book, *Eating Alive.* I began purchasing only whole grains and natural foods, deciding to never again buy highly refined white sugar and flour. The asthma was helped by drinking goat's milk rather than cow's milk. The asthma cleared; we discarded the inhalers and were able to control any signs of bronchitis by natural means— and no antibiotics.

Our family's health has improved. Through your fascinating explanations and diagrams in *Eating Alive,* we are able to see the importance of getting down to the root-cause of any health problem. Also, it is quite obvious to me now how much better it is to eat the local food, and that which is "in season."

Your second book, *The Secrets to Great Health,* has shown us how important it is to have proper liver function. Just recently, when I was diagnosed with a slight hypothyroid, I was able to refer to this book and find very interesting information on the thyroid. After a few blood tests through the medical laboratory services, it was recommended that I start taking a replacement hormone. This is when I started learning all about the dangers of mercury from you, Dr. Matsen.

On your recommendation, I had all my mercury fillings removed. Then you put me on a program of oral chelation to remove any further mercury remaining in my system from vaccinations, etc. Already, there has been an improvement in my pituitary gland, which is not having to work so hard; therefore I am continuing with the chelation. I feel in very good health. Only if my health really deteriorates and all natural ways fail, would I ever dream of taking replacement hormones! My husband and one of my sons are also doing your chelation program.

Now I am going to enjoy this, your third book. I keep all your books handy for reference and study, and for the many interesting recipes. I also lend them to friends, both for the recipes and to help them understand how they, too, can keep healthy, naturally.

Noël Pearce
North Vancouver, BC

PART II

THE
FOOD SECTION

Fats that Heal and Fats that Kill

by Udo Erasmus, PhD

Understand this basic concept: Some fats heal and some fats kill!!
- Some fats promote cancer; other fats inhibit cancer.
- Some fats increase platelet stickiness, making stroke/heart attack more likely; other fats make platelets less sticky, protecting us from heart attacks and strokes.
- Some fats increase blood pressure, and others decrease high pressure
- Some fats result in insulin resistance because they interfere with insulin function, but other fats are required for insulin function.
- Some fats make you fat, and others keep you slim.
- Some fats slow you down, but other fats increase your energy level.
- Some fats make your skin greasy, while others make skin soft, smooth, and velvety.
- Some fats clog your arteries; other fats clean your arteries.
- Some fats increase the highest risk factor for cardiovascular disease, known as LPA; other fats decrease this risk factor.
- Some fats increase fats in the blood (serum triglycerides). Other fats decrease them!!
- Some fats lead to atherosclerosis; others prevent and reverse it
- Some fats improve visual and brain function, and other fats impede it.

95

- Some fats deteriorate kidney function, but others improve kidney function.
- Some fats lead to fatty degeneration of the liver, and other fats benefit the liver, and in fact, can reverse fatty degeneration of the liver.
- Some fats impair adrenal function; others are necessary for it and improve it.
- Some fats inhibit immune function; others are required for it and enhance it.
- Some fats relieve allergies, but other fats worsen them.
- Some fats decrease reproductive function, and others enhance sexual function, required for sperm formation and the female reproductive cycle.
- Some fats can cause mutations; other fats protect our genetic material (DNA) from mutations and other types of damage.
- Some fats depress us; other fats lift depression and elevate mood.
- Some fats increase inflammation; other fats decrease it.
- Some fats interfere with the functions of every cell, tissue, and organ in the body, while other fats enhance, improve, and protect the cells' function.

DIETS

Many people over 50 have grown up on a high fat diet, and are now suffering the well-publicized problems that go along with it: cardiovascular disease, elevated cholesterol, cancer, diabetes, MS, arthritis, PMS, and other degenerative illnesses. These problems are mostly caused by diets where over 40 percent of the calories come from processed and hard fats.

The other extreme that is very popular today—low or no fat diets—have their own health problems: stunted growth in children; dry skin; low energy levels; possible high cholesterol/triglyceride levels; compromised immune system; enhanced likelihood of leaky gut, allergies, and lower testosterone production. That last one is very important for bodybuilders, because muscle development requires testosterone.

Low fat, no fat products are a bad joke. They taste like cardboard (fat gives flavour). To give them taste, manufacturers load them with sugar, which our body turns into the same hard (read: saturated) fats—the very substance we were avoiding when we ate the low or no fats foods to begin with.

KILLER FATS

Several commercial processing methods will turn good fats into killer fats. The three main ones are these.

1. Hydrogenation

This process turns liquid oils into cheap, spreadable, shelf-stable fats. During the process, the essential fatty acids and others are twisted into molecules called "trans-fatty acids" that have never existed in nature in the forms present in margarines, shortenings, shortening oils, partially hydrogenated vegetable oils, and vegetable shortenings.

Research on trans-fatty acids shows a wide range of detrimental side effects.

- They raise the level of LPA, the strongest known risk of cardiovascular disease.
- They change the way our immune system works.
- They decrease testosterone, increase abnormal sperm, and interfere with pregnancy in animals.
- They correlate with low birth weight in human babies.
- They lower the quality of human breast milk.
- They interfere with liver enzymes necessary for detoxification.
- They change the fluidity of cell membranes, making them harder, slowing down their reactions, lowering cell vitality, and making cell membranes more leaky (changing their permeability).

- They change the way our fat cells work.
- They make platelets more sticky.
- They increase cholesterol, increase LDL (bad), and lower HDL (good).
- They interfere with the functions of the essential fatty acids—which we require to be healthy.

Trans-fatty acids (hydrogenated or partially hydrogenated oils) are in breads, candies, cakes, cookies, granola bars, crackers, digestive biscuits, pancake mixes, breakfast cereals, instant soups, chocolate bars, desserts, fruit cakes, chips, convenience and junk foods, peanuts and peanut butter, even in croutons. The law prohibits trans-fatty acids from being used in baby foods. Are they not quite telling us something?

2. Frying
Research consistently shows that fried fats cause cancer and hardening of the arteries. When we fry food, we burn it; we change the chemistry of the oil molecules when smoke develops. These chemically changed molecules do not fit into the precise biochemical architecture of our body. Therefore they interfere with how our cells function—this is how we experience "health problems."

Cancer and hardened arteries are the result of the body's inability to deal with these altered molecules. Recent research showed that cooks who spend time wok or pan frying have a higher incidence of lung cancer.

The oils best for our health—the richest in essential fatty acids—become the most toxic when used for frying. BUT even hard, stable, saturated tropical fats and butter are damaged!

What should we use for frying? WATER. In fact, if health is what we want, water is the ONLY appropriate substance. We are back to braising and steaming!

3. Refining and Deodorizing
These procedures produce colourless, odourless, tasteless, and almost completely nutritionless oils. They are equivalent to white sugar and white flour—products from which most of the nutrients required for human health have been removed.

Except for extra virgin (green) olive oils, which remain UNrefined and UNdeodorized, all oils on supermarket shelves have gone through several of the following harsh processes.

* Degummed: Treated with Drano (sodium hydroxide, an extremely corrosive base for cleaning drains)
* Refined: Treated with window-cleaning acid (Phosphoric acid, an extremely corrosive acid)
* Bleached: Treated with bleaching clays. This process produces rancidity (peroxides), and imparts unpleasant odours and tastes to oils.
* Deodorized: Heated to above frying temperatures to remove the peroxides produced by bleaching. The taste becomes less objectionable, but other chemical changes—tasteless but toxic—take place at high temperatures.

During these processes...
• Perhaps 0.5 to 1.0% of the fatty acid molecules are changed chemically into toxic ones that interfere with normal biochemical interactions between the molecules that are necessary for normal cell functions. This means they interfere with our health.
• Minor ingredients (such as phytochemicals), which make up about 2% of most oils, are removed. These minor ingredients have "major" benefits in our health.
• Some essential fatty acid molecules are destroyed. At least one study showed that in oils heated above 150° C (302° F), these fatty acids are changed from being protective against mutations to being mutation-causing.

We can only speculate about the damage to future generations that fried oils may cause, and on the possible connection between them and the development of new and incurable genetic conditions. Unfortunately, these are being discovered more and more frequently in young children.

OTHER FAT CAUSES OF HEALTH PROBLEMS

4. Excess of hard fats

Fats in pork, beef, lamb, dairy products, and tropical nuts are natural—not synthetic or damaged by processing. Our bodies use these fats in the structure of cell membranes, in fat deposits, and as fuel. They cause problems ONLY when we consume more than we can use. An excess makes platelets more sticky, interferes with insulin function, and interferes with the functions of essential fatty acids—the good stuff from fats.

How much can we safely eat?

If we worked as hard physically as our grandparents did, we could burn (metabolize) quite a lot of hard fats as fuel to produce energy. Since we have become more sedentary, we cannot stay healthy on high hard-fat consumption. The more hard fats we consume, the more essential fatty acids we need to consume.

5. Excess Sugars

This is the fifth fat that kills. Sugar is not a fat, I know, but it just might as well be, because our bodies turn excess sugar into the same hard fats that:
- make platelets sticky;
- interfere with insulin function; and
- interfere with essential fatty acid functions.

In addition, sugar:
- damages teeth and feeds bacteria, yeast, fungus, and cancer cells;
- interferes with vitamin C transport and thereby, with immune function (the colds after Christmas?);
- can increase adrenalin products by up to four times, making this a very powerful internal stressor;
- can cross-link proteins and speed aging; and
- can pull calcium and other minerals from the body.

Although the refined sugars—white, brown, and artificial sugars—are the worst, replacing the 120 lbs of sugar that the average North American consumes every year with the same amount of any other concentrated sweetener—honey, maple syrup, rice syrup, corn syrup, fructose (or any other sugar-word that ends with "-ose")—*will not make that much difference,* because they ALL provide quickly absorbed calories that must be rapidly converted into hard fats, to prevent the toxic effects that "sweet" overload would otherwise have on our bodies.

Okay, so if:
- high-fat diets cause health problems;
- low-fat diets cause health problems;
- oil processing causes health problems;
- excessive hard fats cause health problems; and
- sugars cause health problems . . .

What is left to eat?

Now to the good part!!!

There are 50 essential nutrients that our bodies need in order to function normally—in other words, to be healthy. These are substances our bodies cannot make from other food substances, but *need to take in* as food. Two of these essential nutrients come from fats and oils; the other 48 are vitamins, minerals, and certain amino acids from proteins.

The two nutrients from fats are the "essential fatty acids" (EFAs). One is alpha-linolenic acid or Omega 3 (O-3); the other is linoleic acid or Omega 6 (O-6).

Both of these are VERY sensitive to light, air (oxygen), and high temperatures. This is why they become quite toxic when we fry with them.

The other 48 essential nutrients can be dried, powdered, and stored with little deterioration for several years, but essential fatty acid products must be made carefully, packed carefully, and used fresh, to ensure their health-promoting and maintaining properties. We need more of each Essential Fatty Acid (EFA) every day than of any other nutrient. They are major nutrients we use in tablespoon amounts, not milligram amounts.

ESSENTIAL FATTY ACID FUNCTIONS

- They increase energy production by helping the body obtain more oxygen.
- They increase oxidation rate, metabolic rate, energy levels, and stamina.
- This is most obvious in athletes and elderly, middle-aged, and overweight, people.

When athletes get their essential fatty acid intake balanced and in the right quantities:
- their performance in strength and endurance sports increases; and
- they recover from fatigue quicker, because recovery requires oxygen; EFAs increase the body's ability to metabolize oxygen.

Older or middle-aged people who take in EFA-rich oils notice that:
- Their energy levels pick up noticeably, and they feel more like being active.
- They are able to increase their physical activity, and they stay alert till later in the evening.
- They tire less quickly, and recover faster.
- This energy is not a buzz like you get from coffee or caffeine soft drinks, but a stable, sustained, extended energy.

Essential fatty acids help overweight people in several ways, too.
- They increase the metabolic rate and energy levels. This means we burn more calories. We should not count EFA calories as fat calories, because they increase calorie burning. Instead of being used as fuel, they play a role in the formation of cell membranes, and are converted into hormone-like prostaglandins. These fats keep us slim!

- They help our kidneys dump excess water held in tissues—water that constitutes much of the extra weight some people carry around.
- They help decrease cravings that often result from not getting the nutrients we need. Getting the missing EFAs satisfies the craving.
- They are also mood-elevators, and can lift depression, which is another reason why some people overeat.
- Raised mood and increased energy levels also make us feel like being more active.

BRAIN DEVELOPMENT AND FUNCTION

- Half the weight of our brain, the fat-richest organ in the body, is EFAs.
- The ratio of Omega 3 to 6 in the brain is 1:1.
- EFAs are of special therapeutic usefulness in 3 main areas:
    1. learning problems (dyslexia, hyperactivity, attention deficit, etc.);
    2. correction of criminal behaviour; and
    3. improved functioning in mental illness.

1. • Mother rats deprived of EFA O-3 in their diet produced pups with permanent learning disabilities.
   - Children with dyslexia, dispraxia, attention deficit, hyperactivity, and learning problems have benefitted from taking in oils with correct EFA balance.
   - Hyperactive horses calm down when their EFA intake is corrected. Grass contains more O-3 than O-6 (ratio is about 60:40), but horses are usually fed only refined, cheap corn oil (ratio of 1:100 of O-3:O-6). Corn oil has about 65% O-6 and only 1% O-3. In nature, dogs and cats eat a diet that has both EFAs. Commercial cat food contains no O-3.

2. • Donald Rudin, MD, showed that uncounsellable,
     incorrigible juvenile delinquents became counsellable
     when given O-3 rich oils. Teenagers' food—junk
     food—and food in jails and detention centres lack
     EFAs, so it is no wonder teens may not function right.
   • Inmates could function better when fed a better diet
     than the standard institution food of white sugar,
     white flour, coffee, margarine, white bread, iceberg
     lettuce, pork, beef, and chicken.
   • If our foods are not right for the biological
     requirements of our brains, then our behaviour
     CANNOT be right.
   • Researchers suggest that violent crimes are carried
     out while the perpetrator is suffering from low blood
     glucose. Deprived of its fuel, the brain shifts from
     higher cortical functioning (conceptual, socially
     acceptable, knowing right from wrong) to basic
     functioning (fight or flight). EFAs can stabilize this
     blood glucose problem and maintain more of a
     balance.

3. • EFAs elevate mood and lift depression.
   • Schizophrenics hallucinate less with correct EFA
     intake.

   **If people had a choice, they would not choose criminal
behaviour, mental illness, violence, bizarre behaviour, and
hyperactivity.**

HAIR, SKIN, AND NAILS

EFAs play an important role here.
   • They form a barrier in our skin against loss of
     moisture. This protects us against dehydration.
   • Dehydration can be a cause of many problems
     involving histamines, prostaglandins, and
     inflammation.

- This barrier function of EFAs can also help prevent constipation and its toxic conditions.
- EFAs make skin soft, smooth, and velvety.
- They help you tan better and burn less.
- They help you get relief from eczema, acne, psoriasis, and other skin conditions.
- Oil-soluble toxins leave the body via the skin with sweat, but oils lost by sweating must be replaced to prevent dry skin.
- Dry skin indicates a need for EFAs. In winter, we need more than in summer. Biologically, we can live with dry skin, but not with a dry liver or brain. The internal organs get priority on the EFAs coming into our bodies. Only when they have what they need, do the EFAs get to the skin.

DIGESTIVE SYSTEM HELP FROM EFAs

- EFAs may help prevent "leaky" gut syndrome.
- Good oils have been known to relieve allergies. Allergic reactions to oil are rare, even in allergy-sensitive people; proteins are usually the triggers for allergic reactions, and oils are protein-free.
- EFAs help reduce cravings and addictions to foods, cigarettes, alcohol, and drugs.
- They help the liver, kidneys, adrenals, and pancreas—as well as other glands—to function properly

OTHER INTERNAL SYSTEMS HELPED BY EFAs

- EFAs help sperm formation and prevent PMS in women; certain minerals and vitamins are also necessary.
- EFAs help our kidneys remove excess water, and decrease inflammation in tissues.
- EFAs are required for mineral transport and metabolism.

- EFAs are required for protein metabolism.
- EFAs are essential part of red blood pigmentation, cell growth, and cell division.

Benefits to the Cardiovascular System
- EFAs are necessary for cholesterol transport.
- EFAs lower high triglyceride levels by up to 65% (O-3) and do it better than drugs, without side effects—except that you feel better.
- EFAs produce hormone-like prostaglandins that make our platelets less sticky, thereby decreasing the likelihood of clot formation.
- EFAs help lower high blood pressure.

Benefits to the Immune System
- EFAs protect our genetic material from damage. O-3 EFA has antioxidant functions in the oil-soluble system of our body, similar to vitamin C in the water-soluble system.
- EFAs are used to make "oxygen bullets" to kill infectious foreign invaders.
- EFAs help treat fungus infections (athlete's foot) and yeast overgrowth (Candida).
- Both O-3 and O-6 inhibit tumour growth.

ARE THERE LIMITS ON TAKING EFA-RICH OILS?

- Too close to bedtime, we may have too much energy to sleep; they are best taken before 8 PM.
- If we take more than our liver can handle at one time, we may feel full, heavy, or nauseated.
- The occasional allergic response can be overcome by taking digestive enzymes with the oil.

DEFICIENCY INDICATORS

OMEGA 3	OMEGA 6
growth retardation	eczema-like skin eruptions
behaviour changes	hair loss
weakness	fatty infiltration of the liver
vision & learning problems	behavioural changes
lack of motor coordination	kidney malfunction
tingling sensations in arms/legs	water loss through skin, and thirst
elevated triglyceride levels	glands dry up
high blood pressure	susceptibility to infections
sticky platelets	wounds fail to heal
inflammation in tissues	male sterility
water retention	female miscarriage
dry skin	arthritis-like conditions
mental deterioration	heartbeat abnormalities
low metabolic rate	growth retardation
some immune dysfunctions	dry skin, hair, and eyes
	sometimes increased cholesterol

"MINOR" INGREDIENTS IN OILS

- These make up only a small part of the oil: about 2%.
- They are oil-soluble "phytochemicals": plant-based molecules with major health benefits.
- Extra virgin olive oil (green) still has phytochemicals in it; that is why it is green.
- Phytochemicals improve liver and gallbladder function, digestion, and cardiovascular function.

HOW MUCH, AND PROPORTIONS

- Fats in traditional diets, such as that of the Inuit, contained both EFAs. They were unrefined, and contained the minor ingredients.

- Inuit ratio of O-3 to O-6 was 2.5:1, and this did not produce O-6 deficiency symptoms.
- This ratio serves as nature's measure of the upper limit of safe O-3 richness.
- Mediterranean diets were 1:6, with no O-3 deficiencies.
- The brain of both cultural traditions contains a ratio of 1:1, which indicates that the brain takes what it needs from what the body gets.
- Researchers suggest that the best ratio is 1:4, based on enzyme studies in tissue culture.
- In practice, we find that 2.5:1 provides the best health support and improvement.
- Flax oil is too high in O-3 for long-term use, and can cause O-6 deficit.
- O-6 deficit experiences reported dry eyes, skipped heart beats, and fragile, thin skin
- O-3 and O-6 compete for enzyme space in the cells.

Udo Erasmus is an international authority on fats, oils, cholesterol, and human health. Udo received his B Sc in Honours Zoology from the University of British Columbia, followed by graduate studies in Biochemistry and Genetics. Then, in 1980, his life took a significant turn when he was poisoned by pesticides. When conventional medicine was unable to provide help, he concluded that his health was his own responsibility and he turned his attention to nutrition. Several years of research culminated in his Canadian best-selling book, *Fats That Heal, Fats That Kill*, which earned him a PhD in Nutrition.

In 1987, Udo pioneered technology for pressing and packaging edible, fresh oils made with health in mind, under the exclusion of light, heat, and oxygen—three main factors that can transform nutritious oils into toxic ones. Until that time, oils were highly processed by destructive methods, sacrificing health benefits to attain long shelf life. Udo continues to provide consulting services to health professionals and individuals; he is also expanding "The Right Fat Diet" and working on his third book. Visit Udo at www.udoerasmus.com

Go Organic!

by Jennifer Sieberg, RNC

There's been a lot of talk surrounding the organic industry over the past several years. It can certainly be confusing, so let's start with the basics of what organic means.

Certified organic products are grown without pesticides, antibiotics, hormones, herbicides, fumigants, or artificial colourants. They are also grown without chemical fertilizers or preservatives, and without genetically modified organism inputs such as seed, feed, or raw materials. You didn't want any of that anyway, did you?

Organic farmers certainly have their work cut out for them. But it's worth doing, when you realize that the petrochemicals used in conventional farming can be extremely harmful and dangerous—not only to the farmers' health, but also to *your* health. And no one wants to compromise his or her health just by eating a salad.

If that salad was made with certified organic produce, it would take a great burden off your liver—and your palate would be happier, too. Many top chefs and restaurants are going organic because organic food tastes so much better. In fact, some studies show *certified organic produce* to be higher in nutrient content than conventional produce. (This was the conclusion of a study quoted from *Organic View,* v.2 n.1, January 23, 2000, Organic Consumers Association. The study was done at the University of Copenhagen, funded by Britain's Soil Association.) So organic produce doesn't just *taste better*, it *truly is better* for your health.

The body can withstand a lot of punishment, but often at a cost to our overall health. One punishment we place on our body is the chore of detoxifying petrochemicals from conventional produce. Conventional farmers rely heavily on pesticides and herbicides to get that perfect-looking peach to our fruit basket. A large percentage of herbicides and pesticides—as well as some insecticides used in conventional farming—are considered potentially cancerous. While there is no proven correlation, it may not be a coincidence that cancer has been on the rise since the time traditional farmers began using chemical sprays on their crops.

It's important to mention that children, because of their lower body weight and smaller size, are even more adversely affected by pesticides and toxins. And, during infancy and early childhood, children's cells divide more rapidly, increasing the chance of cell mutation. So you want your children to eat their fruits and veggies, but *make sure they're also organic.*

What happens to the toxic substances we ingest? Once digested, these little monsters and other toxins from coffee, alcohol, nicotine, drugs, and food additives are carried straight to the liver. The liver is an extremely important organ, and deserves a lot of respect because it performs more than 500 different functions for our body. One such function is detoxifying our blood. So when those nasty toxins travel down to the liver, the liver plucks them from our blood and breaks them down.

Depending on your lifestyle and eating habits, your liver may have to do a lot of work simply detoxifying your blood. But remember, the liver has 499 other jobs to do. If your liver is overloaded with toxins, it will be unable to regulate your blood properly, and that situation can cause many symptoms of disease.

It's simple: Organic food = lowered toxic load = healthy liver function = better health.

Conventional food = increased toxic load = compromised liver function = poorer health.

Now let's talk taste! Many believe that nutritionally superior fruits and vegetables have more flavour. A network of tiny rootlets in the soil work to carry essential minerals to a plant. Inorganic fertilizers used in conventional farming can destroy this network, forcing the plant to be reliant upon fertilizers such as NPK (a common fertilizer) for its bare-bones nutrition. Organic farming techniques support this intricate and complex soil network, providing the plants with all the essential nutrients and trace minerals the soil has to offer.

Sometimes it's hard to get kids to eat fruits and vegetables. Kids forced to eat bland, watery-tasting fruit may turn away from fresh produce and reach for a sugary artificial snack. A sweet, full-flavoured certified organic fruit, however, is bound to better satisfy children *and* adults.

Do the taste test yourself. Bite into a sweet, crispy organic apple—and you'll immediately taste the difference!

The key to great health is a healthy, well-functioning liver. By eating *certified organic products*, you are avoiding the toxins in conventional foods that can overload the liver, leading to many symptoms of disease. The bottom line is that organic farming produces great-tasting, nutritionally rich foods that are free of toxic chemicals and other harmful substances.

Jennifer Sieberg is a graduate of the Canadian School of Natural Nutrition, and a professional member of the International Organization of Nutritional Consultants. As a Registered Nutritional Consultant, Jennifer counsels her clients on nutrition and lifestyle. She uses a holistic approach to assess the body systems, taking into consideration the quality and source of the food. Involved in the organics industry, Jennifer works for Green Earth Organics.

Eating Out

When eating in restaurants, select foods that are cooked with little or no added fat; choose foods that are baked, broiled, poached, steamed, or roasted, and avoid fried and deep-fried foods. For protein choices, select chicken breast, fish, or tofu, served with vegetables (lightly cooked in colder weather, raw or salads occasionally in warmer weather), and a moderate amount of pasta, rice, or potatoes.

The following is by no means a complete list; it's just meant to show that you can eat out and still follow this program fairly closely.

- **Greek**
  Chicken (or lamb) souvlaki, tzatziki, cooked vegetables, and a small amount of roast potatoes
- **Japanese**
  Sushi, miso soup, and soybeans steamed in the pod
- **Mexican**
  Chicken or bean tortilla or soft taco. (Go easy on the cheese and avocado, and use <u>mild</u> salsa.)
- **Italian**
  Protein, such as chicken or fish, with steamed vegetables and a small portion of pasta.
- **Indian**
  Mild chicken curry and vegetables, with basmati rice or chapatis

Helpful Hints

Apple Cider Vinegar
Choose raw, unfiltered, organic apple cider vinegar—for example, Bragg brand—that contains beneficial bacteria, trace minerals, and enzymes. It is nutritionally superior and tastes much better than other vinegars. It is available in health food stores and some grocery stores.

Arrowroot Powder
Found in health food stores, it can be substituted for cornstarch as a thickening agent.

Baking Powder
Use nonalum (aluminum-free) baking powder instead of regular, if possible. It's available at health food stores.

Buttermilk
If you'd like to use buttermilk, but don't have any on hand, you can make your own. For each cup of buttermilk that you need, place 1 tablespoon (15 mL) lemon juice or vinegar in a measuring cup. Fill the measuring cup with milk to the 1 cup (250 mL) mark. You can make soy buttermilk in the same way, using soy milk instead of cow's milk.

Chicolin™
Chicolin™ is a powdered food substance derived from the whole tubers of the chicory plant. Chicolin™ contains Inulin (or Oligosaccharides), a soluble fibre found in numerous roots. The Inulin or Oligosaccharides are non-digestible plant sugars; they pass through the digestive system unchanged and slow the absorption of sugars until they reach the large intestine. There they are utilized by the bifidobacteria (your friendly intestinal

flora). Chicolin doesn't cause the same rapid increase in blood sugar levels as regular sugar does. Combine with stevia (see **Stevia**) to use as a sugar replacement.

Cooking with Fats and Oils

There are a number of ways you can avoid adding excess fat when preparing meals. When sautéing or stir-frying vegetables, use water or stock instead of oil, or start with a just small amount of oil (cook over medium-low heat), then add water as needed to prevent food from sticking. In sandwich spreads and casseroles, replace some or all of the mayonnaise that you would normally use with low-fat plain yogurt. When baking muffins, replace some of the oil the recipe calls for with unsweetened applesauce or pureed prunes (baby food); this will also provide natural sweetness and decrease the need for adding sugar.

When fats and oils are heated to high temperatures, their chemical composition is altered and many toxic substances are created. To protect the oil from overheating when sautéing or stir-frying—and thereby minimize the formation of toxic substances—do the following: cook at a low temperature, put water into the saucepan, skillet, or wok first, before adding the vegetables and oil, then put the vegetables into the heated pan before adding any oil. Extra virgin olive oil is a suitable oil to use for light sautéing and stir-frying. Or better yet, omit the oil and use water or stock instead; then you can sauté or stir-fry at a slightly higher temperature. Butter or coconut butter is a suitable fat to use in baked goods such as muffins, and to line baking pans and dishes.

Daikon Radish

Daikon is a member of the Cruciferous family of vegetables and is used in some of the recipes. It has a relatively mild flavour. Avoid the really large ones as they tend to be more fibrous and less tasty. Daikon should be scrubbed and peeled before using. It can be eaten cooked (good in stir-fries) or raw (good grated into salads, or grated and served with just a vinagrette or lemon juice).

Fish
Measure at the thickest portion, and cook for 10 minutes per inch (2.5 cm) of thickness.

Ginger and Garlic
Use only *fresh* garlic and ginger; the dried forms do not compare in taste. Powdered or dried ginger should only be used in baking.

Ground Turkey or Chicken
Make sure these are ground from skinless breast only, to ensure they're low in fat.

Herbs
For the sake of convenience, dried herbs have been used in these recipes, unless otherwise specified. The exceptions are parsley and cilantro; rosemary is another herb that is best used fresh. Use fresh herbs if you have them. When substituting fresh for dried, use 3 times as much fresh herbs; for example, 1 teaspoon (5 mL) of dried herbs is roughly equivalent to 1 tablespoon (15 mL) of chopped fresh herbs. Many different types of fresh herbs are available year-round. They can be found in packages in the produce section of many grocery stores.

Jicama
The jicama is the edible tuber of a plant native to Mexico and Central America. It looks like a turnip with flattened ends. The jicama has a juicy white flesh that's sweet and crisp. It can be eaten raw (children seem to like it this way) or cooked. During cooking, jicama absorbs other flavours yet still remains crisp. Choose small or medium-sized ones and use them chopped up or grated in stews, stir-fries, or salads, or cut into sticks and added to a vegetable platter. Jicama can be used in place of water chestnuts in many recipes. They can be difficult to peel; using a knife, start from either end, cut into the skin, and peel it off.

Lemon Juice
Use the juice of fresh lemons, whenever possible, or use 100%
pure lemon juice from concentrate, available in plastic bottles in
the freezer section of some grocery stores.

Mayonnaise
Use store-bought mayonnaise sparingly—most contain sugar
and unhealthy oils. Try the **Tofu Mayonnaise** recipe, or better
yet, use the **Mayonnaise** recipe contributed by Flora.

Miso
Miso is a rich-tasting fermented bean paste made from
soybeans and grains, such as wheat, barley, or rice. Use it to
flavour soups, sauces, and salad dressings.

Mushrooms
Some of the recipes in the Recipes Section call for mushrooms. If
you know that you have—or if you suspect that you have—an
overgrowth of intestinal yeast, omit the mushrooms.

Organic Foods
Use organically grown foods, whenever possible.

Rice
Brown rice takes longer to cook, but it's more nutritious than
white rice. When you're cooking brown rice, make extra for use
in the following recipes that call for cooked brown rice: **Salmon
Loaf, Fish Roll-Ups, Tofu Patties, Cabbage Rolls, Tofu Bean
Casserole,** and **Chicken, Broccoli, and Rice Casserole.**

Sea Salt
Use unprocessed sea salt; add it at the end of the cooking time
(except in baked products like muffins), to retain the valuable
minerals. Use Celtic Sea Salt® if you can get it.

Spinach
Use fresh, whenever possible. A large bunch of fresh spinach
weighs about 10 ounces (300 g). To cook spinach, wash it well

and remove the stems. Place the spinach leaves in a pot, cover, and cook over medium heat for just a few minutes, until wilted. There's no need to add any water to the pot—there'll be enough water clinging to the spinach leaves.

You can also buy 10 ounce (300 g) plastic bags of *prewashed* spinach in many grocery stores; these cost a little more but save a lot of time since you don't have to wash it. A 10 ounce (300 g) package of frozen spinach, thawed and well drained, can often be substituted for fresh spinach, such as in the **Fish Roll-Ups, Tofu and Veggie Lasagna, Tofu Bean Casserole,** and **Spinach and Feta Cheese Pizza.**

Stevia

Stevia is a plant that grows naturally in South America. Extracts of its leaves have been used for centuries in Brazil and Paraguay as a safe, natural sweetener. Stevia is 200 to 300 times sweeter than sugar and has a slight licorice taste. It doesn't feed yeast and other "Bad Guys," doesn't cause an increase in blood sugar levels, and doesn't promote tooth decay. Stevia is sold in leaf, powder, and liquid forms. The recipes in this book use the white stevia extract, which is a very fine powder.

Because it is very sweet and difficult to measure in small amounts, it can be combined with water—1 teaspoon (5 mL) of stevia powder dissolved in 3 tablespoons (45 mL) filtered or purified water. Put the liquid into a dropper-style bottle and store in the refrigerator. (See *The Stevia Cookbook* by Ray Sahelian, MD, and Donna Gates for more information and recipes.)

Stevia can also be combined with Chicolin™ to create a mixture that can be used to replace sugar in baking, cooking, smoothies, sprinkled on pancakes or waffles, etc. Add a 20 gram container of white stevia powder to a 250 g container of Chicolin™ and shake very well. The mixture is easy to sprinkle but is still very concentrated. Approximately 1 teaspoon (5 mL) of the stevia/Chicolin™ mixture is equivalent to the sweetness of 1 cup (250 mL) of sugar.

Tamari Soy Sauce

The recipes in this book call for tamari soy sauce, a Japanese soy sauce that tends to have a richer taste and that's thicker and less salty than Chinese soy sauces. You can also use Bragg Liquid Aminos, which is made from soybeans and purified water.

Tempeh

Tempeh is a bean cake or patty made from fermented soybeans. Usually sold in 8 ounce (250 g) packages, it can be found in the freezer section in some health food stores. Tempeh has a chewy texture and a slightly nutty, smoky flavour.

Tofu

Tofu or soybean curd is high in protein, low in saturated fat, and a good source of calcium. It's also inexpensive and versatile. Many people complain that tofu is bland-tasting but that's the nice thing about it; it'll take on the flavour of the dish in which it's being used. Tofu can be used to replace other protein sources such as eggs, cottage cheese, chicken, or beef. Use firm or extra-firm tofu in stir-fries, burgers, stews, or casseroles, or as a substitute for ground beef or poultry in chili, spaghetti sauce, lasagna, etc. Silken and soft tofu can be used in dips, dressings, sauces, and soups.

Once the package has been opened, submerge the tofu in fresh water, cover, and store it in the refrigerator for a maximum of 5 days. The water should be changed every day. Tofu can also be frozen for up to 5 months; just drain and wrap well. When thawed, drained, and crumbled, it has a texture similar to ground meat. To drain tofu, press it between 2 pieces of paper towel.

Note: Processed soy products (for example, some soy cheeses) may contain casein, one of the main proteins found in cow's milk. Casein can be allergy-inducing in some people.

Tomatoes

Use fresh, if possible. When fresh tomatoes aren't in season, canned tomatoes can be used in some recipes, such as soups, **Tomato Sauce**, and **Turkey Chili**.

Tortillas
Try to find whole-wheat tortillas that aren't made with yeast, hydrogenated oils, and/or other additives; these are often available in health food stores. Or use the recipe for **Tortillas** in the Recipe section. If you're sensitive to wheat, try substituting other types of flour.

How to
Cook Beans

Besides being low in fat, beans are an excellent source of vegetable protein, B vitamins, fibre, iron, calcium, and other minerals. When cooked beans are listed in a recipe, use dried beans and soak and cook them yourself whenever possible. The beans will be more nutritious, tastier, and less expensive than canned beans. Although the process takes longer than using canned beans, it's really quite easy to soak and cook dried beans; it just takes some planning. Also keep in mind that once cooked, the beans can be stored in the refrigerator for up to 5 days or frozen for up to 6 months. One cup (250 mL) of dried beans will yield 2 to 2½ cups (500 to 625 mL) of cooked beans.

To Cook Dried Beans
First remove any broken or discoloured beans. Place the beans in a sieve and rinse under cold water. Soak them in water using a 3-to-1 ratio: for every cup of beans, add 3 cups of fresh water. Cover and refrigerate overnight for 6 to 10 hours. Drain off the soaking water, place the beans in a sieve or colander, and rinse well under cold running water. This will help to eliminate much of the indigestible sugars that can cause gas. Place the rinsed beans in a large pot and cover with water, again on a 3-to-1 ratio. Add a piece of dried seaweed, such as nori or kombu, if you have it; this will help to degas the beans as well as add flavour. Bring the water to a boil and skim off any foam that rises to the top. Reduce the heat and cover with the lid slightly ajar. Simmer gently—stirring occasionally and skimming off any foam—until the beans are just tender. This will take anywhere from 45 minutes to 1½ hours, depending on the type

of bean. Once cooked, drain off the cooking water and rinse the beans thoroughly; drain well.

Quick-Soak Method
If you don't have time to soak the beans overnight, use the following quick-soak method. Sort through and rinse the dried beans, as directed above. Put the beans into a large pot with 3 times as much water as beans and bring the water to a boil; cook for 2 to 3 minutes. Remove from the heat, cover, and let sit for 1 hour. Drain off the soaking water and rinse the beans well; follow the remaining steps for cooking, as directed above.

   The following recipes call for cooked beans (including chickpeas), so if you're cooking some for one recipe, make extra to use in another recipe: **Bean Dip, Hummus, Minestrone, Bean and Tomato Soup, Bean Salad, Black Bean and Rice Wraps, Turkey Chili**, and **Tofu Bean Casserole**.
   To help reduce the intestinal gas that's often caused by eating beans, be sure to drain and discard the water in which the beans are soaked or cooked, and always rinse the beans with fresh water after soaking or cooking them. Also, if you're not accustomed to eating beans, be sure to introduce them into your diet slowly; eat small amounts at first and slowly increase. Beans are less likely to cause gas when they're eaten on a regular basis.
   If you must use canned beans, be sure to read the label; try to avoid those that contain sugar, MSG, and other additives. Most brands contain salt, but some use seaweed (like kombu) instead. Always drain and rinse canned beans well to help reduce gas. A 14 ounce (398 mL) can is approximately equal to 1½ cups (375 mL) and a 19 ounce (540 mL) can is approximately equal to 2 cups of beans.

How to
Make Yogurt

In the production of yogurt, bacteria eat the lactose sugar in the milk; that makes it easier for your body to digest the yogurt. Yogurt helps reduce the production of cholesterol in your body.

You can use whole, low-fat, or skim milk to make yogurt. Heat 2 cups (500 mL) milk to just below the boiling point, but do not boil. Remove the pot from the heat and place on a thick towel. Let the milk cool until it's lukewarm. If the milk is too hot when adding the yogurt, it may kill the bacterial culture. Add 1 tablespoon (15 mL) of plain yogurt and stir gently. Use a commercial yogurt that contains only milk ingredients and bacterial culture. Cover the pot with a lid and wrap two more thick towels around and on top of the pot. Leave to sit and ferment for several hours, until thickened; this will take anywhere from 8 to 24 hours. The longer you leave it to ferment, the more of the lactose sugar the bacteria will eat. Homemade yogurt will keep in the refrigerator for 7 to 10 days.

It's important that the temperature stay between 80° and 110° F (27° and 45° C) during the fermentation period. If your kitchen is too cool or drafty, you may find that the above method doesn't work for you. Instead, heat the milk as directed above, then cool until it's lukewarm. Place 1 tablespoon (15 mL) plain yogurt in a large, clean jar and pour in the warm milk; stir gently. Cover and keep warm in an oven that is turned on very low (as low as possible) or in an oven with just the light on. Or, wrap the jar in a heating pad set on the lowest setting. Whichever method you decide to use, be sure to check the temperature with a thermometer first to make sure it's close to, but not over, 110° F (45° C).

Strained Yogurt

Homemade yogurt is not as thick as many of the commercial yogurts. If you like a thicker yogurt, place the yogurt in a sieve lined with about 4 layers of cheesecloth; place the sieve over a bowl. Wrap the cheesecloth around the yogurt and give it a slight squeeze. Place a plate over the bowl and sieve and place them in the refrigerator. Let the yogurt drain for 2 to 3 hours, then discard the liquid. One cup (250 mL) yogurt will yield about ¾ cup (175 mL) strained yogurt. You can strain the yogurt even longer to make **Yogurt Cheese** (see Recipes). If you don't have any cheesecloth, you can use a clean tea towel instead; the draining time will be shorter because the tea towel tends to absorb more of the liquid. Small amounts of yogurt can be drained in a coffee filter.

Uses for Yogurt

Low-fat plain yogurt can be used to replace some or all of the mayonnaise in sandwiches, salads, spreads, and casseroles. It can also be used to replace sour cream. If you or your family aren't accustomed to the taste of yogurt, substitute yogurt for *some* of the mayo or sour cream that you would normally use, and gradually increase the amount of yogurt, while decreasing the amount of mayo or sour cream.

Seven Day Sample Menu Plan

The following menu plan is meant to give you an idea of how to create meals and snacks following the nutritional guidelines of THE EATING ALIVE PROGRAM. To save time in the kitchen, you can make extra portions of the dinner suggestions to eat for lunch the next day. The amounts recommended are approximate and can be adjusted according to needs (activity level, metabolism, hunger, etc.).

Make this menu plan work for you; feel free to substitute the breakfast suggestion on one day for that of another; the same applies to snacks, lunches, and dinners. Or see the **Menu Suggestions** Section for alternate choices. Menu suggestions in **bold type** indicate recipes that are included in the **Recipes** Section.

Those people who want to speed up their digestion can omit or limit the starchy carbohydrates (see "A Quick Digestion and Liver Booster" on pages 56 and 57) and include more vegetables instead, until digestion improves.

Please Note: Those who have ileocecal valve problems and yeast in the small intestine will need to avoid/limit crackers and raw fruit and vegetables in the beginning, until the ileocecal valve is repaired. Choose: cooked fruit (applesauce, baked apples or pears, etc) instead of raw fruit, or choose another snack suggestion; steamed vegetables or vegetable soups instead of salads; and yeast-free rye or whole-grain breads instead of rye crackers.

DAY 1

20 to 30 minutes before breakfast: warm lemon and/or ginger drink, and 1 acidophilus capsule (See "A Quick Gallbladder Tonic" on page 58.)

Breakfast: poached egg(s) on 1 slice of rye or whole-grain toast

Snack: ½ cup (125 mL) of low-fat plain yogurt (optional: sweeten with stevia/Chicolin™ to taste)

Lunch: **Salmon Salad** and romaine lettuce rolled up in a small whole-wheat tortilla, and sliced tomatoes

Snack: 1 or 2 yeast-free rye crackers with a small amount of smooth almond butter, pumpkin seed butter, or sesame butter

Dinner: **Chicken with Lemon and Herbs**, barley, and steamed vegetables such as carrots, broccoli, cauliflower, green beans with **Yogurt Herb Dip**. (Make extra chicken, rice, veggies, and dip for tomorrow's lunch; can be eaten hot or cold.)

Make **Bean Salad** for snacks for the next few days.

DAY 2

20 to 30 minutes before breakfast: warm lemon and/or ginger drink, and 1 acidophilus capsule

Breakfast: slow-cooked oatmeal with low-fat milk, rice milk, or soy milk

Snack: fruit in season (apple, pear, berries)

Lunch: leftover chicken, rice, veggies, and dip from last night's dinner

Snack: ½ to 1 cup (125 to 250 mL) of **Bean Salad**

Dinner: **Tuna Casserole** and small green salad with dressing (see **Greek Salad** for dressing recipe) in warmer weather, or steamed veggies in cooler weather. (Make extra for tomorrow's lunch.)

DAY 3
20 to 30 minutes before breakfast: warm lemon and/or ginger drink, and 1 acidophilus capsule
Breakfast: rye toast with smooth almond butter, pumpkin seed butter, or sesame butter
Snack: fruit in season (apple, pear, berries)
Lunch: leftover **Tuna Casserole** from last night's dinner and small green salad with dressing
Snack: ½ to 1 cup (125 to 250 mL) of **Bean Salad**
Dinner: **Turkey Barley Soup** and steamed vegetables with **Tzatziki**

DAY 4
20 to 30 minutes before breakfast: warm lemon and/or ginger drink, and 1 acidophilus capsule
Breakfast: **Yogurt and Tofu Smoothie**
Snack: fruit in season (apple, pear, berries)
Lunch: leftover **Turkey Barley Soup** and steamed vegetables with **Tzatziki**
Snack: 1 or 2 yeast-free rye crackers with a small amount of smooth almond butter, pumpkin seed butter, or sesame butter
Dinner: **Broiled Salmon Steaks**, brown rice, **Sautéed Greens**, and sliced tomatoes

DAY 5
20 to 30 minutes before breakfast: warm lemon and/or ginger drink, and 1 acidophilus capsule
Breakfast: **Scrambled Tofu** or soft-boiled egg(s) and rye toast
Snack: fruit in season (apple, pear, berries)
Lunch: leftover salmon and brown rice from last night's dinner, steamed vegetables and **Tzatziki**
Snack: ½ to 1 cup (125 to 250 mL) of **Bean Salad**
Dinner: **Turkey Burgers** (or **Turkey Loaf**) and **Stir-Fried Vegetables with Yogurt and Cilantro**

DAY 6

20 to 30 minutes before breakfast: warm lemon and/or ginger
drink, and 1 acidophilus capsule

Breakfast: hot cooked cereal (such as barley, spelt, kamut, or
            buckwheat flakes) with low-fat milk or soy milk

Snack: fruit in season (apple, pear, berries)

Lunch: leftover **Turkey Burger/Loaf** on a whole-grain bun
            with sliced tomatoes, romaine lettuce, mustard, and
            a small amount of mayo or mashed avocado

Snack: 1 slice of rye or whole-grain bread with reduced-fat
            cheese or soy cheese

Dinner: **Poached Chicken, Greek Salad**, and steamed
            broccoli and carrots

(Make extra chicken for tomorrow's breakfast.)

DAY 7

20 to 30 minutes before breakfast: warm lemon and/or ginger
drink, and 1 acidophilus capsule

Breakfast: **Chicken Vegetable Hash**

Snack: ½ cup (125 mL) of low-fat plain yogurt (optional:
            sweeten with stevia/Chicolin™ to taste)

Lunch: leftover **Greek Salad** and 1 slice of whole-grain
            bread

Snack: **Yogurt and Tofu Smoothie**

Dinner: **Tofu (or Chicken) and Veggie Stir-Fry** with brown
            rice, barley, or bean thread (vermicelli noodles made
            from beans)

Menu Suggestions

The following menu suggestions will give you an idea of the foods you can eat on this program. Feel free to invent your own, using these as a guideline. Of course, any Lunch and Dinner suggestion may be eaten at breakfast, and vice versa.

Don't go without eating for more than 3 to 4 hours; include Snacks to help regulate your blood sugar levels. In addition to the Snack suggestions listed here, many Lunch and Dinner or Breakfast suggestions may be eaten as a Snack—simply use smaller portions.

Those who want to speed up their digestion can omit or limit the starchy carbohydrates (see "A Quick Digestion and Liver Booster" on pages 56 and 57), and include more vegetables instead, until digestion improves.

Menu suggestions in **bold type** indicate recipes that are included in the Recipe Section. Many of these recipes also have variations, which will increase your options.

BREAKFAST

- Slow-cooked oatmeal with low-fat milk, soy milk, or rice milk
- Hot cooked cereal with low-fat milk, soy milk, or rice milk (Try different types and combinations of cereals, such as: 1 part buckwheat flakes, 2 parts barley flakes, and 2 parts slow-cooking oats, or use a multiflake cereal, sold in packages in health food stores.)
- Dry packaged cereal with low-fat milk, soy milk, or rice milk (Choose whole-grain low-sugar varieties and let the cereal soften in the milk before eating.)
- **Scrambled Tofu** and yeast-free whole-grain toast
- **Chicken Vegetable Hash**

- Yeast-free toast with smooth almond butter, sesame seed butter, or pumpkin seed butter (Use nut and seed butters sparingly, since they are high in fat.)
- Soy cheese melted on yeast-free toast
- Poached or soft-boiled egg on yeast-free toast
- **Steamed Eggs in Spinach "Baskets"** and yeast-free toast
- **Zucchini Bread**, muffin, or scone (see Recipes), and low-fat plain yogurt or soy yogurt
- **Yogurt and Tofu Smoothie** (for larger appetites, include yeast-free toast)

SNACKS

- **Oatcakes** with smooth almond butter, sesame seed butter, or pumpkin seed butter
- **Bean Dip** and whole wheat tortillas
- **Hummus** with one of the following: **Dill Scones, Oatcakes**, rye toast, or occasionally, pita bread
- Yeast-free whole-grain bread or rye crackers with **Quark and Herb Spread, Tofu Spread,** or **Yogurt Cheese**
- **Zucchini Bread**, muffin, or scone (See Recipes for options.)
- Low-fat plain yogurt or soy yogurt
- Boiled egg (preferably soft-boiled) and yeast-free toast
- Small bowl of soup (See Recipes for options.)
- **Bean Dip Burrito**
- **Bean Salad**
- Steamed vegetables (such as broccoli, cauliflower, carrots, zucchini, green beans, snow peas, etc.) and any one of the following dips: **Tzatziki, Bean Dip, Hummus, Yogurt Herb Dip**

LUNCH AND DINNER

- Soup and/or sandwich (Choose from any of those listed in the Recipes Section.)
- **Pasta Salad** with sliced, cooked chicken breast or chunks of salmon or tuna, and sliced tomatoes
- Sandwich and steamed vegetables
- Any of the **Wraps** listed in the Recipes Section, plus some steamed vegetables
- **Bean Salad**, sliced tomatoes, and yeast-free rye toast
- **Poached Fish Fillets, Broiled Tomatoes**, stir-fried vegetables, and brown rice or lentils
- **Broiled Salmon Steaks, Steamed Vegetables with Tofu Parmesan Sauce**, and brown rice or millet
- **Salmon Cakes** with **Yogurt Herb Dip**, steamed asparagus, and **Barley Stew**
- **Tuna Casserole** and steamed green beans, carrots, and cauliflower with **Yogurt Herb Dip**
- **Baked Fish with Black Bean Sauce**, sliced tomatoes, **Sautéed Greens**, and brown rice
- **Breaded Fish Fillets, Stir-Fried Vegetables with Yogurt and Cilantro**, and brown rice or whole-grain pasta
- **Baked Halibut and Vegetables** and **Barley Stew**
- **Fish Roll-Ups**, sliced tomatoes, steamed broccoli, and lentils
- **Fish Fillets in Parchment, Cabbage Casserole**, steamed kale, and brown rice
- Sardines (canned in water) mashed, and mixed with fresh lemon juice and dill, yeast-free toast, and steamed vegetables
- Broiled or baked chicken breast, **Cauliflower Curry**, and brown basmati rice
- **Chicken Vegetable Hash**, poached egg, and steamed broccoli or spinach
- **Chicken, Broccoli, and Rice Casserole** and sliced tomatoes
- **Chicken Kebabs, Tzatziki**, and **Roast Vegetables** or **Greek Salad**

- **Chicken Fajitas** or **Vegetarian Fajitas** and **Sautéed Greens**
- **Chicken Curry**, brown basmati rice, and steamed cauliflower, kale, and peas or **Cauliflower Curry**
- **Breaded Chicken Breasts, Baked Vegetables with Fennel**, and brown rice
- **Chicken with Yogurt and Soy Sauce**, stir-fried vegetables, and whole-grain pasta
- **Chicken with Lemon and Herbs, Barley Stew**, and steamed broccoli and green beans
- **Turkey Burger** or **Tofu Patty** with sliced tomato, sprouts, and mayo on rye bread or whole-grain bun, and **Steamed Vegetables with Tofu Parmesan Sauce**
- **Cabbage Rolls** and steamed vegetables sprinkled with fresh lemon juice and minced fresh herbs
- **Turkey Chili** or **Tofu Chili**, and **Sautéed Greens**
- **Stuffed Zucchini** and **Steamed Vegetables with Tofu Parmesan Sauce**
- **Baked Tofu with Black Bean Sauce**, brown rice, and steamed carrots and Chinese greens
- **Tofu and Veggie Lasagna** and **Sautéed Greens**
- **Tofu and Veggie Stir-Fry** with brown rice, barley, bean thread, or whole-grain pasta
- **Marinated Tofu**, stir-fried vegetables, and brown rice
- **Tofu Bean Casserole** with steamed carrots, brussels sprouts, and green beans
- **Baked Vegetable Frittata**, rye toast, and steamed carrots
- Pizza: choose from **Vegetable Pizza** or **Spinach and Feta Cheese Pizza**
- **Bean Dip Burritos** or **Bean Dip Quesadillas**, and **Sautéed Greens**
- See also the **Asian Recipes Section** for more ideas.

In hotter weather, you can add more cooling foods—in moderation, of course. For example, a serving of fruit grown in season can be eaten as a snack; just make sure that you eat it at least 1 hour before, or 3 to 5 hours after, eating protein foods.

(Heavier proteins, such as chicken and fish, will take longer to digest, compared to lighter proteins such as tofu.) Also, steamed or stir-fried vegetables can occasionally be replaced with raw vegetables or **Greek Salad**, and **Sautéed Greens** can sometimes be replaced with green salads.

Recipes

by Irene Hayton

• For more chicken and turkey dishes, see the following
   recipes for variations: Tofu and Veggie Stir-Fry; Bean
   Dip Burritos; Bean Dip Quesadillas.

MEATLESS MAIN DISHES

- For more tofu and tempeh dishes, see the following
  recipes for variations: Baked Fish with Black Bean
  Sauce; Chicken Fajitas; Chicken Curry; Cabbage Rolls,
  Turkey Chili; Stuffed Zucchini; Lasagna Roll-Ups

VEGETABLES AND SIDE DISHES

QUICK BREADS, MUFFINS, BEVERAGES, ETC.

DIPS, SPREADS, AND SAUCES

Tzatziki

1 large cucumber
2 cups (500 mL) low-fat plain yogurt (see Note)
2 garlic cloves, finely minced
1 teaspoon (5 mL) or more, minced fresh dill (optional)
sea salt, to taste

Peel the cucumber, cut it in half, and remove the seeds; grate it
and then drain it in a sieve. Combine the grated cucumber,
yogurt, garlic, and dill, if using. Season to taste with sea salt.
Mix well and refrigerate. Serve with warm pita bread or
tortillas, steamed vegetables, fish, chicken, beef, or lamb.

Note
For a thicker sauce, buy an extra-thick variety of yogurt or
strain regular yogurt to make it thicker. Place 3 cups (750 mL) of
yogurt into a sieve lined with cheesecloth, and set it over a
bowl; cover and refrigerate. Let it drain for 2 to 3 hours, or until
you have 2 cups (500 mL) of strained yogurt. If you don't have
cheesecloth, you can use a clean tea towel and decrease the
amount of time that you drain the yogurt. For smaller amounts
of yogurt, you can drain it in a coffee filter.

Bean Dip

1½ cups (375 mL) cooked Romano or pinto beans, or a
   14 ounce (398 mL) can, rinsed and drained
½ cup (125 mL) drained and mashed firm tofu (optional)
1 to 2 garlic cloves, minced
2 green onions, chopped
¼ cup (50 mL) chopped fresh cilantro (or parsley or a
   combination)
juice of half a lime (or half a small lemon)
1 teaspoon (5 mL) ground cumin
½ teaspoon (2 mL) sea salt
2 to 4 tablespoons (30 to 60 mL) water

Combine the beans, tofu, 1 of the garlic cloves, green onions, cilantro and/or parsley, lime or lemon juice, cumin, sea salt, and 2 tablespoons of the water in a food processor. Process until smooth, stopping to scrape down the sides, if necessary. Add more of the water, ½ tablespoon (7 mL) at a time, until you achieve the desired consistency. Taste and adjust the seasonings and add the other clove of garlic, if desired. Serve with warmed tortillas or cold steamed vegetables such as broccoli and cauliflower, or use in **Bean Dip Burritos**, **Bean Dip Quesadillas**, or **Tortilla Pinwheels**. Makes about 1½ cups (375 mL).

Tortilla Pinwheels

Spread a thin layer of **Bean Dip** on whole-wheat tortillas and sprinkle with diced sweet red pepper. Top with grated soy cheese, reduced-fat Monterey Jack cheese, and/or Cheddar cheese. Roll the tortillas up tightly, then wrap them in plastic wrap and refrigerate for about 1 hour. Cut into ½ inch (1 cm) slices and arrange on a baking sheet. Bake at 350° F (180° C) for about 10 minutes or until the cheese melts. Serve as an appetizer with low-fat plain yogurt and mild salsa.

Hummus

2 cups (500 mL) cooked chickpeas, or a 19 ounce (540 mL)
    can, rinsed and drained
2 tablespoons (30 mL) tahini (sesame seed paste)
2 large garlic cloves, minced
¼ cup (50 mL) chopped fresh parsley
1 teaspoon (5 mL) ground cumin
¼ teaspoon (1 mL) sea salt
1 tablespoon (15 mL) extra virgin olive oil
3 to 4 tablespoons (45 to 60 mL) fresh lemon juice
2 to 3 tablespoons (30 to 45 mL) water

Combine the chickpeas, tahini, garlic, parsley, cumin, sea salt,
oil, 3 tablespoons (45 mL) of the lemon juice, and 2 tablespoons
of the water in a blender. Process until smooth, stopping to
scrape down the sides, if necessary. If the mixture is too dry,
add more water, ½ tablespoon (7 mL) at a time, while
processing. Taste and adjust the seasonings, and add the rest of
the lemon juice, if desired. Serve with warm pita bread or
tortillas, on **Dill Scones** or toasted rye bread, with steamed
vegetables, or in a sandwich with sliced tomatoes and broccoli
sprouts.

Roasted Eggplant Dip

The seasonings in this dip are similar to those in the **Hummus** *recipe, except the quantities have been adjusted slightly.*

1 large or 2 small eggplants
2 tablespoons (30 mL) tahini (sesame seed paste)
1 large clove garlic, minced
¼ cup (50 mL) chopped fresh parsley
½ teaspoon (2 mL) ground cumin
¼ teaspoon (1 mL) sea salt
3 tablespoons (45 mL) fresh lemon juice

Pierce the eggplant in several places with a fork and place on a baking sheet. Bake at 400° F (200° C) for 25 minutes; turn the eggplant over, and bake for 20 to 30 minutes more, until very tender. Split the eggplant in half and drain in a colander until cool. Scoop out the pulp and discard the skin. Add the remaining ingredients to the pulp and mash well, or process in a food processor until smooth. Use as you would **Hummus**. Makes about 2 cups (500 mL).

Yogurt Herb Dip

½ cup (125 mL) low-fat plain yogurt
½ teaspoon (2 mL) chopped fresh dill, cilantro, or basil
pinch sea salt

Combine all the ingredients and mix well. Serve with fish or
chicken, or with steamed vegetables such as green beans,
broccoli, cauliflower, brussels sprouts, zucchini, snow peas,
potatoes, or carrots.

Notes
- For a thicker dip, use strained yogurt.
- Add Dijon mustard, to taste.
- Omit the fresh herbs and add ground cumin or cumin
  seeds, to taste.
- When using dill, add 1 tablespoon (15 mL) grated
  jicama.

Variation

Tofu Herb Dip
Substitute well-drained silken or soft tofu for the yogurt. Add
½ teaspoon (2 mL) lemon juice and ½ teaspoon (2 mL)
mayonnaise (optional). Process in a blender for a smoother
sauce.

Mayonnaise

This recipe is courtesy of Flora Manufacturing and Distributing, Ltd.

1 egg yolk
1 cup (250 mL) Udo's Choice Ultimate Oil Blend® or flax oil
¼ to ½ teaspoon (1 to 2 mL) dry mustard powder
1 tablespoon (15 mL) fresh lemon juice
cayenne pepper, to taste (optional)

Beat the egg yolk with a wire whip or with a hand blender on medium speed. Slowly add oil. Add lemon juice and mustard to taste.

Tofu Mayonnaise

1 cup (250 mL) drained and mashed firm tofu
2 teaspoons (10 mL) extra virgin olive oil
1 to 2 teaspoons (5 to 10 mL) lemon juice
1 teaspoon (5 mL) rice vinegar
¼ teaspoon (1 mL) finely minced garlic
½ teaspoon (2 mL) Dijon mustard
2 to 3 tablespoons (30 to 45 mL) water
sea salt, to taste

Combine the tofu, oil, lemon juice, vinegar, garlic, mustard, and 1 tablespoon (15 mL) of the water in a blender; process until smooth. Add more water, ½ tablespoon (7 mL) at a time, to achieve the desired consistency. Season to taste with sea salt. Add some finely minced fresh herbs, such as dill or parsley, if desired. Keeps in the refrigerator for up to 3 days. Makes about 1 cup (250 mL).

Note
You can substitute 1 cup (250 mL) of well-drained soft tofu for the firm tofu; this will have a thinner consistency.

Tofu Spread

1 cup (250 mL) drained and mashed firm tofu
1 tablespoon (15 mL) mayonnaise
1 small garlic clove, finely minced (optional)
2 teaspoons (10 mL) lemon juice
2 teaspoons (10 mL) minced green onion
1 tablespoon (15 mL) minced fresh parsley
¼ teaspoon (1 mL) turmeric
sea salt, to taste

Combine all the ingredients and mix well. Use as a sandwich spread or to stuff tomatoes. Makes 2 servings.

Note
Add minced fresh herbs such as basil, cilantro, marjoram, or dill, if you have them.

Yogurt Cheese

Yogurt Cheese is a soft, rich-tasting spreadable cheese you can use in sandwiches and on crackers. To make 1 cup (250 mL) of **Yogurt Cheese**, start with 2 cups (500 mL) yogurt.

Place low-fat plain yogurt in a sieve lined with a clean tea towel or with about 4 layers of cheesecloth; place the sieve over a bowl. Wrap the tea towel or cheesecloth around the yogurt and give it a slight squeeze. Put a light weight (such as a bag of rice or beans) on top, cover with a plate, and leave to drain in the refrigerator for 6 to 8 hours. For a thicker cheese, you can drain the yogurt for up to 24 hours.

Yogurt Cheese and Herb Spread

1 cup (250 mL) **Yogurt Cheese**
1 tablespoon (15 mL) minced green onion
1 tablespoon (15 mL) minced fresh parsley
sea salt, to taste

Combine all the ingredients and mix well. Use as a sandwich spread with tomatoes and sprouts; on baked potatoes instead of sour cream and butter; on rye toast or crackers; or on hot, cooked pasta or steamed veggies. Makes 1 cup (250 mL).

Variations

Yogurt Cheese and Feta Spread
Add 1 cup (250 mL) finely crumbled feta cheese and 1 small garlic clove, finely minced; mix well. Serve on rye toast, rye crackers, or toasted whole-grain bagels. Or serve as an appetizer by spreading it on a plate that has a rim, to contain it. Garnish the spread with diced fresh tomato, chopped green onion, diced cucumber, diced sweet red and/or green pepper, and sliced black olives; serve with whole-grain crackers or pita bread wedges.

Quark and Herb Spread
Substitute quark for the **Yogurt Cheese** in the **Yogurt Cheese and Herb Spread** recipe. Quark is a soft, spreadable cheese available in some grocery stores.

Quark and Feta Spread
Substitute quark for the **Yogurt Cheese** in the **Yogurt Cheese and Feta Spread** recipe.

Yogurt Cheese and Salmon Spread

For those who like the taste of smoked salmon-flavoured cream cheese, use this recipe instead. It tastes similar but has a lower fat content and doesn't contain the nitrates found in smoked salmon.

¼ cup (50 mL) cooked salmon
⅓ cup (75 mL) **Yogurt Cheese**
1 teaspoon (1 mL) minced fresh dill

In a small bowl, flake the salmon well. Add the **Yogurt Cheese** and dill and mix well. Serve on rye crackers, rye or whole-grain toast, or occasionally, on whole-grain bagels.

Variation

Quark and Salmon Spread
Substitute quark for the **Yogurt Cheese**.

Basil Pesto Sauce

Use small portions of this flavourful sauce on cooked pasta,
rice, or vegetables or stir into soups such as **Minestrone**. It can
also be used on pizza or spread over fish fillets before steaming.
To freeze, place a tablespoon of **Basil Pesto Sauce** into each
portion of an ice cube tray; once they're frozen solid, remove
and store the cubes in a plastic freezer bag.

    2 cups (500 mL) fresh basil leaves
    2 to 3 garlic cloves, minced
    ¼ cup (50 mL) pine nuts
    ½ cup (125 mL) freshly grated Parmesan cheese
    3 tablespoons (45 mL) extra virgin olive oil
    ¼ cup (50 mL) water
    ½ teaspoon (2 mL) sea salt

Place all the ingredients in a blender. Process until smooth,
stopping to scrape down the sides, if necessary. Makes about
1 cup (250 mL).

Variation

Parsley Pesto Sauce
If fresh basil is unavailable, use 2 cups (500 mL) fresh parsley,
stems removed, plus 2 tablespoons (30 mL) dried basil.

Tomato Sauce

Tomatoes are high in lycopene, a bioflavonoid that helps protect your membranes from free radicals made from the sun or by your immune system. Cooked tomatoes—such as tomato sauces, tomato paste, and pizza sauce—are a good source of lycopene because the cooking process causes the lycopene to be released.

You can use large, fresh tomatoes (3 to 4) or Roma tomatoes (6 to 8) to make this sauce. Peel the tomatoes only if the skins are tough; this isn't usually necessary with Roma tomatoes. When tomatoes are not in season, substitute a 28 ounce (796 mL) can of tomatoes, and reduce the amount of water to ½ cup (125 mL).

2 teaspoons (10 mL) extra virgin olive oil
1 small onion, chopped, about ½ cup (125 mL)
1 to 2 garlic cloves, minced
3½ cups (875 mL) chopped peeled tomatoes (see Note)
5½ ounce (156 mL) can tomato paste
1 tablespoon (15 mL) chopped fresh basil or 1 teaspoon
   (5 mL) dried
½ teaspoon (2 mL) oregano
½ teaspoon (2 mL) sea salt
1 bay leaf
1 cup (250 mL) water

Heat a large saucepan over medium-low heat. Add the oil, onion, and garlic and cook until the onion is tender. Add the remaining ingredients; bring to a boil, then reduce the heat and simmer, uncovered, for at least 1 hour. Remove the bay leaf. For a smoother sauce, transfer to a blender or food processor. Process with just a few short pulses until the sauce is smooth (do not overprocess). Use in **Tofu and Veggie Lasagna** or **Cabbage Rolls,** or puree the sauce slightly and use it in **Stuffed Zucchini, Lasagna Roll-Ups,** or in **Pizza Sauce.** Makes about 4 cups (1 L).

Note

To peel and seed the tomatoes, put them in boiling water until the skins start to split, up to a maximum of 1 minute. Remove the tomatoes from the water with a slotted spoon and immerse in cold water to stop the cooking process. When they're cool enough to handle, cut out the cores and then remove the skins; they should come off easily. Cut the tomatoes in half and squeeze them gently to remove most of the seeds.

Variation

Pasta Sauce

Add some protein to the sauce—such as tofu, tempeh, chicken, or turkey—and serve over cooked pasta. When sautéing the onion and garlic, just add some crumbled tofu or tempeh or lean ground chicken or turkey breast. Tofu or tempeh should be cooked for about 10 minutes before adding the remaining ingredients; ground chicken or turkey should be cooked until no longer pink, then any fat should be drained off before adding the remaining ingredients.

Tofu Sauce

1 teaspoon (5 mL) extra virgin olive oil
¼ cup (50 mL) chopped onion
1 garlic clove, minced
1 cup (250 mL) mashed firm or medium-firm tofu
¼ teaspoon (1 mL) oregano
½ teaspoon (2 mL) basil
sea salt, to taste

Heat a skillet or saucepan over medium-low heat. Add the oil, onion, and garlic, and sauté until the onion is tender. Add the tofu, oregano, and basil. Cook over medium-low heat for 20 minutes, stirring occasionally and adding a small amount of water, if necessary. Add sea salt, to taste. Use in **Tofu Bean Casserole**, or double the recipe to use in **Tofu and Veggie Lasagna**.

SOUPS

Most of the soup recipes call for stock or water. You can use either **Vegetable Stock** or **Chicken Stock**—these are easy to make and will give the soup much more flavour than if you use water. Stock can be made in advance and frozen for later use. Freeze in 2 cup (500 mL) portions to defrost as needed, or freeze in ice cube trays, then store the cubes in plastic freezer bags to use when stir-frying or sautéing.

Vegetable Stock

10 cups (2.5 L) water
1 large onion, quartered
1 leek, white part only, washed and chopped
2 medium tomatoes, quartered
1 head green leaf or butter lettuce, washed and torn
3 celery stalks with leaves, chopped
2 carrots, chopped
1 bay leaf
1 sprig fresh thyme or ½ teaspoon (2 mL) dried
6 to 8 sprigs fresh parsley, chopped
sea salt, to taste

Combine all the ingredients in a large pot and bring to a boil. Reduce the heat to low and simmer, partially covered, for 1 hour. Strain the stock, and refrigerate for up to 3 days or freeze for later use. Makes about 10 cups (2.5 L).

Chicken Stock

3 to 4 pound (1.5 to 2 kg) chicken or chicken parts
12 cups (3 L) cold water
2 celery stalks with leaves, chopped
2 carrots, chopped
1 onion, chopped
1 leek, white part only, washed and chopped
1 garlic clove, halved
4 sprigs fresh thyme or 1 teaspoon (5 mL) dried
4 sprigs fresh parsley
1 bay leaf
1 teaspoon (5 mL) sea salt

Place the chicken in a large pot with the water. Bring just to a simmer over medium heat and cover partially. Do not boil or stir; this will give a clearer stock. Skim off any foam that rises to the top. Add more water to replace any that may have been removed when skimming the foam. Reduce heat and add remaining ingredients. Simmer, partially covered, for 3 to 4 hours.

Remove the pot from the heat and remove the chicken pieces; set aside. Strain the stock, then cover and refrigerate it until a layer of fat forms on the top. Remove the fat by carefully scooping it off with a spoon, by dragging a clean paper towel over top of it, or by placing a large piece of wax paper on the fat; the fat will stick to the paper towel or wax paper. The stock may be refrigerated for up to 3 days or it can be frozen for later use. Freeze some of the stock in ice cube trays and store the cubes in a plastic bag in the freezer; use for sautéing and stir-frying. Recipe makes 10 to 12 cups (2.5 to 3 L) stock.

Remove the meat from the bones. Use the meat on pizza, in sandwiches, in soups (such as **Chicken Rice Soup**), or in recipes that call for cooked chicken (such as **Chicken Salad, Chicken Vegetable Hash,** and **Wraps**).

Variation

Turkey Stock
Substitute the leftover carcass of a roast turkey for the chicken.

Cabbage Soup

8 cups (2 L) **Vegetable Stock** or water
half a small head of cabbage, chopped, approximately 4 cups
    (1 L)
2 onions, diced
2 garlic cloves, minced
4 celery stalks, sliced
2 carrots, sliced
2 cups (500 mL) chopped green beans
1 leek, white part only, washed and sliced
5½ ounce (156 mL) can tomato paste
28 ounce (796 mL) can tomatoes, chopped
1 teaspoon (5 mL) basil
2 teaspoons (10 mL) oregano
½ teaspoon (2 mL) kelp powder
2 tablespoons (30 mL) chopped fresh parsley (optional)
1 tomato, chopped (optional)
sea salt, to taste

Combine all the ingredients, except the sea salt, in a large pot and bring to a boil. Reduce the heat, cover, and simmer until the vegetables are tender. Season to taste with sea salt. Makes 8 to 10 servings.

Creamy Broccoli Soup

2 cups (500 mL) **Chicken Stock**, **Vegetable Stock**, or water
1 small onion, chopped
1 garlic clove, minced
1 carrot, sliced
1 celery stalk, sliced
1 tablespoon (15 mL) chopped fresh parsley (optional)
4 cups (1 L) chopped broccoli
1 cup (250 mL) low-fat milk, soy milk, or rice milk
sea salt, to taste
grated reduced-fat Cheddar cheese (optional)

Combine the stock or water, onion, garlic, carrot, celery, and parsley in a large saucepan. Bring to a boil, then reduce the heat to medium-low. Cover and cook for 10 minutes, stirring occasionally. Add the broccoli and stir well. Continue cooking, stirring occasionally, for 10 to 15 minutes, or until the vegetables are tender. Puree the soup, in batches, in a blender or food processor until smooth. Return the soup to the saucepan and stir in the milk. (For a thicker soup, use less milk or omit it altogether, if you wish.) Cook over medium-low heat just until heated through; add sea salt. Optional: add a small amount of grated reduced-fat Cheddar cheese just before serving. Makes 4 servings.

Linda's Lentil Spinach Soup

1 tablespoon (15 mL) extra virgin olive oil
2 onions, chopped
3 garlic cloves, chopped
1½ cups (375 mL) red lentils
7 cups (1.75 L) **Chicken Stock, Vegetable Stock,** or water
1 to 3 teaspoons (5 to 15 mL) chili powder, to taste
1 to 3 teaspoons (5 to 15 mL) ground cumin, to taste
½ to 1 teaspoon (2 to 5 mL) cinnamon, to taste
5½ ounce (156 mL) can tomato paste
1 bunch fresh spinach, washed, stems removed, and torn,
    about 8 cups (2 L)
a few sprigs of fresh parsley, chopped
sea salt, to taste

Heat a large saucepan over medium-low heat. Add the oil,
onion, and garlic, and sauté until the onion is tender. Add the
lentils, stock or water, chili powder, cumin, and cinnamon.
Bring to a boil, then reduce the heat to low. Cover and simmer
until the lentils are tender, about 40 minutes. Add the tomato
paste, spinach, and parsley, and simmer for 10 minutes more.
Season to taste with sea salt. Makes 8 to 10 servings.

Turkey Barley Soup

When buying ground turkey (or chicken), make sure it's ground from skinless breast to ensure it's low in fat.

2 teaspoons (10 mL) extra virgin olive oil
1 small onion, chopped
1 garlic clove, minced
2 celery stalks, diced
2 carrots, diced
1 pound (500 g) lean ground turkey (or chicken) breast
5 cups (1.25 L) **Chicken Stock**, **Vegetable Stock**, or water
½ cup (125 mL) pot barley
19 ounce (540 mL) can tomatoes, chopped
3 tablespoons (45 mL) tomato paste (see Note)
1 bay leaf
½ teaspoon (2 mL) celery seed
½ teaspoon (2 mL) sea salt

Heat a skillet over medium-low heat. Add the oil, onion, garlic, celery, and carrots, and cook for 5 minutes. Transfer the cooked vegetables to a large soup pot and return the skillet to the heat. Add the ground turkey to the skillet and cook until it's no longer pink, breaking it up with a fork. Drain off any fat, then add the turkey to the soup pot. Add the stock or water, barley, tomatoes, tomato paste, bay leaf, and celery seed to the pot. Bring to a boil, then reduce the heat to low. Cover and simmer for about 1 hour, until the barley is cooked. Remove the bay leaf and add the sea salt. Makes about 8 servings.

Note
Leftover tomato paste can be frozen for later use. Put 1 tablespoon (15 mL) tomato paste into each section of an ice cube tray, cover, and place in the freezer. Once they're frozen, transfer the cubes to a plastic freezer bag and seal. Use the cubes to flavour soups (like this recipe and **Turkey Barley Soup**) and other dishes (such as **Turkey Chili** and **Pizza Sauce**).

Minestrone

2 teaspoons (10 mL) extra virgin olive oil
1 small onion, chopped
2 garlic cloves, minced
½ cup (125 mL) diced celery
½ cup (125 mL) diced carrots
1 cup (250 mL) chopped peeled tomatoes
4 cups (1 L) **Chicken Stock, Vegetable Stock,** or water
½ cup (125 mL) diced zucchini
½ teaspoon (2 mL) basil
½ teaspoon (2 mL) oregano
3 tablespoons (45 mL) chopped fresh parsley
½ cup (125 mL) uncooked short whole-grain pasta
1 cup (250 mL) cooked kidney beans (red or white)
3 cups (750 mL) fresh spinach leaves, washed, stems
    removed, and torn
sea salt, to taste
freshly grated Parmesan cheese (optional)
Pesto Sauce (optional)

Heat a large saucepan over medium-low heat. Add the oil, onion, garlic, celery, and carrots, and sauté until the onion is tender. Add the tomatoes, stock or water, zucchini, basil, oregano, and parsley, and bring to a boil. Reduce the heat to low, add the pasta, and cook for 5 minutes. Add the beans and spinach and cook 5 minutes more, or until the spinach is softened. Season to taste with sea salt. Top each serving with freshly grated Parmesan cheese and/or a dollop of **Basil Pesto Sauce** or **Parsley Pesto Sauce**, if desired. Makes 6 servings.

Chicken Rice Soup

2 teaspoons (10 mL) extra virgin olive oil
1 leek, white part only, washed and chopped, or 1 small
    onion, chopped
1 carrot, chopped
1 celery stalk, chopped
4 cups (1 L) **Chicken Stock** or **Vegetable Stock**
⅓ cup (75 mL) uncooked brown rice
½ teaspoon (2 mL) EACH basil, thyme, and marjoram
⅛ teaspoon (0.5 mL) ground sage
1 bay leaf
1½ cups (375 mL) chopped cooked chicken
¼ cup (50 mL) chopped fresh parsley
sea salt, to taste

Heat a large saucepan over medium-low heat. Add the oil, leek
or onion, carrot, and celery, and sauté until the onion is tender,
about 5 minutes. Add the stock, rice, herbs, and bay leaf. Bring
to a boil, then reduce the heat to low. Cover and simmer for 30
minutes. Add the chicken and simmer for another 10 minutes,
or until the rice is done. Remove the bay leaf, add the parsley,
and season to taste with the sea salt. Makes 4 servings.

Note
For a quicker version, omit the uncooked rice and simmer the
stock and seasonings for 10 minutes instead of 30 minutes. Add
1 cup (250 mL) cooked rice or ½ cup (125 mL) uncooked whole-
grain pasta, when adding the chicken.

Miso Soup

This soup is very quick and easy to make. The amounts of miso, tofu, green onion, and ginger can be adjusted according to taste. Wakame seaweed can be found in the dried form in health food stores. It contains calcium, B vitamins, and minerals, and it adds a nice flavour to this soup. Wakame expands quite a bit, so cut it into very small pieces. Firm tofu can be substituted for soft or silken tofu.

4 inch (10 cm) piece of wakame seaweed (optional)
4 cups (1 L) water
4 tablespoons (60 mL) miso
½ cup (125 mL) finely cubed silken or soft tofu
2 green onions, sliced
½ teaspoon (2 mL) finely minced or grated fresh ginger
   (optional)

Cut the seaweed into small pieces using scissors. In a medium saucepan, combine the seaweed and water. Bring to a boil, then reduce the heat to low. Remove ½ cup (125 mL) of the water from the saucepan and combine with the miso in a small bowl; mix with a fork until the miso is dissolved. Pour the miso mixture back into the saucepan and add the tofu, green onion, and ginger, if using. Simmer for a few minutes until heated through, but do not boil. Makes 4 servings.

Variation

Miso Vegetable Soup
When the water comes to a boil, add ½ cup (125 mL) EACH sliced snow peas, and finely sliced bok choy and carrots. Reduce the heat to medium, and simmer for about 5 minutes or until the vegetables are just tender. Add the remaining ingredients, as described above.

Bean and Tomato Soup

2 teaspoons (10 mL) extra virgin olive oil
1 onion, chopped
1 garlic clove, minced
1 celery stalk, chopped
1 teaspoon (5 mL) ground cumin
½ teaspoon (2 mL) ground coriander
2 cups (500 mL) **Chicken Stock**, **Vegetable Stock**, or water
3 cups (750 mL) chopped peeled tomatoes, or a 28 ounce
    (796 mL) can
1½ cups (375 mL) cooked red kidney beans, or a 14 ounce
    (398 mL) can
1½ cups (375 mL) cooked pinto beans or white kidney beans,
    or a 14 ounce (398 mL) can
4 cups (1 L) fresh spinach or kale, washed, stems removed,
    and torn
1 tablespoon (15 mL) fresh lemon juice (optional)
½ teaspoon (2 mL) sea salt

Heat a saucepan over medium-low heat. Add the oil, onion,
garlic, celery, cumin, and coriander, and sauté until the onion is
tender. Add the stock or water and the tomatoes. Bring to a boil,
then reduce the heat to low. Cover, and simmer for 15 minutes.
Add the beans, spinach, and lemon juice, if using, and simmer
for 5 minutes more. Add the sea salt. Makes 6 servings.

Creamy Vegetable Soup

2 teaspoons (10 mL) extra virgin olive oil
1 onion, chopped
1 garlic clove, minced
1 carrot, chopped
1 celery stalk, chopped
2 cups (500 mL) **Chicken Stock, Vegetable Stock,** or water
1 cup (250 mL) cauliflower florets
1 cup (250 mL) chopped tomatoes
2 tablespoons (30 mL) chopped fresh parsley, divided
½ teaspoon (2 mL) oregano
½ teaspoon (2 mL) ground cumin
¼ teaspoon (1 mL) thyme
2 cups (500 mL) packed fresh spinach leaves, washed, stems
    removed, and torn
1 cup (250 mL) soft or silken tofu
½ teaspoon (2 mL) sea salt

Heat a large saucepan over medium-low heat. Add the oil,
onion, garlic, carrot, and celery; sauté until the onion is tender,
about 5 minutes. Add the stock or water, cauliflower, tomatoes,
1 tablespoon (15 mL) of the parsley, oregano, cumin, and thyme.
Bring to a boil, then reduce the heat to low. Cover and simmer
for 20 minutes. Add the spinach and continue simmering until
the vegetables are tender, about 5 to 10 minutes. Puree the soup,
in batches, in a blender or food processor until smooth. Return
the soup to the saucepan. Puree the tofu until smooth, then stir
slowly into the soup. Heat through, then add the sea salt.
Garnish with the remaining 1 tablespoon (15 mL) parsley.
Makes 4 servings.

Tomato Soup

When tomatoes aren't in season, use three 14 ounce (398 mL) cans of good plum tomatoes.

- 2 teaspoons (10 mL) extra virgin olive oil
- 1 small onion, chopped
- 1 garlic clove, minced
- 1 celery stalk, chopped
- 1 carrot, chopped
- 6 medium tomatoes, peeled, seeded, and chopped, about
    5 cups (1.25 L) (see Note)
- 1 tablespoon (15 mL) chopped fresh basil
- 1 tablespoon (15 mL) chopped fresh parsley
- 1 bay leaf
- 1 cup (250 mL) **Chicken Stock**, **Vegetable Stock**, or water
- ¼ teaspoon (1 mL) sea salt

Heat a large saucepan over medium-low heat. Add the oil, onion, garlic, celery, and carrot, and sauté until the onion is tender, about 5 minutes. Add the tomatoes, basil, parsley, bay leaf, and stock or water. Bring to a boil, then reduce the heat to low. Cover and simmer for 20 to 30 minutes, or until the carrots are tender. Remove the bay leaf and add the sea salt. Use a blender to puree the soup, in batches, until smooth. Makes about 4 servings.

Note
To peel and seed the tomatoes, put them in boiling water until the skins start to split, up to a maximum of 1 minute. Remove from the water with a slotted spoon and immerse the tomatoes in cold water to stop the cooking process. When they're cool enough to handle, cut out the cores and then remove the skins; they should come off easily. Cut the tomatoes in half and squeeze them gently to remove most of the seeds.

SALADS

Salads that contain raw vegetables, like green salads, **Coleslaw**, and **Greek Salad**, should be eaten in moderation, and in warm weather when you are out in the sunshine. Cooked salads, such as **Bean Salad**, **Potato Salad**, **Salmon Salad**, **Tuna Salad**, **Chicken Salad**, and **Egg Salad**, can be eaten in cool weather.

Greek Salad

Dressing
¼ cup (50 mL) extra virgin olive oil
1 tablespoon (15 mL) lemon juice
1 tablespoon (15 mL) apple cider vinegar or red wine vinegar
1 garlic clove, minced
½ teaspoon (2 mL) oregano
¼ teaspoon (1 mL) sea salt

2 large or 3 medium tomatoes
1 cucumber (peeled, unless using long English cucumber)
2 small sweet green and/or red peppers
half a red onion
½ cup (125 mL) crumbled feta cheese
Calamata olives (optional)

Combine all the dressing ingredients and mix well. Cover and let stand at room temperature for at least 1 hour before serving.

Cut the tomatoes, cucumber, peppers, and red onion into bite-size pieces. Toss gently with the feta and olives in a large glass bowl. Allow each person to add the dressing to his/her salad; you don't need to use a lot of dressing because the chopped vegetables create a lot of juice. Any leftover dressing can be kept for a few days. Makes 6 to 8 servings.

Optional: Omit the peppers and red onion. Add torn Romaine lettuce, chopped fresh cilantro, and chopped green onions.

Potato Salad

1 pound (500 g) small new potatoes, white or red (about 10 to
　12 potatoes)
½ cup (125 mL) low-fat plain yogurt (use extra-thick or
　strained yogurt)
1 teaspoon (5 mL) Dijon mustard
1 teaspoon (5 mL) minced fresh dill
1 teaspoon (5 mL) minced fresh parsley
¼ teaspoon (1 mL) sea salt
1 small celery stalk, diced
3 radishes, diced
3 green onions, sliced

Cut the potatoes in quarters and boil them until just tender, but
not mushy. Drain and rinse under cold water; drain well and set
aside.

　While the potatoes are cooking, combine the yogurt, mustard,
dill, parsley, and sea salt; set aside.

　Combine the potatoes, yogurt mixture, celery, radishes, and
green onions. Mix gently and refrigerate for at least 1 hour
before serving. Makes 4 to 6 servings.

Note
Add chopped hard-boiled egg, if desired.

Bean Salad

1½ cups (375 mL) fresh green beans, cut into 1 inch (2.5 cm)
   pieces
1½ cups (375 mL) fresh wax beans, cut into 1 inch (2.5 cm)
   pieces
2 cups (500 mL) cooked red kidney beans, or a 19 ounce
   (540 mL) can, rinsed and drained
2 cups (500 mL) cooked chickpeas, or 19 ounce (540 mL) can,
   rinsed and drained
¾ cup (175 mL) diced red onion
1 small sweet green or red pepper, diced
1 celery stalk, diced

Dressing
¼ cup (50 mL) apple cider vinegar
¼ cup (50 mL) fresh lemon juice
⅓ cup (75 mL) Udo's Choice Ultimate Oil Blend®, sunflower,
   or safflower oil
1 teaspoon (5 mL) Dijon mustard
1 tablespoon (15 mL) chopped fresh parsley
1 garlic clove, minced
½ teaspoon (2 mL) oregano
½ teaspoon (2 mL) basil
½ teaspoon (2 mL) celery seed
½ teaspoon (2 mL) sea salt

Blanch the green beans and the wax beans in boiling water for 4
minutes. Rinse thoroughly in cold water to stop the cooking
process. Drain well and place in a large bowl; add the kidney
beans, chickpeas, red onion, green pepper, and celery.

For the dressing, combine all the dressing ingredients and
pour over the bean mixture; mix well. Cover and refrigerate for
several hours or overnight, stirring occasionally. Makes about
10 servings.

Pasta Salad

Dressing
  ⅓ cup (75 mL) extra virgin olive oil or Udo's Choice Ultimate
    Oil Blend®
  2 tablespoons (30 mL) apple cider vinegar
  1 tablespoon (15 mL) fresh lemon juice
  1 large garlic clove, minced
  1 teaspoon (5 mL) basil
  ¼ teaspoon (1 mL) sea salt

  3 cups (875 mL) whole-grain rotini pasta, uncooked
  ½ cup (125 mL) grated carrot
  1 cup (250 mL) broccoli florets
  1 cup (250 mL) cauliflower florets
  1 small sweet red pepper, chopped
  1 cup (250 mL) artichoke hearts, drained and chopped
  4½ ounce (125 mL) can sliced black olives
  ½ to 1 cup (125 to 250 mL) crumbled feta cheese
  2 tablespoons (30 mL) chopped fresh dill

Mix together all the dressing ingredients and let stand at room temperature for at least 2 hours before serving the salad.

Cook the rotini according to package directions, until just tender. Rinse under cold water and drain well, then toss with a small amount of the dressing to keep it from sticking together. In a large bowl, combine the pasta with the remaining ingredients. Add the dressing just before serving and mix well. Makes 8 to 10 servings.

Notes
- To add more protein, gently stir in chunks of salmon, cooked chicken, or cubed firm tofu (marinate the tofu in some of the dressing before adding it to the salad).
- In cooler weather, lightly cook the broccoli and carrots by steaming them for 3 minutes. Rinse under cold water to stop the cooking process.

Coleslaw

Indole-3-carbinol is the most active ingredient of the cruciferous vegetables; it's found in especially high quantities in broccoli, cabbage, and brussels sprouts. Its ability to stimulate the liver enzymes to break down your steroid hormones and eliminate chemicals gives it strong anticancer properties. Cabbage juice also has very strong anti-ulcer properties.

4 cups (1 L) finely shredded green cabbage
2 cups (500 mL) finely shredded red cabbage
½ cup (125 mL) shredded carrot
½ cup (125 mL) minced red onion or sweet Bermuda onion

Dressing
½ cup (125 mL) Udo's Choice Ultimate Oil Blend®
⅓ cup (75 mL) apple cider vinegar
1 teaspoon (5 mL) Dijon mustard
½ teaspoon (2 mL) celery seed
½ teaspoon (2 mL) sea salt

In a large salad bowl, combine the cabbage, carrot, and onion. Combine all the dressing ingredients and mix well. Pour over the cabbage mixture, stir well, and refrigerate for a few hours before serving, stirring occasionally. Makes 6 to 8 servings.

Cabbage Juice

This recipe requires a juicer. It's important to use only very fresh cabbage and carrots when making this juice.

½ cup (125 mL) cabbage juice (approximately half a small head)
¼ to ½ cup (50 to 125 mL) carrot juice (approximately 2 to 4 carrots)

Combine cabbage and carrot juices, to taste. Serve immediately, and sip slowly.

Sauerkraut Salad

2 cups (500 mL) chopped sauerkraut
¼ cup (50 mL) grated carrot
3 tablespoons (45 mL) finely chopped sweet red pepper
2 to 3 tablespoons (30 to 45 mL) grated or finely chopped red or white onion, to taste
¼ teaspoon (1 mL) paprika
sliced green onions (optional)

Place the sauerkraut in a sieve and rinse with cold water to remove some of the salt; this step is optional as you may wish to use the sauerkraut as is. Drain off some of the liquid and place the sauerkraut in a large glass bowl. Add the remaining ingredients and mix well. Makes 4 servings.

MORE SALADS

The following salad recipes use low-fat plain yogurt to replace much of the mayonnaise that's traditionally used in these recipes. Those who cannot eat yogurt can use the recipe for **Mayonnaise** or **Tofu Mayonnaise**. These salads can used as sandwich fillings; or in hot weather, these salads can occasionally be served on lettuce leaves as part of a salad plate, with raw and/or steamed veggies.

Salmon Salad

6 ounces (170 g) cooked salmon, about 1 cup (250 mL), or a
   7½ ounce (213 g) can, drained
1 tablespoon (15 mL) chopped green onion
2 teaspoons (10 mL) chopped fresh dill or 1 teaspoon (5 mL)
   dried
2 teaspoons (10 mL) mayonnaise
1 tablespoon (15 mL) low-fat plain yogurt
1 to 2 teaspoons (5 to 10 mL) lemon juice

Flake the salmon, then add the remaining ingredients and mix well. Use as a sandwich spread on yeast-free whole-grain bread, rye crackers, or tortillas, or stuff into pita bread with broccoli sprouts. Makes 2 servings.

Variation

Tuna Salad
Substitute a can of water-packed tuna for the salmon.

Chicken Salad

*You can poach 1 whole chicken breast (see recipe for **Poached Chicken Breasts**) to use in this recipe.*

> 1 cup (250 mL) diced cooked chicken (approximately 1 whole chicken breast)
> 1 tablespoon (15 mL) finely chopped celery
> 1 tablespoon (15 mL) chopped green onion
> 1 tablespoon (15 mL) minced fresh parsley (optional)
> 2 teaspoons (10 mL) mayonnaise
> 2 tablespoons (30 mL) low-fat plain yogurt
> pinch sea salt

Combine all the ingredients and mix well. Use as a sandwich spread on yeast-free rye bread, stuff into a pita (yeast-free variety, if you have yeast problems), wrap in a warmed whole-wheat tortilla, or use the salad to stuff tomatoes. Makes 2 servings.

Variation

Turkey Salad
Substitute turkey for the chicken.

Curried Chicken Salad

1 cup (250 mL) cubed cooked chicken
1 tablespoon (15 mL) finely chopped celery
1 tablespoon (15 mL) chopped green onion
1 tablespoon (15 mL) minced fresh cilantro
2 teaspoons (10 mL) mayonnaise
2 tablespoons (30 mL) low-fat plain yogurt
¼ to ½ teaspoon (1 to 2 mL) curry powder, to taste
pinch ground cumin
pinch sea salt

Combine all the ingredients and mix well. Use as a sandwich spread. Makes 2 servings.

Egg Salad

4 hard-boiled eggs
1 tablespoon (15 mL) finely chopped celery
1 tablespoon (15 mL) chopped green onion
2 teaspoons (10 mL) mayonnaise
3 to 4 teaspoons (15 to 20 mL) low-fat plain yogurt
½ teaspoon (2 mL) Dijon mustard
sea salt, to taste

Peel and mash the eggs. Add the remaining ingredients and mix well. Use as a sandwich spread. Makes 2 to 3 servings.

Note
Optional: discard 2 of the yolks to reduce the fat content of this recipe.

SANDWICHES AND WRAPS

Sandwiches

Here's a list of suggestions for sandwich fillings; serve on yeast-free rye or whole-grain bread. Add sliced tomatoes and/or sprouts (try broccoli sprouts), if desired. For smaller appetites, or for those wishing to reduce the amount of bread they eat, serve open-face on 1 slice of bread. Many of these sandwich fillings can also be served in pita bread (if you don't have yeast problems), or rolled up in whole-wheat tortillas.

Fillings
(Those in **bold type** indicate recipes included in this book.)
- **Hummus**
- **Tofu Spread**
- **Yogurt Cheese and Herb Spread; Quark and Herb Spread**
- **Salmon Salad; Tuna Salad**
- **Chicken Salad; Turkey Salad**
- **Curried Chicken Salad**
- **Egg Salad**
- Slices of **Turkey** (or **Chicken**) **Loaf** (see **Turkey Burgers** recipe)
- Slices of **Marinated Tofu**
- Sliced cooked chicken or turkey breast (not the processed kind!), with a small amount of mayo mixed with yogurt

Wraps

Wraps make a nice change from sandwiches. To assemble the wraps, place the listed ingredients in the middle of a whole-wheat tortilla, fold one end over the filling, then fold both sides over and wrap tightly. The amount of each ingredient will depend on personal taste and on the number of servings you wish to make. If you're taking the wrap for lunch at work, package the tortilla separately from the filling ingredients, and assemble the wrap just before eating.

If possible, use whole-wheat tortillas that aren't made with yeast or hydrogenated oils; be sure to read labels. Or make your own, using the **Tortillas** *recipe. To warm the tortillas, wrap them tightly in parchment paper and place in a 300° F (150° C) oven for 10 to 15 minutes, or heat in a skillet for about 1 minute per side.*

For those who are limiting the amount of starchy carbohydrates they eat, any of the following food suggestions can be eaten without the tortilla.

Black Bean and Rice Wraps

In a small baking dish, mix together basmati rice (preferably brown basmati), black beans, ground cumin, and lime juice. Cover and place in the oven for 15 minutes with the tortilla(s). Place the rice/bean mixture on the tortilla(s) and add diced tomato, chopped green and/or red onion, minced fresh cilantro, mild salsa, and low-fat plain yogurt. Additional toppings include cooked chicken, sliced avocado, and grated reduced-fat cheese (such as Cheddar and/or Monterey Jack) or soy cheese.

Chili and Feta Wraps

Wrap up warmed **Turkey Chili** (or **Tofu Chili** or **Tempeh Chili**), feta or goat cheese, diced tomato, and brown rice.

Chicken and Veggie Pesto Wraps

Sauté sliced chicken breast plus some sweet green and/or red pepper until the chicken is no longer pink inside; add torn, fresh spinach, cover, and continue cooking until the spinach is wilted (about 2 minutes). Combine with brown rice and a small amount of **Basil Pesto Sauce** or **Parsley Pesto Sauce** in a whole-wheat tortilla.

Chicken Souvlaki Wraps

Wrap up **Chicken Kebabs** (remove the skewer!), **Tzatziki**, diced tomato, and any of the following optional toppings: feta cheese or goat cheese, diced onion, steamed or sautéed greens (such as spinach or kale).

Roast Vegetable Wraps

Follow the recipe for **Roast Vegetables** using eggplant instead of the carrots, the rutabaga, and the potatoes (see Variation). Combine the **Roast Vegetables** with feta cheese or goat cheese, **Tzatziki**, and steamed or sautéed greens (optional).

FISH

Broiled Salmon Steaks

2 tablespoons (30 mL) lemon juice
1 tablespoon (15 mL) Tamari soy sauce
1 teaspoon (5 mL) minced or grated fresh ginger
1 garlic clove, minced
2 salmon steaks

Mix together the lemon juice, soy sauce, ginger, and garlic. Pour over the salmon steaks and marinate in the refrigerator for 20 minutes, turning the steaks over after 10 minutes.

Place the salmon on a lightly buttered broiler pan. Measure steaks at their thickest portion, and broil for 10 minutes per inch (2.5 cm) of thickness, or until the salmon flakes easily when tested with a fork. Turn the steaks over halfway through the cooking time, basting with the marinade. Good hot or cold. Makes 2 servings.

Salmon Cakes

6 ounces (170 g) cooked salmon, about 1 cup (250 mL), or a
    7½ ounce (213 g) can, drained
1 egg
3 tablespoons (45 mL) fine dried whole-grain bread crumbs
1 tablespoon (15 mL) minced green onion
1 tablespoon (15 mL) minced red onion
1 tablespoon (15 mL) minced sweet red pepper
1 tablespoon (15 mL) minced fresh parsley
1 tablespoon (15 mL) minced fresh dill or 1 teaspoon (5 mL)
    dried
1 teaspoon (5 mL) lemon juice
¼ teaspoon (1 mL) sea salt
1 teaspoon (5 mL) extra virgin olive oil

Combine all the ingredients except the oil, and mix well. On a
plate, shape the mixture into 4 small or 2 large patties, about
½ inch (1 cm) thick.

    Heat a skillet over medium-low heat. Add the oil, then add
the patties (use a lifter as they will be quite moist). Cook for 3 to
4 minutes per side, or until lightly browned. Alternatively, place
the salmon cakes on a lightly buttered baking sheet and broil
for 3 to 4 minutes per side. Good served with lemon juice and
low-fat plain yogurt, or with **Yogurt Herb Dip** (made with dill).
Makes 2 to 4 servings.

Variation

Tuna Cakes
Substitute a can of water-packed tuna for the salmon.

Salmon Loaf

This is good made with brown basmati rice and Mozzarella cheese.

6 ounces (170 g) cooked salmon, about 1 cup (250 mL), or a
  7½ ounce (213 g) can, drained
1 cup (250 mL) cooked brown rice
½ cup (125 mL) grated reduced-fat cheese or soy cheese
2 tablespoons (30 mL) chopped green onion
2 tablespoons (30 mL) chopped celery
1 egg
¼ cup (50 mL) chopped fresh parsley
1 tablespoon (15 mL) minced fresh dill or 1 teaspoon (5 mL)
  dried
¼ teaspoon (1 mL) sea salt

Flake the salmon, then add the remaining ingredients and mix
well. Press into a lightly buttered small loaf pan and bake at
350° F (180° C) for 25 to 30 minutes, or until firm. This tastes
good served with **Yogurt Herb Dip** or with low-fat plain
yogurt. Serve hot or cold. Makes 2 to 4 servings.

Variation

Tuna Loaf
Substitute a can of water-packed tuna for the salmon.

Tuna Casserole

Try using pasta made from spelt, quinoa, kamut, soy, or whole-wheat flour.

¾ cup (175 mL) short whole-grain pasta, such as macaroni or rotini
2 cups (500 mL) broccoli florets
6½ ounce (184 g) can water-packed tuna, drained
3 tablespoons (45 mL) sliced green onion
¼ cup (50 mL) finely chopped celery
½ cup (125 mL) low-fat plain yogurt
2 tablespoons (30 mL) mayonnaise
1 teaspoon (5 mL) lemon juice
1 tablespoon (15 mL) chopped fresh parsley
¼ teaspoon (1 mL) thyme
¼ teaspoon (1 mL) sea salt
1 tomato, sliced
½ cup (125 mL) grated reduced-fat cheese (optional)

Cook the pasta according to the package directions, but undercook it slightly; add the broccoli during the last 2 minutes of cooking time. Drain and rinse under cold water; drain again and set aside.

In a large bowl, flake the tuna. Add the green onion, celery, yogurt, mayonnaise, lemon juice, parsley, thyme, and sea salt; mix well. Gently stir in the pasta and broccoli. Spoon the mixture into a lightly buttered baking dish, arrange the tomato slices on top, and sprinkle with the cheese, if using. Cover and bake at 350° F (180° C) for 30 minutes, until hot. Makes 2 large or 4 small servings.

Poached Fish Fillets

Poaching is a quick, low-fat method for cooking chicken as well as fish. Other vegetables—such as onion, celery, tomato, sweet green pepper— and herbs such as thyme, bay leaf, etc., can be substituted or added to the poaching liquid.

2 firm fish fillets, about 4 ounces (125 g) each
water
juice of half a lemon
1 garlic clove, cut in half
1 carrot, chopped
2 sprigs fresh parsley
1 sprig fresh dill or fennel

Fill a deep skillet or wok with enough water to cover the fish (but don't add the fish yet). Add the lemon juice, garlic, carrot, parsley, and dill or fennel; bring just to a boil. Reduce the heat to a very gentle simmer, and using a slotted spatula, add the fish. Cover and cook for 5 to 10 minutes, until the fish flakes easily when tested with a fork. Carefully remove the fillets with a slotted spatula and drain before serving. Discard the poaching liquid and other ingredients. Makes 2 servings.

Baked Fish with Black Bean Sauce

2 fish fillets, about 4 ounces (125 g) each (use snapper, cod,
    halibut, sole, etc.)
¼ cup (50 mL) water
1 garlic clove, minced
2 teaspoons (10 mL) minced fresh ginger
2 tablespoons (30 mL) Chinese salted black beans, rinsed,
    drained, and chopped
1 tablespoon (15 mL) Tamari soy sauce
2 green onions, sliced
½ to 1 teaspoon (2 to 5 mL) sesame oil, to taste (optional)

Place the fish in a baking dish and set aside.

Heat a small saucepan or skillet over medium heat. Add 1 to
2 tablespoons (15 to 30 mL) of the water, plus the garlic, ginger,
and black beans; sauté until fragrant, about 1 minute. Add the
remaining water and the soy sauce, reduce the heat, and
simmer for 3 minutes. Spread the sauce over the fish fillets, then
sprinkle the green onions over top. Bake at 425° F (210° C) for 7
to 10 minutes or until the fish flakes easily when tested with a
fork. Drizzle with sesame oil, if using, and serve. Makes 2
servings.

Variations

Baked Tofu with Black Bean Sauce
Substitute half a 12 ounce (350 g) package of firm tofu for the
fish fillets. Cut the tofu into ½ inch (1 cm) slices and arrange in a
single layer in a baking dish.

Baked Tempeh with Black Bean Sauce
Substitute an 8 ounce (250 g) package of tempeh for the fish
fillets. Cut the tempeh in half, crosswise, then into ½ inch (1 cm)
slices lengthwise; arrange in a single layer in a baking dish.

Stir-Fry Tofu and Veggies in Black Bean Sauce
Substitute half a 12 ounce (350 g) package of firm tofu for the
fish fillets. Cut the tofu into ½ inch (1 cm) cubes and set aside.

Heat a wok or skillet over medium-high heat. Sauté the garlic, ginger, and black beans in the water as instructed above. Add the remaining water and the soy sauce, plus 2 thinly sliced small carrots, 1 cup trimmed snow peas, and 1 small bunch broccoli, cut into bite-size pieces. Cover and cook for 2 minutes, stirring occasionally and adding more water to prevent sticking, if necessary. Remove the cover and add the cubed tofu and green onion. Gently stir-fry for 3 minutes, or until the vegetables are tender-crisp. Drizzle with sesame oil, if using, before serving.

Breaded Fish Fillets

½ cup (125 mL) **Oat and Whole-Grain Coating** or ½ cup
   (125 mL) fine whole-wheat bread crumbs
1 tablespoon (15 mL) freshly grated Parmesan cheese, rice
   cheese, or soy cheese (optional)
1 tablespoon (15 mL) minced fresh parsley
¼ teaspoon (1 mL) basil
1 teaspoon (5 mL) finely grated lemon rind
pinch sea salt
1 egg
¼ cup (50 mL) low-fat plain yogurt
4 skinless, boneless fish fillets, about 4 ounces (125 g) each

Combine the **Oat and Whole-Grain Coating** or bread crumbs
with the cheese, parsley, basil, lemon rind, and sea salt in a
shallow dish or pie plate. In a separate dish, beat together the
egg and yogurt. Dip each fillet into the yogurt mixture, then
into the bread crumb mixture. Place the coated fillets in a lightly
buttered baking dish. Bake at 425° F (210° C) for 8 to 10 minutes,
or until the fish flakes easily when tested with a fork. Makes 4
servings.

Oat and Whole-Grain Coating
⅓ cup (75 mL) oats
⅔ cup (150 mL) fresh whole-grain bread crumbs
1 teaspoon (5 mL) dry mustard powder

In an ungreased skillet, cook the oats, stirring frequently, over
medium-low heat for 5 to 10 minutes, until lightly toasted. Set
aside to cool.
   Combine the oats, bread crumbs, and mustard powder. Use
in **Breaded Fish Fillets** or **Breaded Chicken Breasts**. The
Coating can be stored in the refrigerator in a tightly closed jar
for about 1 week.

Note
To make the bread crumbs, finely chop or grate (by hand or in a
food processor) 1 slice of bread.

Baked Halibut and Vegetables

You can substitute other types of fish (snapper, cod, etc.) for the halibut and/or you can use fillets instead of steaks. Just remember to cook the fish for approximately 10 minutes per inch (2.5 cm) of thickness (measure the thickest portion of the fish), adding the vegetables and seasoning during the last 5 minutes.

1 pound (500 g) halibut steaks
water or stock
1 small zucchini, cut into ¼ inch (6 mm) slices
1 tomato, chopped
1 cup (250 mL) snow peas, trimmed
2 green onions, chopped
½ teaspoon (2 mL) basil or 2 teaspoons (10 mL) minced fresh
  dill
¼ teaspoon (1 mL) sea salt

Place the fish in a single layer in a baking dish. Add just enough water or stock to cover the bottom of the dish, about ¼ cup (50 mL). Cover and bake at 450° F (230° C) for 5 minutes. Remove from the oven and arrange the zucchini, tomato, snow peas, and green onion around the fish. Sprinkle with the basil or dill and sea salt. Cover and bake for 5 to 10 minutes more, or until the fish flakes easily when tested with a fork. Makes 4 servings.

Fish Roll-Ups

*You can use any type of white fish in this recipe. Choose long, thin
fillets suitable for rolling.*

> 4 boneless sole fillets, about 4 ounces (125 g) each
> 2 teaspoons (10 mL) lemon juice
> 2 teaspoons (10 mL) extra virgin olive oil
> ¼ cup (50 mL) diced onion
> ¼ cup (50 mL) diced celery
> half a bunch fresh spinach, washed, steamed, well drained,
>   and chopped
> ½ cup (125 mL) cooked brown rice
> ¼ cup (50 mL) low-fat plain yogurt
> ¼ teaspoon (1 mL) sea salt

Sprinkle ½ teaspoon (2 mL) of the lemon juice along the length
of each fillet and set the fillets aside.

Heat a small saucepan over medium-low heat. Add the oil,
onion, and celery and sauté until tender. Add the spinach and
cook for 2 minutes more to remove any excess moisture.
Remove from the heat and add the rice, yogurt, and sea salt.
Spoon an equal amount of the mixture onto each fillet; roll up
and secure with toothpicks. Place the fillets in a lightly buttered
baking dish. Cover and bake at 375° F (190° C) for about 15
minutes, or until the fish flakes easily when tested with a fork.
Serve plain or with lemon wedges and/or **Yogurt Herb Dip**
(made with dill). Makes 4 servings.

Note
The roll-ups can be steamed instead of baked in the oven; see
Steamed Fish Fillets for instructions.

Fish Fillets in Parchment

4 fish fillets, about 4 ounces (125 g) each
2 teaspoons (10 mL) mayonnaise
1½ teaspoons (7 mL) chopped fresh dill or ½ teaspoon (2 mL) dried
1 tablespoon (15 mL) chopped fresh parsley
¼ teaspoon (1 mL) sea salt
8 thin slices of onion
8 thin slices of lemon or lime

Place each fillet on a piece of parchment paper. Spread each fillet with ½ teaspoon (2 mL) of mayonnaise, then sprinkle with the dill, parsley, and sea salt. Place 2 onion slices and 2 lemon slices on top of each one. Bring the front and back edges of the parchment together and seal tightly using a triple fold, then fold the left and right sides under using a double fold. Place the packets on a baking sheet and bake at 375° F (190° C) for 15 to 20 minutes, until the fish flakes easily when tested with a fork. Serve with fresh lemon and/or **Yogurt Herb Dip**. Makes 4 servings.

Note
Parchment paper is available in grocery stores where the plastic wrap, sandwich bags, etc. are found.

Steamed Fish Fillets

Steaming is a quick, low-fat method for cooking fish and chicken, as well as vegetables. If you don't have a folding metal steaming rack, you can use one of the following: a bamboo steamer, a pasta pot with an accompanying perforated steaming basket, or an electric steamer. Or you can make your own steamer by placing a cooling or roasting rack inside a wok, roasting pan, or electric frying pan; just make sure that whatever container you use has a tight-fitting lid.

To steam fish, set a folding metal steaming rack into a large saucepan so that the rack is fully open. Add about 1 inch (2.5 cm) of water to the saucepan. The water shouldn't touch the fish; add enough water to keep the saucepan from boiling dry. Place each fish fillet (use any type of fish) on a piece of parchment paper. You can add herbs to the water or you can sprinkle them directly onto the fish. Bring the water in the saucepan to a boil, then place each piece of parchment paper (with the fish) into the steaming rack. Cover with a tight-fitting lid and steam for about 5 minutes (depending on the thickness of the fillet) or until the fish flakes easily when tested with a fork.

Variations

Steamed Fish with Pesto
Spread a thin layer of **Basil Pesto Sauce** or **Parsley Pesto Sauce** over the fish fillets before steaming.

Steamed Fish with Black Bean Sauce
Follow the recipe for **Baked Fish with Black Bean Sauce**, except steam the fish instead of baking it.

Steamed Fish with Ginger and Soy Sauce
Follow the recipe for **Broiled Salmon Steaks**, substituting salmon fillets for the steaks; steam the salmon instead of baking.

Steamed Fish Roll-Ups
Follow the recipe for **Fish Roll-Ups**, except steam the roll-ups instead of baking them.

POULTRY

Poached Chicken Breasts

Chicken Stock, approximately 2 cups (500 mL)
2 teaspoons (10 mL) chopped fresh rosemary
1 garlic clove, quartered
1 whole boneless, skinless chicken breast, cut in half

Fill a deep skillet or wok with just enough **Chicken Stock** to cover the chicken. Add the rosemary and garlic and bring just to a boil. Reduce the heat to a very gentle simmer, and, using tongs or a slotted spatula, add the chicken. Cover and simmer for 12 to 15 minutes, until the chicken is no longer pink inside, turning the chicken over after 6 minutes. Remove the chicken and drain before serving. Discard the poaching liquid and other ingredients. Serve with **Tzatziki** or **Yogurt Herb Dip**. Makes 2 servings.

Notes
- If you don't have **Chicken Stock** on hand, use water instead and add some fresh lemon juice—about 1 tablespoon (15 mL).
- The poached chicken can also be used in sandwiches or in recipes that call for cooked chicken, such as **Chicken Salad, Chicken Rice Soup, Black Bean and Rice Wraps, Chicken and Veggie Pesto Wraps, Chicken Vegetable Hash, Chicken Burritos,** and **Chicken Quesadillas**.

Chicken Vegetable Hash

2 teaspoons (10 mL) extra virgin olive oil
½ cup (125 mL) chopped onion
½ cup (125 mL) chopped sweet red pepper
1 small potato, diced
¼ cup (50 mL) **Chicken Stock, Vegetable Stock,** or water
1 cup (250 mL) cubed cooked chicken (or turkey)
1 tomato, chopped
sea salt, to taste

Heat a large skillet over medium-low heat. Add the oil, onion, and pepper, and sauté until the onion is almost tender. Add the potato and stock or water. Cover and simmer until the potato is tender, about 10 to 15 minutes, stirring occasionally and adding a small amount of water, if necessary. Add the chicken and tomato; sauté for 2 minutes more. Season to taste with sea salt. Serve with poached eggs, if desired. Makes 2 to 3 servings.

Chicken, Broccoli, and Rice Casserole

1 teaspoon (5 mL) extra virgin olive oil
1 whole boneless, skinless chicken breast, cut into 1 inch
   (2.5 cm) pieces
¾ cup (175 mL) rice milk
1 tablespoon (15 mL) cornstarch or arrowroot powder
½ teaspoon (2 mL) curry powder
¼ teaspoon (1 mL) sea salt
1½ cups (375 mL) cooked brown rice (use basmati rice, if you
   have it)
2 cups (500 mL) broccoli florets, cut into bite-size pieces
¼ cup (250 mL) grated reduced-fat Cheddar cheese (optional)

Heat a skillet over medium-low heat. Add the oil and chicken;
sauté for 1 to 2 minutes on each side, adding a small amount of
water to prevent sticking, if necessary. Remove from the heat
and drain off any liquid; set aside.

In a small saucepan, whisk together the rice milk, cornstarch
or arrowroot powder, and curry powder; bring just to a boil,
stirring constantly. Remove from the heat and add the sea salt.

Combine the chicken, sauce, and rice in a small lightly
buttered baking dish. Cover and bake at 350° F (180° C) for 15
minutes. Meanwhile, steam the broccoli for 2 minutes. Once the
casserole has cooked for 15 minutes, remove it from the oven
and gently stir in the steamed broccoli. Top with the cheese,
if using, and bake uncovered for 5 minutes more. Makes
2 servings.

Chicken Kebabs

2 whole boneless, skinless chicken breasts
1 tablespoon (15 mL) extra virgin olive oil
1 tablespoon (15 mL) lemon juice
1 tablespoon (15 mL) apple cider vinegar
1 teaspoon (5 mL) chopped fresh oregano or ½ teaspoon
  (2 mL) dried
1 teaspoon (5 mL) chopped fresh rosemary
1 garlic clove, minced

Cut the chicken into 1 inch (2.5 cm) cubes, place on metal or wooden skewers, and arrange in single layer in a large glass baking dish. Mix the remaining ingredients together and spoon over the chicken. Cover and refrigerate for 1 hour. Place the kebabs on a broiler pan and broil for 3 to 5 minutes. Turn the kebabs over and continue broiling until the chicken is no longer pink inside. Alternatively, cook the kebabs in the baking dish at 350° F (180° C) for 15 to 20 minutes, or until done. Serve with **Tzatziki** or **Yogurt Herb Dip**. Makes 4 servings.

Chicken with Yogurt and Soy Sauce

1 whole boneless, skinless chicken breast, cut in half
½ cup (125 mL) low-fat plain yogurt
1 tablespoon (15 mL) Tamari soy sauce
1 teaspoon (5 mL) Dijon mustard
1 tablespoon (15 mL) chopped fresh parsley

Place the chicken in a baking dish. In a small bowl, combine the yogurt, soy sauce, and mustard; mix well, then spoon over the chicken. Bake uncovered at 350° F (180° C) for 30 to 35 minutes, until the chicken is no longer pink inside. Remove the chicken to a serving plate. Whisk the sauce, then spoon it over the chicken and sprinkle with the parsley. Makes 2 servings.

Chicken Fajitas

8 whole-wheat tortillas
2 teaspoons (10 mL) extra virgin olive oil
1 sweet red pepper and 1 sweet yellow pepper, cut into thin
    strips
1 red or yellow onion, sliced thin, then cut into halves
2 garlic cloves, minced
½ teaspoon (2 mL) oregano
½ teaspoon (2 mL) ground cumin
pinch cayenne (optional)
2 whole boneless, skinless chicken breasts, cut into thin strips
1 small tomato, chopped
juice of 1 lime
2 tablespoons (30 mL) minced fresh cilantro
¼ teaspoon (1 mL) sea salt

Wrap the tortillas in parchment paper and bake at 300° F
(150° C) for 10 to 15 minutes, until warm.

Heat a large skillet over medium-low heat. Add 1 teaspoon
(5 mL) of the oil, plus the peppers, onion, and garlic; sauté for
about 5 minutes, adding water to prevent sticking, if necessary.
Add the oregano, cumin, and cayenne (if using), and sauté for
2 minutes more. Remove the vegetables from the skillet and set
aside. Add the remaining 1 teaspoon (5 mL) of the oil plus the
chicken to the skillet; sauté until the chicken is no longer pink
inside. Drain off any fat. Return the vegetables to the skillet and
add the tomato, lime juice, cilantro, and sea salt. Cook for 2
minutes more.

Place an equal amount of the chicken/vegetable mixture
down the centre of each tortilla. Add optional toppings, if
desired, and roll up the tortillas. Makes 8 fajitas.

Optional Toppings
    Chopped tomatoes
    Grated reduced-fat cheese
    Low-fat plain yogurt
    Mild salsa
    Sliced or mashed avocado

Variation

Vegetarian Fajitas
Omit the chicken and use some **Bean Dip** as an additional topping, or add sliced tempeh when sautéing the peppers, onions, and garlic.

Breaded Chicken Breasts

½ cup (125 mL) low-fat plain yogurt
¼ teaspoon (1 mL) sea salt
1 tablespoon (15 mL) minced fresh parsley
1 tablespoon (15 mL) minced fresh herbs (such as basil, oregano, thyme, dill, or chives) or 1 teaspoon (5 mL) dried
2 whole chicken breasts, skinned and cut in half
1 cup (250 mL) **Oat and Whole-Grain Coating** (see **Breaded Fish Fillets**) or 1 cup fine whole-grain bread crumbs
2 tablespoons (30 mL) freshly grated Parmesan cheese, soy cheese, or rice cheese (optional)

Combine the yogurt, sea salt, parsley, and other herbs in a glass bowl and mix well. Add the chicken and toss to coat. Cover and marinate in the refrigerator for 1 hour, if time permits.

On a pie plate, combine the **Oat and Whole-Grain Coating** with the cheese, if using. Coat the chicken with the breading mixture and place on a lightly buttered baking sheet. Bake at 350° F (180° C) for 30 to 35 minutes for boneless, or 40 to 45 minutes for bone-in chicken, until chicken is no longer pink inside. Makes 4 servings.

Chicken Curry

For those with dairy sensitivities, the use of yogurt is optional.
   2 teaspoons (10 mL) extra virgin olive oil
   2 whole skinless chicken breasts (bone-in), cut into halves
   1 large onion, chopped
   2 garlic cloves, minced
   1 tablespoon (15 mL) minced fresh ginger
   1 tablespoon (15 mL) ground cumin
   1 tablespoon (15 mL) ground coriander
   2 teaspoons (10 mL) turmeric
   2 large tomatoes, chopped
   ¾ cup (175 mL) low-fat plain yogurt (optional)
   ¼ to ½ teaspoon (1 to 2 mL) garam masala, to taste
   ½ teaspoon (2 mL) sea salt
   chopped fresh cilantro, to taste

Heat a large skillet over medium-low heat. Add the oil and
chicken. Sauté for about 5 minutes, until the chicken is lightly
browned on both sides, adding a small amount of water to
prevent sticking, if necessary. Remove the chicken from the
skillet and keep it warm. Add the onion, garlic, and ginger to
the skillet. Sauté for about 5 minutes, or until the onion is
tender, adding more water, if necessary. Add the cumin,
coriander, and turmeric, and sauté for 1 minute. Add the
tomatoes and mix well. Return the chicken to the skillet and
reduce the heat to low. Cover and simmer for 20 minutes,
stirring occasionally. Stir in the yogurt, if using, then cover and
simmer for another 5 to 10 minutes, until the chicken is tender
and no longer pink inside. Remove from the heat and stir in the
garam masala, sea salt, and cilantro. Serve with basmati rice
and/or chipatis. Makes 4 servings.

Note
For a smoother sauce, transfer the sauce (in batches, if
necessary) to a blender, and process until smooth.

Variations

Chicken Curry with Spinach
Add 1 to 2 cups (250 to 500 mL) chopped fresh spinach when adding the yogurt. Puree the sauce in a blender, if desired.

Tofu and Chickpea Curry
Omit the chicken and sauté the onion, garlic, and ginger as directed above. Add the cumin, coriander, and turmeric and cook for 1 minute more. Add the tomatoes, then cover and simmer for 5 minutes, stirring often. Stir in the yogurt, if using. (Sauce may be pureed in a blender at this point, then returned to the skillet.) Add a 12 ounce (350 g) package of firm tofu—cut into ½ inch (1 cm cubes)—and 2 cups (500 mL) cooked chickpeas. Cover and simmer 5 minutes more. Remove from the heat and stir in the garam masala, sea salt, and cilantro. Makes 4 to 6 servings.

Chicken with Lemon and Herbs

1 whole skinless chicken breast, cut in half
1 garlic clove, minced
1 teaspoon (5 mL) extra virgin olive oil
1 tablespoon (15 mL) lemon juice
1 tablespoon (15 mL) water
½ teaspoon (2 mL) oregano
½ teaspoon (2 mL) basil
pinch sea salt

Place the chicken in a baking dish. Combine the remaining ingredients and pour over the chicken. Bake uncovered, basting occasionally, at 350° F (180° C) for 30 to 35 minutes for boneless, 40 to 45 minutes for bone-in, or until chicken is no longer pink inside. Makes 2 servings.

Cabbage Rolls

1 large or 2 medium heads green cabbage
1 teaspoon (5 mL) extra virgin olive oil
1 large onion, chopped
1 pound (500 g) lean ground turkey (or chicken) breast
2 cups (500 mL) cooked brown rice
1 teaspoon (5 mL) EACH sage, thyme, ground rosemary,
    marjoram, celery seed, and sea salt
2 to 3 cups (500 to 750 mL) tomato sauce (see recipe for
    Tomato Sauce or use canned tomato sauce), or a 28 ounce
    (796 mL) can tomatoes, chopped

Core the cabbage(s) and gently place in a large pot of boiling water. Lower the heat and simmer, removing the leaves as they become soft and pliable (but NOT mushy). This will take about 10 to 15 minutes. You'll need approximately 16 leaves; set them aside to drain well on towels. Remove the cabbage from the water. Set aside a few extra cabbage leaves to place on top of the cabbage rolls. Leftover cabbage can be chopped and used in soups or stir-fries.

Heat a skillet over medium-low heat. Add the oil and onion, and sauté for 2 minutes. Add the ground turkey and cook until the turkey is no longer pink. Drain off any fat. Transfer to a large bowl and add the rice and seasonings; mix well.

Place 2 to 3 spoonfuls of the rice mixture onto each cabbage leaf, depending on the size of the leaf. Roll up from the base, tucking in the sides as you roll. You may need to cut out the centre rib at the base of the leaf to make the cabbage leaf easier to roll. Place the cabbage rolls in a baking dish and pour some tomato sauce or chopped tomatoes over them. Cover the rolls with the extra cabbage leaves; pour the remaining tomato sauce over top. Cover and bake at 350° F (180° C) for about 1 hour. Makes approximately 16 cabbage rolls.

Variations

Tofu Cabbage Rolls
Substitute 2 cups (500 mL) mashed or crumbled firm tofu for the ground turkey.

Quick Cabbage "Rolls"
Use this method if you don't have the time to roll the cabbage leaves. Do not boil the cabbage; instead, carefully remove a few of the outer leaves and set them aside (to place on top of the finished casserole). Chop the rest of the cabbage. In a large casserole dish, put a layer of chopped cabbage, then a layer of rice mixture. Continue alternating layers like this until all of the rice mixture is used. Spread some tomato sauce over top. Cover with the reserved cabbage leaves and pour the remaining tomato sauce over top. Cover and bake at 350° F (180° C) for about 1 hour. Makes 6 to 8 servings.

Turkey Chili

If you don't have time to soak and cook the beans, use canned beans; just be sure to rinse and drain them first. Omit the mushrooms if you have yeast problems.

2 teaspoons (10 mL) extra virgin olive oil
1 onion, chopped
2 garlic cloves, minced
1 celery stalk, chopped
half a sweet green pepper, chopped (optional)
1 pound (500 g) lean ground turkey or chicken breast
3½ cups (875 mL) chopped peeled tomatoes, or a 28 ounce
  (796 mL) can
2 cups (500 mL) cooked red kidney beans, black beans, or
  pinto beans (or a combination)
6 large mushrooms, sliced (optional)
2 tablespoons (30 mL) tomato paste
1 teaspoon (5 mL) oregano
2 to 3 teaspoons (10 to 15 mL) chili powder, to taste
1 teaspoon (5 mL) ground cumin
½ teaspoon (2 mL) celery seed
1 teaspoon (5 mL) sea salt
1 teaspoon (5 mL) vinegar (optional)
chopped fresh cilantro (optional)

Heat a large saucepan over medium-low heat. Add the oil, onion, garlic, celery, and green pepper (if using), and sauté for 2 minutes. Add the ground turkey and cook until the turkey is no longer pink. Drain off any fat. Add the remaining ingredients, except the sea salt, vinegar, and cilantro. Bring to a boil, then reduce the heat to low, cover, and simmer for at least 1 hour, stirring occasionally. Add the sea salt and vinegar, if using; taste and adjust the seasonings, if necessary. Sprinkle each serving with chopped fresh cilantro, if desired. Makes 6 to 8 servings.

Variations

Tofu Chili
Substitute a 12 ounce (350 g) package of firm tofu, mashed or crumbled, for the ground turkey. (If you want the tofu to have more of a ground meat texture, freeze it first, then thaw, drain well, and crumble.)

Tempeh Chili
Substitute an 8 ounce (250 g) package of tempeh for the tofu.

Stuffed Zucchini

3 medium zucchini, about 7 inches (18 cm long)
2 teaspoons (10 mL) extra virgin olive oil
½ pound (250 g) lean ground turkey breast
1 small onion, diced
1 garlic clove, minced
half a bunch fresh spinach, washed, steamed, well drained,
    and chopped
¼ to ½ cup (50 to 125 mL) freshly grated Parmesan cheese,
    soy cheese, or rice cheese (optional)
2 cups (500 mL) tomato sauce (see recipe for **Tomato Sauce** or
    use canned tomato sauce), divided
½ teaspoon (2 mL) basil
½ teaspoon (2 mL) oregano
¼ teaspoon (1 mL) sea salt
½ cup (125 mL) grated low-fat cheese (optional)

Slice the ends off each zucchini and cut in half lengthwise.
Scoop out the centres, leaving a shell at least ¼ inch (6 mm)
thick. Chop the scooped-out zucchini and set aside. Place the
zucchini shells in boiling water for 2 to 3 minutes, just until they
are slightly tender. Remove from the water and drain on paper
towels.

Heat a skillet over medium-low heat. Add the oil, ground
turkey, onion, garlic, and chopped zucchini. Cook until the
vegetables are tender. Drain off any fat. Add the spinach, cheese
(if using), 1 cup (250 mL) of the tomato sauce, and the basil,
oregano, and sea salt; mix well. Spoon some of the mixture into
each zucchini shell.

Spread the remaining 1 cup (250 mL) tomato sauce onto the
bottom of shallow baking dish(es). Place the stuffed zucchini
shells on top of the sauce and bake at 350° F (180° C) for 20 to 30
minutes, until heated through. Sprinkle with cheese, if using,
and cook for 5 minutes more. Spoon some tomato sauce from
the baking dish over the stuffed zucchini and serve. Makes 3
large servings or 6 small servings.

Variations

Stuffed Eggplant
Use 1 large eggplant instead of the zucchini. Increase the baking time to 35 to 45 minutes, or until the eggplant is tender.

Stuffed Peppers
Use 3 medium sweet red or yellow peppers instead of the zucchini. Cut each one in half lengthwise, and remove the seeds and membranes.

Tofu Stuffed Vegetables
Use half a 12 ounce (350 g) package of firm tofu, well drained and mashed, instead of the ground turkey.

Lasagna Roll-Ups

Follow the recipe for **Stuffed Zucchini**, omitting the zucchini. The stuffing mixture can then be rolled up in lasagna noodles. Cook 8 lasagna noodles until *al dente*. Spread an equal amount of the stuffing mixture along the length of each lasagna noodle, leaving the last quarter section bare; roll up. Spread ½ cup (125 mL) of the tomato sauce on the bottom of a baking dish. Arrange the lasagna roll-ups on top of the sauce and cover with the remaining tomato sauce. Cover and bake at 350° F (180° C) for 20 to 30 minutes, until hot and bubbly. If using the cheese, sprinkle it on top of the roll-ups during the last 5 minutes of baking time. Makes about 4 servings.

Notes
- Follow the recipe for **Stuffed Zucchini**, using only half the zucchini called for in the recipe. Use the leftover stuffing to make half a batch of **Lasagna Roll-Ups** for the next day's lunch or dinner.
- Use half a 12 ounce (350 g) package of firm tofu, well drained and mashed, instead of the ground turkey.

Turkey Burgers

1 pound (500 g) lean ground turkey breast
2 tablespoons (30 mL) oat flakes
1 egg white
2 tablespoons (30 mL) freshly grated Parmesan cheese, soy
   cheese, or rice cheese (optional)
2 teaspoons (10 mL) extra virgin olive oil
1 green onion, finely chopped
1 small garlic clove, minced
½ teaspoon (2 mL) basil
½ teaspoon (2 mL) oregano
¼ teaspoon (1 mL) sea salt

In a large bowl, combine all the ingredients and mix well. Shape
the mixture into 4 patties and place on a lightly buttered broiler
pan. Broil for 5 to 7 minutes on each side, until cooked. Serve
with **Tzatziki** or on whole-grain buns with tomatoes, sprouts,
and a small amount of mayonnaise. Makes 4 servings.

Variation

Turkey Loaf
Add 1 more tablespoon (15 mL) oat flakes, plus ¼ cup (50 mL)
packed grated carrot, and a 10 ounce (300 g) package of frozen
chopped spinach, thawed and well drained. Mix well and press
into a lightly buttered loaf pan. Bake at 350° F (180° C) for about
45 minutes, or until no longer pink in the centre. Pour off any
liquid and let stand for a few minutes before serving. Makes
4 servings.

Note
• Use slices of leftover **Turkey Loaf** in sandwiches. Add
  mustard (regular or Dijon), sliced tomatoes, lettuce or
  sprouts, a sprinkle of sea salt, and a small amount of
  mayo or avocado (sliced or mashed).

Chicken Burgers
Substitute lean ground chicken breast for the turkey breast.

MEATLESS MAIN DISHES

Tofu Patties

1 cup (250 mL) well-drained and mashed firm tofu
1 cup (250 mL) cooked brown rice
2 tablespoons (30 mL) flour
½ cup (125 mL) grated carrot
1 garlic clove, minced
¼ teaspoon (1 mL) sea salt
1 tablespoon (15 mL) Tamari soy sauce
½ teaspoon (2 mL) basil
½ cup (125 mL) grated, reduced-fat Cheddar cheese or soy
 cheese (optional)

In a large bowl, mix together all the ingredients. Using your hands, shape the mixture into 4 patties and place them on a lightly buttered baking sheet. Bake at 350° F (180° C) for 15 minutes. Gently turn the patties over and bake for 10 to 15 minutes more, until lightly browned. Makes 2 to 4 servings.

Variation

Curried Tofu Patties
Omit the soy sauce, basil, and cheese. Add 1 teaspoon (5 mL) minced fresh ginger and 1 teaspoon (5 mL) curry powder. If the mixture is too dry to form patties, add 1 to 2 tablespoons (15 to 30 mL) water.

Tofu and Veggie Lasagna

This version of lasagna is lower in fat than traditional lasagna recipes—it uses less cheese, and tofu replaces the cottage cheese and ground beef.

1 batch **Tomato Sauce**
2 batches **Tofu Sauce** or 2 cups (500 mL) well-drained and
   mashed firm tofu
8 lasagna noodles, preferably whole grain
1 bunch fresh spinach, washed, steamed, well drained, and
   chopped
2 tablespoons (30 mL) chopped fresh parsley
½ cup (125 mL) freshly grated Parmesan cheese, soy cheese,
   or rice cheese, divided
1 medium zucchini, cut into ¼ inch (6 mm) slices
1 cup (250 mL) grated reduced-fat Mozzarella cheese

Make the **Tomato Sauce** and the **Tofu Sauce**, if using, then set them aside.

Cook the lasagna noodles until just tender. Do not overcook; it's better to slightly undercook the noodles. Drain and rinse under cold water to stop the cooking process; drain again and set aside.

In a large bowl, combine the **Tofu Sauce** or tofu, spinach, parsley, and ¼ cup (50 mL) of the cheese; mix well and set aside.

Spread ½ cup (125 mL) **Tomato Sauce** on the bottom of a 9 x 13 inch (23 x 33 cm) baking dish. Top with 4 lasagna noodles, half the tofu mixture, half the sliced zucchini, half the Mozzarella cheese, and half the remaining **Tomato Sauce**. Repeat the layers and sprinkle the remaining cheese on top. Bake at 325° F (160° C) for 40 to 45 minutes, until hot and bubbly. Remove from the oven and let stand for 10 minutes before serving. Makes 6 to 8 servings.

Notes
- Half-a-pound (250 g) lean ground turkey or chicken breast can be added to the **Tomato Sauce** recipe when

sautéing the onion and garlic. Drain off any fat before adding the remaining ingredients.

- For those who don't have yeast problems, add 1 cup (250 mL) sliced fresh mushrooms to the **Tomato Sauce** recipe.
- Replace half or all of the zucchini with sliced eggplant.
- Replace the Parmesan cheese that goes on the top with ¼ cup (50 mL) grated reduced-fat Cheddar cheese.
- For those who are sensitive to dairy products, replace the Parmesan and Mozzarella cheeses with soy cheese and/or rice cheese.

Variations

Quick Tofu and Veggie Lasagna
Shorten the preparation time by using any combination of the following.

- A good store-bought tomato or pasta sauce instead of the **Tomato Sauce** recipe
- Well-drained and mashed firm tofu instead of the **Tofu Sauce** recipe
- A 10 ounce (300 g) package of frozen spinach, thawed and well drained, instead of the fresh spinach
- Fresh or "no-cook" lasagna noodles instead of the dried variety. When using "no-cook" noodles, adjust the cooking time and add extra water, if called for on the package.

Scrambled Tofu

1 to 2 teaspoons (5 to 10 mL) extra virgin olive oil
¼ cup (50 mL) chopped onion
¼ cup (50 mL) chopped sweet red pepper
1 cup (250 mL) well-drained and mashed firm tofu
¼ teaspoon (1 mL) turmeric
½ teaspoon (2 mL) oregano
1 small tomato, diced
sea salt, to taste

Heat a skillet over medium-low heat. Add the oil, onion, and pepper, and sauté until tender. Add the tofu, turmeric, and oregano, and cook for about 5 minutes, or until any extra moisture evaporates. Add the tomato and cook for 2 minutes more. Season to taste with sea salt. Serve with rye toast or rolled up in warmed whole-wheat tortillas. Makes 2 servings.

Tofu Bean Casserole

This is a good recipe for using up any leftover cooked brown rice and/or beans. Use whatever type of beans you have on hand. You can also substitute whatever type of cheese you prefer for the feta, such as soy cheese, rice cheese, or Cheddar.

1 batch **Tofu Sauce**
1 to 1½ cups (250 to 375 mL) cooked beans (Romano, pinto, black beans, etc.)
1 cup (250 mL) cooked brown rice (preferably basmati)
½ cup (125 mL) crumbled feta cheese or goat cheese
half a bunch fresh spinach, washed, steamed, well drained, and chopped
6 canned artichoke hearts, halved (optional)
1 teaspoon (5 mL) Tamari soy sauce
1 tomato, sliced
¼ cup (50 mL) freshly grated Parmesan cheese, soy cheese, or rice cheese (optional)

In a large bowl, combine all the ingredients except the tomatoes and Parmesan cheese; mix well. Press into a lightly buttered casserole. Arrange the tomato slices on top and sprinkle with the cheese, if using. Cover and bake at 350° F (180° C) for 20 to 30 minutes, until heated through. Makes 2 to 4 servings.

Tofu and Veggie Stir-Fry

Stir-frying is usually done over high heat. To reduce the risk of toxic fats, this recipe (like all others that involve sautéing or stir-frying in this book) uses a lower temperature to cook the food. Chicken Stock, Vegetable Stock, or water can be used in place of the oil—in which case a slightly higher temperature can be used.

The following vegetables and amounts are suggestions only. You can use fewer varieties of vegetables than those called for here. Feel free to use others, such as zucchini, celery, onion, cabbage, green beans, asparagus, tomato, daikon radish, or spinach and other leafy greens. Just remember that the harder, firmer vegetables should be cooked longer than the softer vegetables. Be sure to have all of the vegetables chopped and ready before you start to cook.

1 tablespoon (15 mL) cornstarch or arrowroot powder
1 tablespoon (15 mL) Tamari soy sauce
2 teaspoons (10 mL) rice vinegar
1½ cups (375 mL) well-drained and cubed firm tofu

Sauce
¼ cup (50 mL) water
1 tablespoon (15 mL) Tamari soy sauce
2 teaspoons (10 mL) cornstarch or arrowroot powder
¼ to ½ teaspoon (1 to 2 mL) sesame oil (optional)

2 teaspoons (10 mL) extra virgin olive oil
½ cup (125 mL) sliced carrots
¾ cup (175 mL) broccoli florets
¾ cup (175 mL) cauliflower florets
¼ cup (50 mL) **Chicken Stock, Vegetable Stock,** or water
1 garlic clove, minced
1 to 2 teaspoons (5 to 10 mL) minced fresh ginger
½ cup (125 mL) snow peas, trimmed
¾ cup (175 mL) bok choy stalks
1 cup (250 mL) bok choy leaves, chopped
½ cup (125 mL) bean sprouts
1 green onion, chopped

In a small bowl, mix together the cornstarch or arrowroot powder, soy sauce, and rice vinegar. Add the tofu and mix well, to coat. Marinate in the refrigerator for 1 hour.

Combine all the sauce ingredients and set aside.

Heat a large skillet or wok over medium-low heat. Add the olive oil, carrots, broccoli, and cauliflower; stir-fry for 1 minute. Add the stock or water, cover, and cook for 1 minute more. Add the garlic, ginger, snow peas, and bok choy stalks; stir-fry for 2 minutes. Small amounts of stock or water may be used at any time to prevent sticking. Add the bok choy leaves, bean sprouts, green onion and tofu; stir-fry for 2 minutes more. Stir the sauce, then pour into the skillet; stir-fry until the sauce thickens. Serve over brown rice, barley, pasta, or bean thread (vermicelli noodles made from beans). Makes 2 to 3 servings.

Variations

Stir-Fry with Black Bean Sauce
Omit the sauce. When adding the garlic and ginger to the wok, also add 1 tablespoon (15 mL) Chinese salted black beans that have been rinsed, drained, and chopped.

Tempeh and Veggie Stir-Fry
Substitute an 8 ounce (250 g) package of tempeh for the tofu. Use black beans as directed above, if desired.

Chicken and Veggie Stir-Fry
Substitute 1 whole boneless, skinless chicken breast, cut into 1 inch (2.5 cm) pieces, for the tofu. Cook the chicken in the oil first (before adding the carrots and other vegetables), then remove it and set aside. Follow the remaining directions, returning the chicken to the wok just before adding the sauce at the end. Use black beans, if desired.

Marinated Tofu

12 ounce (350 g) package of firm tofu, cut into ½ inch (1 cm) slices
¼ cup (50 mL) Tamari soy sauce
1 tablespoon (15 mL) water
1 tablespoon (15 mL) minced or grated fresh ginger
1 garlic clove, minced

Arrange the tofu slices in a single layer in a baking dish. Combine the soy sauce, water, ginger, and garlic, and pour over the tofu. Cover and marinate in the refrigerator for 30 minutes or longer. (If possible, marinate for several hours or overnight; the longer it marinates, the more flavourful it'll be.) Turn the slices over at least once while marinating. Cover and bake at 350° F (180° C) for 10 minutes. Turn the tofu slices over and bake, uncovered, for 10 minutes more. Serve with stir-fried vegetables and brown rice, or use in sandwiches. Good hot or cold. Makes 2 to 4 servings.

Curried Lentils and Rice

2 teaspoons (10 mL) extra virgin olive oil
1 small onion, diced
1 garlic clove, minced
1 teaspoon (5 mL) minced fresh ginger
½ teaspoon (2 mL) curry powder
¼ teaspoon (1 mL) ground cumin
2 cups (500 mL) **Chicken Stock**, **Vegetable Stock**, or water
½ cup (125 mL) brown basmati rice, rinsed and drained
½ cup (125 mL) brown lentils, sorted, rinsed, and drained
2 tablespoons (30 mL) chopped fresh cilantro
¼ teaspoon (1 mL) sea salt

Heat a saucepan over medium-low heat. Add the oil, onion, garlic, and ginger, and sauté until the onion is tender. Add the curry powder and cumin and cook for 1 minute more. Add the stock or water, rice, and lentils. Bring to a boil, then reduce the heat to low. Cover and simmer for about 40 minutes, or until the rice and lentils are cooked. Remove from the heat, and stir in the cilantro and sea salt. Makes 4 main-course servings.

Variation

Herbed Lentils and Rice
Omit the ginger, curry powder, and cumin and add 1 teaspoon (5 mL) oregano and 1 teaspoon (5 mL) basil. Substitute parsley for the cilantro and add ¼ cup (50 mL) freshly grated Parmesan cheese, soy cheese, or rice cheese when adding the sea salt and parsley.

Steamed Eggs in Spinach "Baskets"

5 cups (1.25 L) packed fresh spinach leaves, washed and
    stems removed
2 eggs
2 tablespoons (30 mL) finely crumbled feta cheese or goat
    cheese
tomato slices (optional)
sea salt, to taste

Place a folding metal steaming rack in a large saucepan and add
water. The water shouldn't touch the food that will be sitting in
the steaming rack, but add enough water so that the saucepan
doesn't boil dry. Place the spinach in the steaming rack, cover
with a tight-fitting lid, and bring to a boil. Steam the spinach
until it just starts to wilt; this takes about 1 to 2 minutes once
the water has come to a boil. Turn off the heat, and remove the
steaming rack from the saucepan.
    Inside the steaming rack, separate the spinach into 2 equal
parts, then form it into 2 small "baskets" by creating sides and
bottoms that won't leak. Carefully crack an egg into each
spinach "basket."
    Return the saucepan to the heat and bring to a boil again.
Turn the heat down to medium-high, then place the steaming
rack—with the spinach baskets—inside the saucepan. Cover
and steam until the egg whites are almost set, about 3 minutes.
Place 1 tablespoon (15 mL) of the cheese on top of each egg.
Replace the lid and simmer for 1 minute more, or until the egg
whites are set and the cheese is melted. Sprinkle with sea salt, to
taste. Serve on top of tomato slices and/or yeast-free rye toast.
Makes 1 to 2 servings.

Notes
- If you don't have a folding metal steaming rack, see
  Steamed Fish Fillets for options.
- For additional flavour, use **Chicken Stock** or **Vegetable
  Stock** as a steaming liquid instead of water, and/or add
  garlic to the steaming liquid.

Baked Vegetable Frittata

You may add or substitute other vegetables such as spinach, sweet red pepper, asparagus, leeks, or mushrooms. Other herbs such as basil, dill, or marjoram can be used instead of, or in combination with, the oregano.

2 whole eggs
2 egg whites
¼ cup (50 mL) low-fat milk
½ cup (125 mL) reduced-fat Mozzarella cheese
2 tablespoons (30 mL) diced onion (use green, white, or red onion)
½ teaspoon (2 mL) oregano
¼ teaspoon (1 mL) sea salt
½ cup (125 mL) water
2 cups (500 mL) chopped broccoli
1 teaspoon (5 mL) extra virgin olive oil
1 garlic clove, minced
1 cup (250 mL) chopped zucchini
1 tomato, diced or sliced

Mix together the eggs, egg whites, milk, cheese, green onion (if using), oregano, and sea salt; set aside.

In a skillet, bring the water to a boil. Reduce the heat slightly and add the broccoli; cover and cook for 2 minutes, stirring occasionally. Add the oil, white or red onion (if using), garlic, and zucchini; cook over medium heat for 2 minutes more. Remove from the heat and stir into the egg mixture. Pour the mixture into a lightly buttered 9 inch (23 cm) pie plate and arrange the tomato on top. Bake at 350° F (180° C) for 20 to 25 minutes, or until the eggs are set. Makes 4 servings.

Vegetable Pizza

Feel free to add or substitute other toppings, such as roasted sweet red pepper, roasted garlic, artichokes, onion, zucchini, sun-dried tomatoes, black olives, or grated carrot. Increase the protein content by adding chopped cooked chicken, cooked lean ground turkey breast, or sautéed tempeh or tofu. If you have yeast problems, omit the mushrooms. Reduced-fat Cheddar cheese can be substituted for some or all of the Mozzarella cheese.

Pizza Dough (see Note)
  2 cups (500 mL) flour, e.g., 1 cup (250 mL) whole-wheat flour
    + 1 cup (250 mL) unbleached flour or 2 cups spelt or kamut
    flour
  1 teaspoon (5 mL) nonalum baking powder
  ½ teaspoon (2 mL) baking soda
  ¼ teaspoon (1 mL) sea salt
  2 tablespoons (30 mL) extra virgin olive oil
  1 cup (250 mL) low-fat plain yogurt

Pizza Sauce
  7½ ounce (213 mL) can tomato sauce or 1 cup (250 mL) of the
    Tomato Sauce recipe, slightly blended
  2 tablespoons (30 mL) tomato paste
  1 garlic clove, finely minced
  1 teaspoon (5 mL) basil
  1 teaspoon (5 mL) oregano
  (This makes enough for 2 pizzas; leftover sauce can be frozen
    for later use.)

Toppings
  2 cups (500 mL) broccoli florets, cut into small pieces and
    steamed for 2 minutes
  1 small green or red pepper, sliced or chopped
  1 cup (250 mL) sliced mushrooms
  1 tomato, sliced
  1½ cups (375 mL) grated reduced-fat Mozzarella cheese or
    soy cheese

To make the **Pizza Dough**, combine all the dry ingredients in a large bowl. Stir together the yogurt and oil, then add to the dry ingredients. Mix well, then knead the dough on a lightly floured surface. Roll into a ball, cover, and set aside while preparing the sauce and toppings.

To make the **Pizza Sauce**, mix together all the ingredients and set aside. Have all the topping ingredients ready before rolling out the dough.

Roll out the dough on a lightly floured surface to fit into a lightly buttered 12 inch (30 cm) pizza pan, or press into a lightly buttered baking sheet. Prick the dough with a fork several times. Prebake at 425° F (210° C) for about 7 minutes or until the crust begins to brown. Remove from the oven and spread half the **Pizza Sauce** over the crust. Arrange the broccoli, then the green/red pepper, mushrooms, and tomatoes on top. Sprinkle with the cheese, then bake for 8 to 10 minutes, until the cheese is bubbly and the crust is browned. Makes one 12 inch (30 cm) pizza.

Note
The **Pizza Dough** will make a fairly thick crust. If you prefer a thinner crust, roll out the dough to the desired thickness, then use the leftover dough to make another smaller pizza; just use more toppings.

Alternatively, you can make just half of the **Pizza Dough** (the recipe is easily halved) and roll out the dough to make a 10 or 12 inch (25 to 30 cm) pizza crust.

Variation

Tortilla Pizzas
Instead of using **Pizza Dough**, use whole-wheat tortillas as pizza crusts. Place the tortillas on baking sheets; broil for about 1 minute on each side (watch carefully to make sure they don't burn). Preheat the oven to 400° F (200° C) while putting the sauce and toppings on the tortillas. Bake for 10 minutes or until the cheese is melted.

Spinach and Feta Cheese Pizza

1 batch **Pizza Dough** and 1 batch **Pizza Sauce**
  (see recipe for **Vegetable Pizza**)
1 bunch fresh spinach, washed, steamed, well drained and
  chopped
1 cup (250 mL) crumbled feta cheese
1 tomato, diced
½ cup (125 mL) grated reduced-fat Mozzarella cheese

Prepare **Pizza Dough** and **Pizza Sauce** according to
instructions.

Prebake the **Pizza Dough** at 425° F (210° C) for about 7
minutes until the crust begins to brown. Spread half the **Pizza
Sauce** over the crust. Arrange the spinach on top of the sauce,
then sprinkle with the feta cheese and tomatoes. Top with the
Mozzarella cheese and bake for 8 to 10 minutes, until the cheese
is bubbly and the crust is browned. Makes 1 pizza.

Bean Dip Burritos

Place some **Bean Dip**—about ¼ cup (50 mL)—in the middle of an 8 inch (20 cm) whole-wheat tortilla. Top with some diced fresh tomato and any of the optional toppings listed below. Fold one end of the tortilla over the filling, fold both sides over, and roll up tightly. Repeat with additional tortillas, depending on the number of servings you want to make. Place the tortillas seam-side down in a lightly buttered baking dish. Bake at 350° F (180° C) for 10 to 15 minutes, until heated through.

Optional Toppings
   Plain low-fat yogurt
   Mild salsa
   Grated reduced-fat Cheddar or Mozzarella cheese or soy
      cheese
   Diced mild green chilies (fresh or canned)
   Diced white or green onion
   Mashed or sliced avocado
   Chopped sweet green or red pepper
   Steamed chopped vegetables, such as zucchini, broccoli,
      spinach
   Minced fresh cilantro

Variation

Chicken Burritos
Substitute sliced cooked chicken breast for the **Bean Dip**.

Bean Dip Quesadillas

Place an 8 inch (20 cm) whole-wheat tortilla on a baking sheet. Spread some **Bean Dip**—about ¼ cup (50 mL)—over the entire tortilla. Top with some diced tomato and any other optional toppings listed in the **Bean Dip Burritos** recipe. Place another tortilla on top and press down firmly. Bake at 425° F (210° C) for about 5 minutes, or until the cheese is melted and the top begins to turn brown. Cut into wedges and serve with low-fat plain yogurt and mild salsa. Makes 1 to 2 servings.

Variation

Chicken Quesadillas
Substitute sliced cooked chicken breast for the **Bean Dip**.

VEGETABLES AND SIDE DISHES

All vegetables are high in potassium and therefore have a cooling effect on the body. This can be offset somewhat by cooking and salting them. It's important not to use too many cooling foods, especially in cool weather, or you may weaken your ileocecal valve enough to permit your intestinal bacteria to travel from your large intestine up into your small intestine. The cooking process helps break down the tough fibres of the vegetables and improves the absorption of bioflavonoids, which can be 100 times more powerful free-radical scavengers than vitamin C. Excess cooking, however, can cause a loss of vitamin C and folic acid.

A quick and easy way to cook many types of vegetables is by steaming them in a steaming rack over boiling water until they're tender-crisp. You can add flavour to the vegetables by adding herbs, ginger, onion, and/or garlic to the steaming water. Instead of butter or margarine, season steamed vegetables with minced fresh herbs and/or a squeeze of fresh lemon juice. Or use **Yogurt Herb Dip, Tofu Herb Dip, Tzatziki,** or **Tofu Parmesan Sauce**.

Baked Beets

Baking the beets enhances their colour and retains their flavour. Since they take a long time to bake, cook a lot of them at once—they can also be eaten cold. Try them grated in salads or use in Borscht. Beets have so much flavour, all they need is a bit of sea salt before eating. If possible, buy beets whole, with the greens attached, and cook the greens as well, using the **Sautéed Greens** *recipe.*

Cut off the beet greens, if attached, leaving about 1 inch of stem. Wash the beets under running water. Leave them whole, with a bit of root and stem attached. Wrap beets in parchment paper: bring the front and back edges of the parchment together and seal tightly using a triple fold, then fold the left and right sides under using a double fold. Bake at 375° F (190° C) for about 45 minutes for small beets (60 to 75 minutes for larger beets). The beets are done if they're soft when pierced. Remove skins and slice or chop. (They are easier to peel when they're cold.) Serve hot or cold, sprinkled with sea salt.

Sautéed Greens

Use any combination of greens that you like in this recipe; even some lettuces, such as Romaine, can be used. Some of the sturdier greens, such as collard, mustard, and dandelion greens, may need to be blanched first. To do this, add the greens to a large pot of boiling water, and cook for approximately 3 minutes.

1 tablespoon (15 mL) extra virgin olive oil
1 medium shallot or ¼ cup (50 mL) finely chopped onion
1 to 2 garlic cloves, minced
2 to 3 teaspoons (10 to 15 mL) minced or grated fresh ginger
8 to 10 cups (2 to 2.5 L) washed, torn greens with stems
    removed (Choose from swiss chard, spinach, cabbage, bok
    choy, kale, dandelion greens, watercress, broccoli rabe,
    mustard greens, collard greens, or beet greens.)
Chicken Stock, Vegetable Stock, or water
sea salt, to taste
fresh lemon juice, rice vinegar, or soy sauce (optional)

Heat a large skillet or wok over medium-low heat. Add the oil, shallot or onion, garlic, and ginger, and sauté for about 2 minutes. Add the sturdier greens (cabbage, mustard greens, kale, collard greens, beet greens, etc.) and toss well. Add a small amount of water or stock; cover and cook for 2 minutes. Add the remaining greens (lettuce, spinach, swiss chard, watercress) and toss well; cover and cook for 3 to 5 minutes more or until the greens are tender, stirring occasionally and adding more water or stock, if necessary. Sprinkle with sea salt and lemon juice, vinegar, or soy sauce, to taste. Makes 4 servings.

Baked Vegetables with Fennel

Use as much of each vegetable as desired, depending on the number of servings you wish to make. Add or substitute other vegetables, if you wish.

Celery
Carrots
Eggplant
Zucchini
Fennel bulb
Snow peas
Pinch of basil
Water

Cut the celery, carrots, eggplant, zucchini, and fennel bulb into ½ inch (1 cm) pieces and place in a baking dish. Trim the snow peas and add to the remaining vegetables. Add enough water to just cover the bottom of the baking dish. Sprinkle with basil. Cover and bake at 350° F (180° C), stirring occasionally, for 30 minutes, or until the vegetables are tender.

Stir-Fried Vegetables with Yogurt and Cilantro

Use as much of each of the listed ingredients as needed, depending on the number of servings you wish to make. Other greens, such as bok choy, swiss chard, beet greens, collard greens, etc., can be added or substituted for the spinach. If you choose to stir-fry the vegetables using stock or water instead of oil, you can cook them at a higher temperature.

Extra virgin olive oil
Sliced carrots
Cauliflower florets
Minced fresh ginger
Minced garlic
Snow peas
Broccoli florets
Fresh spinach, washed and torn into pieces
Chopped tomato
Chopped fresh cilantro
Low-fat plain yogurt (at room temperature)

Heat a skillet or wok over medium-low heat. Add a small amount of oil and the carrots and cauliflower; stir-fry for 2 minutes, adding water to prevent sticking, if necessary. Add the garlic, ginger, snow peas, and broccoli, and stir-fry for 2 minutes more. Add the spinach and tomatoes; stir until the tomatoes are heated through and the spinach is cooked. Turn the heat down to low, add the cilantro and a few tablespoons of yogurt, and heat through.

Cabbage Casserole

2 teaspoons (10 mL) extra virgin olive oil
1 onion, chopped
1 garlic clove, minced
½ cup (125 mL) **Chicken Stock** or **Vegetable Stock**
2 tablespoons (30 mL) cornstarch or arrowroot powder
19 ounce (540 mL) can tomatoes, chopped
¼ cup (50 mL) chopped fresh parsley
½ teaspoon (2 mL) sea salt
1 medium head green cabbage, chopped
1 carrot, grated

Heat a large skillet over medium-low heat. Add the oil, onion, and garlic, and sauté until the onion is tender. Whisk together the stock and cornstarch or arrowroot powder, and stir into the skillet. Add the tomatoes, parsley, and sea salt and mix well.

Place the cabbage and carrots in a large, lightly buttered casserole. Add the onion/tomato mixture and mix well. Cover and bake at 350° F (180° C) for 1 to 1¼ hours, until tender, stirring every 15 minutes. Makes about 8 servings.

Roast Vegetables

1 teaspoon (5 mL) chopped fresh rosemary
1 teaspoon (5 mL) chopped fresh thyme or ½ teaspoon (2 mL) dried
1 tablespoon (15 mL) extra virgin olive oil
¼ teaspoon (1 mL) sea salt
2 carrots, cut into 1 inch (2.5 cm) pieces
½ small rutabaga, cut into 1 inch (2.5 cm) pieces
4 small red or white potatoes, unpeeled and cut in half
1 red onion, cut into 8 wedges
2 garlic cloves, slivered
¼ cup (50 mL) **Chicken Stock, Vegetable Stock**, or water
1 small zucchini, cut into 1 inch (2.5 cm) pieces
1 medium sweet red pepper, cut into 8 wedges

Combine the rosemary, thyme, oil, and sea salt in a roasting pan or large glass baking dish. Add the carrots, rutabaga, potatoes, onion, and garlic, and toss well to coat. Add the stock or water. Cover and bake at 375° F (190° C) for 25 minutes. Remove the cover and add the zucchini and red pepper. Stir well, adding a small amount of water, if necessary. Bake uncovered, stirring occasionally, for 15 to 20 minutes more, until the vegetables are tender and golden. Makes 4 servings.

Variation

Roast Eggplant
Substitute 1 large eggplant, cut into 1 inch (2.5 cm) cubes, for the carrots, rutabaga, and potatoes. Cook for only 5 minutes before adding the zucchini and red pepper.

Barley Stew

1 tablespoon (15 mL) extra virgin olive oil
1 small onion, finely chopped
1 garlic clove, minced
1 carrot, grated
1 celery stalk, finely chopped
1 cup (250 mL) pot barley
3 medium tomatoes, peeled and chopped (see Note)
1½ cups (375 mL) **Chicken Stock**, **Vegetable Stock**, or water
2 tablespoons (30 mL) chopped fresh parsley
¼ teaspoon (1 mL) sea salt

Heat a saucepan over medium-low heat. Add the oil, onion, garlic, carrot, and celery, and sauté until the onion is tender. Rinse the barley, then drain it and add to the saucepan. Cook for 3 minutes, stirring constantly and adding a small amount of stock or water to prevent sticking, if necessary. Add the tomatoes, stock, and parsley. Bring to a boil, then reduce the heat to medium-low. Cover and cook for 40 to 45 minutes, until the liquid is absorbed and the barley is tender. Let sit for 10 minutes, then season with the sea salt. Sprinkle with more chopped fresh parsley before serving, if desired. Makes 6 to 8 servings.

Note
To peel and seed the tomatoes, put them in boiling water until the skins start to split, up to a maximum of 1 minute. Remove the tomatoes from the water with a slotted spoon and immerse in cold water to stop the cooking process. When they're cool enough to handle, cut out the cores and then remove the skins; they should come off easily. Cut the tomatoes in half and squeeze them gently to remove most of the seeds.

Steamed Vegetables with Tofu Parmesan Sauce

The sauce can be used over any steamed vegetables or over rice or pasta.

1 carrot, sliced
¾ cup (175 mL) cauliflower florets
¾ cup (175 mL) broccoli florets
half a small zucchini, cut into ¼ inch (6 mm) slices
¼ cup (50 mL) silken or soft tofu, mashed
2 tablespoons (30 mL) low-fat plain yogurt
2 tablespoons (30 mL) freshly grated Parmesan cheese, soy
    cheese, or rice cheese
pinch sea salt

Steam the vegetables until tender-crisp. (Steam the carrots and cauliflower for about 2 minutes, then add the broccoli and zucchini and steam for 2 minutes more.) Mix together the remaining ingredients and pour over the steamed vegetables. Makes 2 servings.

Note
For a creamier sauce, process the tofu, yogurt, cheese, and sea salt in a blender until smooth.

Broiled Tomatoes

2 large tomatoes
½ cup (125 mL) finely crumbled feta cheese or goat cheese
¼ cup (50 mL) low-fat plain yogurt
1 tablespoon (15 mL) chopped fresh basil or 1 teaspoon
    (5 mL) dried
1 green onion, chopped

Cut the tomatoes in half and scoop out some of the centres. In a small bowl, combine the remaining ingredients; spoon into the tomato halves. Broil for about 5 minutes. Makes 2 to 4 servings.

Cauliflower Curry

1 tablespoon (15 mL) extra virgin olive oil
1 large onion, finely chopped
1 garlic clove, minced
1 teaspoon (5 mL) minced fresh ginger
1 teaspoon (5 mL) curry powder
1 small head cauliflower, cut into bite-size florets
½ cup (125 mL) water
1 cup (250 mL) peas, fresh or frozen
1 teaspoon (5 mL) garam masala
¼ teaspoon (1 mL) sea salt
2 tablespoons (30 mL) chopped fresh cilantro

Heat a large skillet over medium-low heat. Add the oil, onion, garlic, and ginger, and sauté until the onion is tender, about 5 minutes. Add the curry powder; stir well, and sauté for 1 minute. Add the cauliflower and sauté for 2 minutes. Add the water and peas and reduce the heat to low. Cover and cook for 10 to 12 minutes, stirring occasionally, until the cauliflower is tender. Remove from the heat and stir in the garam masala, sea salt, and cilantro. Makes 4 to 6 servings.

QUICK BREADS, MUFFINS, BEVERAGES, ETC.

Those who wish to lose weight should be mindful of the glycemic ratings of grains, especially processed grains. The higher the glycemic rating, the faster the starch will be released into your body. Excess sugar will be stored as fat, particularly in the abdominal area. Generally, those who wish to lose weight, or who are having problems with high blood sugar, should choose carbohydrates that have no GI/GL values (such as cruciferous and other non-starchy vegetables) and those with low GL values.

Use whole-grain flours whenever possible. For those who are sensitive to wheat, a variety of alternate flours can be used, such as barley, rye, oats, rice, soy, millet, bean, etc. Keep in mind, however, that not all of these flours can replace wheat flour on a 1-to-1 ratio; you will need to experiment with different amounts and combinations to find what works best for you. (Spelt and kamut flours are two that *can* be used to replace wheat flour on a 1-to-1 ratio.) For those who require gluten-free baked goods, try experimenting with soy, bean, rice, or millet flours.

Hearth Bread

1 cup (250 mL) slow-cooking oats
3 cups (750 mL) flour, e.g., 2 cups (500 mL) rye flour + 1 cup
(250 mL) unbleached flour
2 teaspoons (10 mL) baking soda
1 teaspoon (5 mL) nonalum baking powder
1 teaspoon (5 mL) sea salt
2 tablespoons (30 mL) molasses or ½ teaspoon (2 mL)
stevia/Chiclolin™ (optional)
¼ cup (50 mL) melted butter
1 egg
1½ cups (375 mL) soy milk, buttermilk, low-fat milk, or water

Combine the oats with 1 cup (250 mL) of the milk or water. Mix
well and let stand in the refrigerator for 1 hour, or overnight.
Mix the dry ingredients together and add to the oat mixture.
Mix the wet ingredients together, including the remaining ½
cup (125 mL) of milk or water. Add to the oat/flour mixture,
stirring as little as possible. Place in a lightly buttered loaf pan
or form into a round shape on a baking sheet. Bake at 375° F
(190° C) for 50 to 60 minutes.

Note
If you'd like to use buttermilk, but don't have any on hand, you
can make your own. For each cup of buttermilk that you need,
place 1 tablespoon (15 mL) lemon juice or vinegar in a
measuring cup. Fill the measuring cup with milk to the 1 cup
mark. You can make soy buttermilk in the same way, using soy
milk instead of cow's milk.

Zucchini Bread

1 cup (250 mL) whole-wheat pastry flour
1 cup (250 mL) unbleached flour
1 cup (250 mL) slow-cooking oats
1 tablespoon (15 mL) nonalum baking powder
1 teaspoon (5 mL) baking soda
1 teaspoon (5 mL) sea salt
1 teaspoon (5 mL) cinnamon
1 teaspoon (5 mL) nutmeg
1 teaspoon (5 mL) powdered ginger
2 eggs
½ cup (125 mL) melted butter
½ cup (125 mL) unsweetened applesauce
¼ cup (50 mL) low-fat milk, soy milk, or rice milk
1½ cups (375 mL) packed grated zucchini
½ cup (125 mL) packed grated carrot

In a bowl, combine the flour, oats, baking powder, baking soda, salt, cinnamon, nutmeg, and ginger. In another large bowl, beat together the eggs and butter. Add the applesauce, milk, zucchini, and carrot, and mix well. Stir into the dry ingredients. Place the batter into 2 buttered 8 x 4 inch (1.5 L) loaf pans. Bake at 350° F (180° C) for 45 to 50 minutes or until a toothpick comes out clean when inserted into the centre. Cool on a wire rack before serving. Makes 2 loaves.

Blueberry Muffins

Berries are the fruit of the north and are loaded with healthy lignans. Some can be easily dried for winter use. Cranberries, lingonberries, and blueberries are the least cooling. Raspberries, strawberries, and blackberries are a little more cooling. Apples, pears, plums (prunes), etc., are grown in warmer weather, while peaches, grapes, melons, etc., are grown in hotter weather. Oranges, papaya, pineapple, and bananas are a few of the fruits of the very hot tropics. Eating the fruits in season in your area is one way to let your kidneys know what climate you live in so they can help adjust your body's mineral levels to suit your weather.

1 cup (250 mL) slow-cooking oats
1 cup (250 mL) low-fat buttermilk, soy milk, or rice milk
3 tablespoons (45 mL) melted butter
¼ cup unsweetened applesauce
2 egg whites
2 tablespoons (30 mL) molasses
1 tablespoon (15 mL) finely grated lemon peel (optional)
1¼ cups (300 mL) whole-wheat pastry flour
1 tablespoon (15 mL) nonalum baking powder
¼ teaspoon (1 mL) sea salt
1 cup (250 mL) fresh or frozen blueberries

In a large bowl, combine the oats and milk; mix well and let stand for at least 15 minutes. Add the butter, applesauce, egg whites, molasses, and lemon peel, if using; mix well. In a separate bowl, mix together the flour, baking powder, and sea salt. Pour into the wet ingredients and mix just until moistened. Gently stir in the berries. Spoon into a lightly buttered or paper-lined muffin pan. Bake at 375° F (190° C) for 20 to 25 minutes, or until firm. Place the muffin pan on a wire rack to cool for 10 minutes before removing the muffins. Makes 12 muffins.

Notes
- Substitute other berries such as raspberries, blackberries, or cranberries (fresh or dried) for the blueberries.
- Whole-wheat pastry flour gives baked goods a lighter

texture than regular whole-wheat flour. Whole-wheat pastry flour can be found in some health food stores. If you don't have any, use ¾ cup (175 mL) whole-wheat flour and ½ cup (125 mL) unbleached flour.

- Muffins are best if eaten within 2 days, or they can be frozen for later use.
- If using canned applesauce in this recipe, leftover sauce can be frozen in ¼ cup (50 mL) packages for future batches of muffins, or for use in **Zucchini Bread**.

Variation

Apple Muffins
Omit the lemon peel and add 1½ teaspoons (7 mL) cinnamon to the dry ingredients. Substitute 1 cup (250 mL) of chopped peeled apple for the berries.

Carrot Oat Muffins

1 cup (250 mL) slow-cooking oats
1 cup (250 mL) low-fat buttermilk, soy milk, or rice milk
4½ ounce (128 mL) jar strained prunes (baby food)
½ cup (125 mL) packed grated carrot
3 tablespoons (45 mL) molasses
1 egg white
1¼ cups (300 mL) whole-wheat pastry flour
1 tablespoon (15 mL) nonalum baking powder
1½ teaspoons (7 mL) cinnamon
½ teaspoon (2 mL) nutmeg
½ teaspoon (2 mL) sea salt

In a large bowl, combine the oats and milk; mix well and let
stand for at least 15 minutes. Add the prunes, carrot, molasses,
and egg white; mix well. In another bowl, combine the flour,
baking powder, cinnamon, nutmeg, and sea salt; mix well, then
add to the wet ingredients. Mix just until moistened. Spoon into
a lightly buttered or paper-lined muffin pan. Bake at 375° F
(190° C) for 15 to 18 minutes, or just until a toothpick inserted in
the centre of a muffin comes out clean; do not overcook. Place
the muffin pan on a wire rack to cool for 10 minutes before
removing the muffins. Makes 12 muffins. (Muffins are best if
eaten within 2 days, or they can be frozen for later use.)

Variation

Zucchini Oat Muffins
Substitute ½ cup (50 mL) packed grated zucchini for the carrot.

Pumpkin Spice Muffins

1 cup (250 mL) slow-cooking oats
¾ cup (175 mL) low-fat buttermilk, soy milk, or rice milk
1 cup (250 mL) mashed cooked pumpkin
3 tablespoons (45 mL) pure maple syrup
3 tablespoons (45 mL) butter, melted
1 egg white
2 cups (500 mL) oat flour
1 tablespoon (15 mL) nonalum baking powder
1 teaspoon (5 mL) cinnamon
½ teaspoon (2 mL) nutmeg
½ teaspoon (2 mL) ground (powdered) ginger
½ teaspoon (2 mL) sea salt

In a large bowl, combine the oats and milk; mix well and let stand for at least 15 minutes. Add the pumpkin, maple syrup, butter, and egg white; mix well. Combine the flour, baking powder, cinnamon, nutmeg, ginger, and sea salt, then add to the other ingredients. Mix just until moistened. Spoon into a lightly buttered or paper-lined muffin pan. Bake at 375° F (190° C) for about 20 minutes, or just until a toothpick inserted in the centre of a muffin comes out clean. Place the muffin pan on a wire rack to cool for 10 minutes before removing the muffins. Makes 12 muffins. (Muffins are best if eaten within 2 days, or they can be frozen for later use.)

Dill Scones

1 cup (250 mL) flour, e.g., ½ cup (125 mL) whole-wheat flour
    + ½ cup (125 mL) unbleached flour
1 tablespoon (15 mL) nonalum baking powder
¼ teaspoon (1 mL) sea salt
¼ cup (50 mL) soft butter
1 cup (250 mL) slow-cooking oats
3 tablespoons (45 mL) chopped fresh dill or 1 tablespoon
    (15 mL) dried
⅔ cup (150 mL) low-fat plain yogurt

Mix together the flour, baking powder, and salt. With a fork,
blend in the butter until the mixture resembles coarse crumbs.
Add the oats and dill; mix well and then stir in the yogurt.
Knead the dough several times on a lightly floured surface, then
shape into a circle about ½ inch (1 cm) thick. Cut into 12
wedges, place on baking sheet, and bake at 425° F (220° C) for
12 to 15 minutes. Makes 12 scones.

Variations

Blueberry Scones
Omit the dill and add ¼ teaspoon (1 mL) stevia/Chicolin™ to
the flour mixture. Gently stir ½ cup (125 mL) blueberries (or
other berries) into the mixture, after stirring in the yogurt.

Cheese Scones
Omit the dill and add ¾ cup (175 mL) grated reduced-fat
Cheddar cheese when adding the yogurt. (Use aged Cheddar, if
you have it.)

Oatcakes

Oatcakes are available in some stores, but they are often made with hydrogenated vegetable oil. Use this easy recipe to whip up a batch yourself. Use oatmeal, not oat flakes, available in health food stores and some grocery stores. Alternatively, you can use a coffee grinder to make your own oatmeal; just grind old-fashioned large oat flakes, in batches, until they're the consistency of oatmeal. This takes only about 3 short (1 second) pulses in the coffee grinder—be sure not to grind them too fine.

> 3 to 4 tablespoons (45 to 60 mL) boiling water
> 1½ tablespoons (22 mL) butter, softened
> 1 cup (250 mL) oatmeal (or ground oat flakes)
> ¼ teaspoon (1 mL) baking powder
> ¼ teaspoon (1 mL) sea salt

In a cup or small bowl, combine 3 tablespoons (45 mL) of the boiling water with the butter. Stir and let stand until the butter is melted.

Meanwhile, combine the oatmeal, baking powder, and sea salt in a large bowl. Add the water/butter mixture and mix well. Add more hot water, a few drops at a time, until you have a stiff dough. Knead the dough, then roll out on a lightly floured surface (use oat flour, if you have it) until very thin, about ⅛ inch (3 mm) thick.

Cut the dough into squares or triangles, or use the mouth of a drinking glass to cut the dough into circles. Place on a baking sheet and bake at 350° F (180° C) for about 20 minutes, or until crisp but not brown. Makes 8 to 10 round oatcakes, each about 3 inches (8 cm) in diameter.

Tortillas

Use 1 cup (250 mL) kamut or spelt flour instead of whole-wheat and unbleached flours if you like.

½ cup (125 mL) whole-wheat flour
½ cup (125 mL) unbleached flour
¼ teaspoon (1 mL) sea salt
⅓ cup (75 mL) water
1 teaspoon (5 mL) olive oil

Stir together the flour and salt. Add the water and mix well. Knead the dough well, adding extra flour if needed, then divide into 4 equal-size balls. Roll out each ball on a lightly floured surface as thin as possible, about ⅛ inch (3 mm) thick.

Heat a large skillet over medium-high heat. Add ¼ teaspoon (1 mL) of the oil and spread it evenly over the skillet. Add 1 of the tortillas and cook for about 3 minutes per side, until lightly brown. Repeat for remaining tortillas. Use immediately, or cool completely and store in the refrigerator in a tightly sealed plastic bag. Makes 4 tortillas.

Apple Berry Crisp

2 medium apples, sliced
1 tablespoon (15 mL) fresh lemon juice
2 cups (500 mL) blueberries, fresh or frozen
2 cups (500 mL) raspberries, fresh or frozen

Topping
1 cup (250 mL) slow-cooking oats
2 tablespoons (30 mL) flour
1 teaspoon (5 mL) cinnamon
stevia powder or stevia/Chicolin™, to taste (optional)
2 tablespoons (30 mL) softened butter

Spread the apple slices in a lightly buttered 9 x 13 inch (23 x 33 cm) baking dish. Sprinkle the lemon juice over the apples, then layer the blueberries and raspberries on top. Mix together the topping ingredients and sprinkle over the raspberries. Bake at 350° F (180° C) for 25 to 30 minutes, until hot and bubbly. Makes 6 to 8 servings.

Notes
- Other fruits such as pears, apricots, and blackberries can be used.
- The topping ingredients can be doubled for those who like more topping.

Yogurt and Tofu Smoothie

Don't be afraid to add the oil in this recipe—it's a great way to supply your body with the essential fatty acids that it needs to keep you healthy. (See the article on pages 95 to 108, Fats That Heal and Fats That Kill, by Udo Erasmus.) You can substitute yogurt or water for the tofu and vice versa in this recipe, depending on what you like and what you have on hand.

Normally Dr. Matsen advises against combining proteins (the soy and the yogurt) with sweets (the blueberries, in this case) because proteins require hydrochloric acid (HCl) for digestion in the stomach, and sweets can inhibit HCl production. Combining sweets and proteins, therefore, results in a slower rate of digestion, allowing yeast and bacteria more time to create toxins. However, the proteins in the yogurt and tofu do not require as much HCl as more complex proteins (for example, fish or chicken). Also, the blueberries are not very sweet so the HCl production may not be affected in most people.

1 tablespoon (15 mL) Udo's Choice Ultimate Oil Blend®
½ cup (125 mL) plain low-fat yogurt
½ cup (125 mL) soft tofu
½ cup (125 mL) fresh or frozen blueberries
vanilla extract or stevia/Chicolin™ to taste (about ½ teaspoon or 2 mL)

Combine all ingredients in a blender and process until well mixed.

Note
For additional flavour, substitute a few raspberries for some of the blueberries.

Lemonade

¾ cup (175 mL) freshly squeezed lemon juice (see Note)
4 cups (2 L) spring or filtered water
¼ teaspoon (1 mL) stevia powder
Garnish: strawberry slices and/or blueberries; lemon slices
and/or mint leaves

Combine the first three ingredients and mix well to dissolve the stevia. Add more lemon juice, or stevia, to taste. (Because stevia is so sweet, be sure to add it only a pinch at a time.) Pour over ice, add a garnish, if you wish, and enjoy.

Note
This lemonade tastes best when you use fresh lemons. If you don't have fresh lemons, you can use 100% pure lemon juice from concentrate, available in plastic bottles in the freezer section of some grocery stores.

Variation

Iced Green Tea Lemonade (by Carol Song)
Substitute 4 cups (2 L) of room-temperature green tea for the water. Use Japanese green tea and steep for only 5 minutes or the tea will be bitter. To dissolve the stevia, premix it in a small amount of warm water.

Asian Recipes

by Carol Song

OTHERS

SOUPS

Cornish Game Hen and Ginseng Soup

Ingredients
- 1 cup (250 mL) sweet brown rice
- 2 Cornish game hens
- 6 cups (1.5 L) filtered water
- 3 cloves garlic, whole
- 1 piece fresh ginseng, about 3 to 4 inches (7.5 to 10 cm) in length, peeled and sliced
- grated peel from 1 orange
- 2 teaspoons (10 mL) sea salt (to taste)

Directions:
1. Wash the rice and soak overnight in enough cold water to cover the rice. Drain well.
2. Rinse the Cornish game hens and stuff the cavities with the rice. Secure with skewers or tie the legs together securely.
3. Place the hens and the water in a large pot; bring the water to a boil, skimming off any foam that rises to the top.
4. Add ginseng, garlic, and the grated orange peel. Reduce the heat to low and simmer for 3 to 4 hours.
5. Add sea salt to taste and you have yourself a delicious and nutritious meal.

Serves 2 people as an entrée. (Add some steamed brown rice to the soup for a heartier meal.)

Miso Soup

Ingredients:

5 cups (1.25 L) filtered water

2 tablespoons (30 mL) miso

8 knots konnyaku and/or 1 small package bean thread noodles

12 oz (350 g) package of medium tofu, cut into ½ inch (1 cm) cubes

4 small pieces dulse and/or wakame seaweed
   (4 small pieces = the size of the palm of your hand)

Directions:

1. If you are going to use wakame, soak it in warm water for 10 minutes and rinse 3 or 4 times in a bowl of water until there is no trace of sand. Squeeze out excess water and chop into bite-size pieces. If you are using dulse, it usually is ready to eat, so soaking and rinsing is unnecessary.

2. Bring the water to a boil in a medium pot. Reduce the heat to medium and add the miso; stir until dissolved. Simmer for 5 minutes.

3. Add the konnyaku and/or bean thread. Add the wakame and/or dulse and bring to a boil.

4. Evenly distribute the tofu between 4 or 5 bowls, then add the soup. You may want to use tongs to evenly distribute the noodles.

Serves 4 to 5 people.

Goes well with almost anything.

Winter Melon Soup

Ingredients:
  1 whole chicken leg
  5 cups (1.25 L) filtered water
  1 slice winter melon (see Note)
  2 teaspoons (10 mL) sea salt (to taste)
  8 knots konnyaku
  1 small package bean thread noodles
  1 tablespoon (15 mL) fish sauce
  12 oz (350 g) package of medium tofu, cut into bite-size cubes
  2 eggs, whisked (optional)

Directions:
  1. Remove the meat from the chicken leg and cut it into slices. Place the chicken meat, chicken bone, water, winter melon, and sea salt in a large pot and bring to a boil. Skim off any foam that rises to the top. Reduce heat to medium-low and simmer for 10 minutes.
  2. Wash the melon and remove the seeds; cut into bite-size cubes then add to the pot. Cook for 10 minutes more.
  3. Add the konnyaku, bean thread, fish sauce, and tofu; simmer for 5 minutes.
  4. If using the eggs, bring the soup to a boil; add the eggs while stirring the soup fast to feather the egg because it instantly cooks in the soup.

Serves 6 people as an appetizer, or 4 to 5 people as an entrée.

Note:
Winter melon is usually found in the grocery section in large slices, or quarters because the whole vegetable is large. It is dark green on the outside and white on the inside. You can leave the skin on or you can peel it off, but don't forget to remove the seeds.

Vietnamese Noodle Soup

Ingredients:
- 1 whole chicken
- 8 cups (2 L) filtered water
- 1 medium onion (whole), peeled and washed
- 2 tablespoons (30 mL) Asian fish sauce
  (Watch out: it's stinky, so don't sniff it directly.)
- 1 tablespoon (15 mL) sea salt
- 3 cloves star anise
- 2 packages rice noodles
- 3 cups (750 mL) bean sprouts, washed
- 1 bunch cilantro, washed and minced
- 1 lime, washed and quartered

Directions:
1. Wash the chicken, place in a large pot with the water, and bring to a boil. Reduce the heat to low, cover, and simmer for 2 hours; skim off any foam that rises to the top.
2. Add the onion, fish sauce, sea salt, and star anise; cover and simmer for another hour.
3. Remove the chicken from the pot. Remove the meat from the bones and chop.
4. Cook the rice noodles according to the instructions on the package (be careful not to overcook), and set aside.
5. Bring the soup to a boil.
6. Portion the noodles into large bowls; add the sprouts and the chicken. Sprinkle a generous amount of the cilantro on the top, then add the soup until it covers the noodles. Squeeze the lime over the soup before eating.

Serves 6 people as an entrée.

Goes well with **Pickled Vegetable Medley**.

SALADS

Watercress Salad

Ingredients:
  1 English cucumber
  4 teaspoons (20 mL) sea salt
  2 cups (500 mL) water
  2 pinches sea salt
  1 bunch watercress, washed
  1 teaspoon (5 mL) soy sauce
  1 tablespoon (15 mL) sesame oil
  ½ teaspoon (2 mL) minced garlic
  ½ teaspoon (2 mL) stevia/Chicolin™
  1 teaspoon (5 mL) apple cider vinegar

Directions:
  1. Cut the cucumber in half lengthwise, then slice. Place the slices in a small bowl, one layer at a time, and sprinkle evenly with the 4 teaspoons of sea salt. Let sit for 10 minutes.
  2. Bring the water to a boil, then add the 2 pinches of sea salt and the watercress. Blanch the watercress for 3 minutes, drain it thoroughly, then coarsely chop it.
  3. Rinse the cucumber and drain well.
  4. In a large bowl, combine the watercress, cucumber, soy sauce, sesame oil, garlic, stevia/Chicolin™, and apple cider vinegar; mix well.

Optional additions: pinch of roasted sesame seeds, or ½ teaspoon (2 mL) of sesame paste.

Serves 2 to 3 people as a side dish.

Goes well with rice dishes and/or chicken.

Daikon-Wakame Salad

Ingredients:
- 1½ cups (375 mL) wakame seaweed
- 1 cup (250 mL) julienned daikon radish or jicama (cut into matchsticks about 2 inches/5 cm long and ¼ inch/6 mm thick)
- ½ cup (125 mL) julienned carrot (cut like the daikon radish)
- ½ cup (125 mL) julienned cucumber (cut like the daikon radish)
- ¼ cup (50 mL) sea salt
- 2 tablespoons (30 mL) rice vinegar
- ½ teaspoon (2 mL) stevia/Chicolin™
- 1 tablespoon (15 mL) sesame oil
- ½ teaspoon (2 mL) minced garlic
- 1 pinch sea salt

Directions:
1. Soak the wakame in warm water for 30 minutes then blanch it in boiling water for about 1 minute. Chop it into pieces that are no larger than 2 inches x 2 inches (5 cm x 5 cm) then set aside.
2. Put the daikon (or jicama), carrot, and cucumber in a large bowl; sprinkle the sea salt evenly over all the vegetables. Mix well and let sit for 10 minutes.
3. Rinse the salted vegetables then drain well.
4. In a large bowl, combine the vegetables and the wakame with the remaining ingredients; mix well and enjoy.

Serves 4 people as an appetizer or a side dish.

Pickled Vegetable Medley

Ingredients:
- 1 small diakon radish, peeled and cut into matchsticks about 2 inches/5 cm long and ¼ inch/6 mm thick
- 2 to 3 medium carrots, peeled and cut into matchsticks about 2 inches/5 cm long and ¼ inch/6 mm thick
- half a small head of cabbage, cut into 1½ inch/4 cm cubes
- 2 stalks green onion, thinly sliced
- 4 to 5 sprigs cilantro, cut into 2 inch/5 cm lengths
- 4 cloves garlic, sliced
- 2 tablespoons (30 mL) grated ginger
- ¼ cup (50 mL) sea salt
- 2 tablespoons (30 mL) apple cider vinegar
- 1 teaspoon (5 mL) stevia/Chicolin™ (add a pinch more if you prefer a sweeter taste)
- 1 teaspoon (5 mL) fish sauce
- 2 pinches sea salt
- 1 tablespoon (15 mL) sesame oil
- 1 teaspoon (5 mL) roasted sesame seeds (see Note on page 256)

Directions:
1. Put the daikon, carrots, and cabbage in a large bowl; sprinkle with the ¼ cup (50 mL) sea salt, while stirring well to evenly distribute the salt. Let sit for 30 minutes.
2. Rinse and drain the salted vegetables.
3. Add the green onion, cilantro, garlic, ginger, apple cider vinegar, and stevia/Chicolin™ to the pickled vegetables; stir until well mixed.
4. Drizzle the sesame oil and sprinkle the roasted sesame seeds on top.
3. Place in the refrigerator to chill for 20 minutes.

Serves 6 people as a decorative side dish to be eaten with an entrée.

Goes well with the **Curry, Bee Bim Bhup, Vietnamese Noodle Soup,** or any meat dish.

Sunomono Salad

Ingredients:
   1 cucumber, peeled and seeds removed
   3 tablespoons (45 mL) rice vinegar
   1 tablespoon (15 mL) distilled water
   ½ teaspoon (2 mL) stevia/Chicolin™
   1 pinch sea salt
   ½ teaspoon (2 mL) grated ginger
   1 clove garlic, minced
   1 small package of bean thread noodles
   1 teaspoon (5 mL) roasted sesame seeds (see Note)

Directions:
   1. Slice the cucumber thinly crosswise.
   2. In a medium bowl, combine the vinegar, water,
      stevia/Chicolin™, sea salt, ginger, and garlic; mix well.
      Marinate the cucumber in this mixture for about an hour.
   3. Cook the bean thread according to the package directions
      and drain. Put the bean thread into bowls; add the
      cucumber and sauce to the bean thread, sprinkle sesame
      seeds on top and serve.

Serves 2 to 3 as an appetizer

Note:
You can buy sesame seeds roasted or you can roast them
yourself. Rinse the sesame seeds in water, then roast in a pan
over medium heat, stirring slowly until lightly browned. Cool
completely and store in a tightly sealed jar.

FISH AND SEAFOOD

Curried Sole Fillets

Ingredients:
  1 large egg
  2 tablespoons (30 mL) water
  2 tablespoons (30 mL) flour
  2 tablespoons (30 mL) plain yogurt
  ½ teaspoon (2 mL) sea salt (or more, to taste)
  1 tablespoon (15 mL) curry powder
  1 pinch garam masala
  6 sole fillets
  half a sweet red pepper, thinly sliced
  2 tablespoons (30 mL) olive oil
  1 lemon, cut into 6 wedges

Directions:
  1. In a medium bowl, mix the egg and water, then add the flour, yogurt, salt, curry powder, and garam masala.
  2. Lay the sole fillets on a plate. Spread the sauce evenly over the fillets. Cover and place in the refrigerator for about an hour.
  3. Heat a large skillet over medium-high heat. Add the oil and half the fillets; cook for 2 minutes on each side. Remove and cook the remaining 3 fillets. Add the other 3 fillets and the red peppers to the skillet. Cover and let simmer for 4 to 5 minutes.
  4. Serve with lemon wedges.

Serves 3 to 4 people as an entrée.

Goes well with any veggies, rice, or pasta.

Steamed Rock Cod

Ingredients:
  1 medium-size rock cod, about 2 to 3 lbs/1 kg (as fresh as
    possible)
  3 tablespoons (45 mL) minced cilantro
  1 tablespoon (15 mL) of packed, thinly sliced ginger
  2 stalks green onion, thinly sliced
  ⅓ cup (75 mL) soy sauce
  ⅓ cup (75 mL) extra virgin olive oil

Directions:
  1. Rinse the fish; cut deep slits about 1 inch (2.5 cm) apart
     into both sides of the fish. Insert the ginger into the slits.
  2. Place the fish in a shallow bowl or deep plate (one that's
     deep enough to hold the sauce.)
  3. Put about 2 inches (5 cm) of water into a steamer and bring
     to a boil. Place the bowl or plate containing the fish into
     the steamer, cover, and cook for 15 minutes. Check the fish
     inside; the colour should be opaque by the spine, not
     translucent. (see Note)
  4. Remove the fish from the steamer; sprinkle the green onion
     and cilantro over top.
  5. Drizzle the soy sauce over the fish.
  6. Heat the olive oil until hot, and drizzle over the fish.

Serves 3 to 4.

Goes great with a stir-fry, rice, noodles, or a grilled salad.

Note:
If you don't have a steamer, use a covered skillet or wok that's
large enough to hold the bowl or plate that contains the fish.
Put about 1 inch (2.5 cm) of water into the bottom of the skillet
or wok.

Mackerel Medley

Ingredients:
2 cups (500 mL) cubed daikon radish
1 whole Pacific mackerel (remove head and tail and cut fish
    into slices about 1½ inches/3.5 cm thick)
1 medium onion, chopped
3 cloves garlic, minced
1 tablespoon (15 mL) minced ginger
¾ cup (175 mL) soy sauce
2 teaspoons (10 mL) stevia/Chicolin™
2 sprigs cilantro, chopped
1 tablespoon (15 mL) roasted sesame seeds (see Note)

Directions:
1. Place the daikon in the bottom of a medium-size pot. Lay
   the mackerel slices on top of the daikon, and arrange the
   onions over top of the fish.
2. Mix together the garlic, ginger, soy sauce, and
   stevia/Chicolin™; pour this mixture evenly over top of the
   mackerel and vegetables.
3. Heat the pot over medium-high heat until the soy sauce
   mixture comes to a boil; reduce heat to low. Simmer for 20
   minutes, using a turkey baster to baste the onions with the
   soy sauce mixture every five minutes, for an even
   flavouring.
4. Arrange the fish and vegetables on serving plates, pour the
   sauce over top, and sprinkle with the cilantro and sesame
   seeds.

Serves 3 to 4.
Goes great with a stir-fry, rice, noodles, or a grilled salad.

Note:
You can buy sesame seeds roasted or you can roast them
yourself. Rinse the sesame seeds in water, then roast in a pan
over medium heat, stirring slowly until lightly browned. Cool
completely and store in a tightly sealed jar.

Broiled Black Bean Salmon

Ingredients
 ½ cup (125 mL) salted Chinese black beans
 6 cloves garlic
 1 tablespoon (15 mL) minced fresh ginger
 1 bunch cilantro
 1 small onion, chopped
 ½ cup (125 mL) extra virgin olive oil
 1 tablespoon (15 mL) stevia/Chicolin™
 ¾ cup (175 mL) soy sauce
 1 large salmon fillet, deboned (about 1 lb/500g)
 1 tablespoon (15 mL) roasted sesame seeds (see Note)

Directions:
 1. Soak the black beans in hot water for 10 minutes then
    drain off the water.
 2. Place the black beans, garlic, ginger, cilantro, onion, olive
    oil, stevia/Chicolin, and soy sauce in a food processor and
    process until minced.
 3. Place the salmon in a roasting pan or a large oval casserole
    dish. Spread the black bean mixture evenly over top of the
    fish. Cover and bake at 350° F (180° C) for 10 minutes, then
    reduce the oven temperature to 325° F (165° C) for 30
    minutes. Turn the oven off; let the fish sit in the oven for
    another 15 minutes. Sprinkle with sesame seeds before
    serving.

Serves 3 to 4 as an entrée.

Goes great with a stir-fry, rice, noodles, or on a grilled salad.

Note:
You can buy sesame seeds roasted or you can roast them
yourself. Rinse the sesame seeds in water, then roast in a pan
over medium heat, stirring slowly until lightly browned. Cool
completely and store in a tightly sealed jar.

Stuffed Squid

Ingredients:
2 large squid (available in most fish stores or in the freezer
  section of some grocery stores)
3½ oz (100 g) bean sprouts
12 oz (350 g) package of medium tofu, crumbled
3 small sweet red peppers, diced
1 green onion, minced
1 tablespoon (15 mL) minced garlic
¼ teaspoon (1 mL) sea salt

Directions:
1. Thaw the squid, if frozen, and wash. Separate the legs
   from the body.
2. Blanch the squid legs in boiling water for 3 minutes; drain
   and dice.
3. Blanch the bean sprouts in 2 cups of boiling water with 2
   pinches of salt for 2 minutes; drain well.
4. In a large bowl, combine the squid legs, bean sprouts, tofu,
   red pepper, green onion, garlic, and sea salt; mix well.
5. Place the mixture into the squid tubes (bodies) and close
   the openings with skewers.
6. Place the squid in a steamer over boiling water and cook
   for 20 minutes. Optional: Steam for only 10 minutes, then
   cook on the barbeque, over medium heat, for the
   remaining 10 minutes.
7. Allow the squid to cool for 5 minutes, then cut into 1 inch
   (2.5 cm) slices and serve.

Serves 2 people as an entrée, or 6 as an appetizer.

Seafood Stew

Ingredients:
  2½ cups (675 mL) filtered water
  ½ lb (250 g) salmon, washed and cut into 1 inch (2.5 cm)
    cubes
  ½ lb (250 g) halibut, washed and cut into 1 inch (2.5 cm)
    cubes
  ½ lb (250 g) sea bass or black cod, washed and cut into 1 inch
    (2.5 cm) cubes
  ½ cup (125 mL) cubed zucchini (¾ inch/1.5 cm cubes)
  1½ cups (375 mL) watercress, cut 2 inches/5 cm in length
  1 cup (250 mL) soybean sprouts
  1 cup (250 mL) cubed daikon (½ inch/1 cm cubes)
  1 cup (250 mL) cubed medium tofu (¾ inch/1.5 cm cubes)
  1 green onion, cut 2 inches/5 cm in length
  1 teaspoon (5 mL) minced garlic
  2 slices (⅛ inch/3 mm) ginger
  1 teaspoons (5 mL) sea salt (to taste)

optional for those who don't have shellfish allergies
  2 live clams in the shell, washed
  3 prawns with the head on, washed
  ½ cup (125 mL) frozen or canned butter clams, drained

Directions:
  1. Place the water, all the seafood, zucchini, watercress,
     soybean sprouts, and daikon into a large pot and bring to a
     boil.
  2. Reduce heat to medium-low and simmer for 10 minutes.
  3. Add the tofu, green onion, garlic, ginger, and sea salt (to
     taste). Bring to a boil again and serve immediately.

Serves 6 people as a side dish or 4 as an entree.

Goes well with any rice dish.

EGG DISHES

Chowanmushi (Egg Soufflé)

Ingredients:
   5 large eggs
   3 tablespoons (45 mL) tobiko eggs (flying fish roe)
   1 cup (250 mL) filtered water, chicken stock, or fish stock
   1 teaspoon (5 mL) sea salt (to taste)

Directions:
   1. Put about 2 inches (5 cm) of water into a steamer and bring to a boil; reduce the heat to low as you are preparing the dish (see Note).
   2. Beat the eggs, then add the water or stock and the sea salt; beat thoroughly.
   3. Divide the egg mixture between 2 soufflé or rice bowls, leaving at least ½ inch/1 cm between the mixture and the rim. Sprinkle the tobiko evenly over top.
   4. Place the bowls in the steamer, cover and steam on <u>low</u> with the lid slightly ajar, for 15 to 20 minutes (depending on the size of the bowl) until the eggs are set. Important: Steaming on low and keeping the lid slightly ajar is what gives the soufflé a light, even consistency; if the temperature is too high and the steam is too hot, the egg mixture will boil and the texture will change.
   5. Optional: if you have nori or wakame seaweed, cut some into small strips and sprinkle on top of the soufflés before serving.

Serves 2 as an appetizer.

Goes well with **Zaru Soba** and **Sunomono Salad**.

Note:
If you don't have a steamer, use a covered skillet or wok that's large enough to hold bowls that contain the egg mixture. Put about 1 inch (2.5 cm) of water into the bottom of the skillet or wok.

Bee Bim Bhup

This recipe is actually really easy to make, so don't let the long lists of ingredients and directions scare you off.

Ingredients:
   3 cups (750 mL) brown rice
   5 cups (1.25 L) filtered water
   2 bunches spinach, washed and stems removed
   5 cloves garlic, minced (divided)
   3 tablespoons (45 mL) sesame oil (divided)
   6 pinches sea salt (divided)
   3 tablespoons (45 mL) extra virgin olive oil (use 1
      tablespoon/15 mL per stir-fry)
   4 medium carrots, coarsely grated
   2 small zucchini, coarsely grated
   10 oz (300 g) ground turkey or chicken
   2 cups (500 mL) blanched soy bean sprouts or mung bean
      sprouts
   6 eggs

Sauce
   ⅓ cup (75 mL) sesame oil
   2 tablespoons (30 mL) soy sauce
   ¼ teaspoon (1 mL) stevia/Chicolin™
   1 stalk green onion, minced
   2 tablespoons (30 mL) minced cilantro (optional)

Directions:
   1. Wash the rice and drain completely. Put the filtered water
      and the rice in a large pot or a rice cooker and cook
      according to package directions.
   2. Blanch the spinach in boiling water for 3 minutes, squeeze
      out the excess water, and chop. Put the spinach in a
      medium bowl and add 1 of the minced garlic cloves,
      2 tablespoons/30 mL of the sesame oil, and 2 pinches of the
      sea salt. Mix thoroughly and set aside.
   3. Heat a large skillet over medium heat; add 1
      tablespoon/15 mL of the olive oil, 1 of the minced garlic

cloves, the carrots, and 1 pinch of the sea salt. Stir-fry for about 5 to 6 minutes, until the carrots are tender. Place in a bowl and drizzle 1 tablespoon of the sesame oil over top; set aside.

4. Follow the directions in step 3, substituting the zucchini for the carrots.
5. Follow the directions in step 3, substituting the ground turkey or chicken for the carrots (cook until no longer pink.)
6. Place the soy or mung bean sprouts in a medium bowl and 1 of the minced garlic cloves, 1 tablespoon/15 mL of sesame oil, and 1 pinch of the sea salt. Mix thoroughly and set aside.
7. For the sauce, place the sesame oil and soy sauce in a small bowl and, using a whisk, add the stevia/Chicolin™ until blended. Sprinkle the green onion on top of the sauce.
8. Fry the eggs sunny side up and place on a plate.
9. To arrange the Bee Bim Bhup: For each serving, put a cup of rice in the middle of a large bowl. Arrange some spinach, carrots, zucchini, ground turkey, and sprouts on top of the rice, placing each ingredient in a separate section (like the sections of a pie). Place an egg in the centre of each bowl, on top of the other ingredients. Drizzle 1 to 2 teaspoons (5 to 10 mL) of sauce over top of each, and serve.

You could either eat as is, or mix everything together, which is the Korean way.

Serves 6 people as an entree. Goes well with **Miso Soup.**

OTHERS

Zaru Soba

Ingredients:
- 1 sheet nori seaweed
- 14 oz (400 g) buckwheat noodles
- 5 cups (1.25 L) water
- 2 tablespoons (30 mL) grated horseradish or daikon radish
- 1 stalk green onion, sliced thinly
- 1 teaspoon (5 mL) wasabi powder or ½ teaspoon (2 mL) wasabi paste

Sauce
- 1 piece kombu seaweed, about 4 inches/10 cm in length
- ½ cup (125 mL) filtered water
- 5 tablespoons (75 mL) Tamari soy sauce
- ⅓ teaspoon (1.5 mL) stevia/Chicolin™
- 1 teaspoon (5 mL) rice vinegar

Directions:
1. To make the sauce, put the kombu into a small pot with the ½ cup (125 mL) of water and bring to a boil. Remove from the heat and stir in the soy sauce, stevia/Chicolin™, and vinegar. Put the sauce in the refrigerator to cool.
2. In a skillet over medium heat, lightly cook the nori seaweed until the colour changes to light green (about 2 minutes.) Use scissors to cut the nori into thin strips (about 2 inches/5 cm long and ¼ inch/½ cm wide) and set aside.
3. Bring the 5 cups of water to a boil; add the buckwheat noodles and cook according to the directions on the package, stirring often. Rinse thoroughly in cold water and drain well.
4. Put the noodles onto 2 plates and sprinkle the nori seaweed over top. Place the horseradish or daikon radish on the side of each plate so that each person can add it to their noodles as they wish.

5. Remove the sauce from the refrigerator; add the wasabi and green onion and then pour the sauce into 2 small bowls to be used as a dipping sauce for the noodles.

Serves 2 as an entrée.

Goes well with the **Chowanmushi** or the **Sunomono Salad**.

Rice with Soy Sprouts

Ingredients:
   6 cups (1.5 L) filtered water
   1 teaspoon (5 mL) sea salt
   10 oz (300 g) soy bean sprouts, washed and drained
   3 cups (750 mL) brown rice, washed and drained

Sauce
   2 tablespoons (30 mL) soy sauce
   2 tablespoons (30 mL) green onion, minced
   1 tablespoon (15 mL) minced garlic
   2 tablespoons (30 mL) sesame oil

Directions:
   1. Put the water and the sea salt in a large pot and bring to a boil. Blanch the soy bean sprouts in the boiling water for 5 minutes with the lid on. Using a pasta scoop or a slotted spoon, remove the soy bean sprouts and set aside to cool.
   2. Put the rice into the water that was used to blanch the sprouts. Bring the water back to a boil, then reduce the heat to low. Cover and simmer for 25 minutes.
   3. Add the sprouts to the pot, stir in gently, cover and cook for 20 minutes longer.
   4. Combine all the sauce ingredients in a small bowl, mix well and then stir into the rice.

Serves 4 people as an entrée, or 6 as a side dish.

Try with **Miso Soup** or **Daikon-Wakame Salad.**

Curry

Ingredients:
 2 cups (500 mL) filtered water
 2 medium potatoes, cut into 1 inch (2.5 cm) cubes
 2 medium carrots, cut into 1 inch (2.5 cm) cubes
 1 small jicama, cut into 1 inch (2.5 cm) cubes
 1 medium onion, cut into 1 inch (2.5 cm) cubes
 ½ cup (125 mL) cooked, diced chicken meat (optional)
 2 cloves garlic, minced
 ½ teaspoon (2 mL) grated ginger
 1 tablespoon (15 mL) extra virgin olive oil
 3 tablespoons (45 mL) curry powder
 ½ teaspoon (2 mL) garam masala
 1 tablespoon (15 mL) flour
 ½ cup (125 mL) coconut milk
 2 tablespoons (30 mL) plain yogurt
 1 teaspoon (5 mL) sea salt (or more to taste)

Directions:
 1. Place the water, all the veggies, the chicken (if using), garlic, and ginger in a large pot and bring to a boil. Reduce the heat to medium-low and simmer, uncovered, for 15 minutes, stirring occasionally.
 2. Heat a small skillet over medium heat; add the olive oil, curry powder, garam masala, and flour. Stir-fry until clumped together; then add the mixture to the pot, stirring until the curry is evenly distributed. Simmer for 10 minutes, stirring every couple of minutes.
 3. Add the coconut milk, yogurt, and salt to the pot; simmer for another 10 minutes.

Serves 3 to 4 people as an entrée.

Goes well with rice, flat breads, or steamed veggies.

5-Grain Porridge

Ingredients:
    2 cups (500 mL) filtered water
    1 cup (250 mL) 5-grain mixture (see below)
    pinch sea salt
    1 tablespoon (15 mL) flax seeds, freshly ground

5-grain mixture
    2 cups (500 mL) organic slow-cooking oats
    1 cup (250 mL) organic raw buckwheat groats
    1 cup (250 mL) organic pearl barley
    1 cup (250 mL) organic rye flakes
    ½ cup (125 mL) organic quinoa (well rinsed and dried)

Directions:
1. In a medium pot, bring the water to boil then turn down the heat to medium. Add the 1 cup of the 5-grain mixture and cook for 10 minutes, stirring occasionally.
2. Turn off the heat, cover the pot, and let sit for 15 minutes.
3. Stir in the sea salt. (Add more, to taste, if desired.)
4. Sprinkle the ground flax seed over the porridge before eating.

Variations

-with miso-
Instead of adding the sea salt, stir in 1 tablespoon (5 mL) of miso; stir well until the miso is distributed evenly.

-with cinnamon and stevia/Chicolin™-
When adding the sea salt, stir in the following, as well.
    ½ teaspoon (2 mL) cinnamon
    1 teaspoon (5 mL) stevia/Chicolin™ (or more)
    2 tablespoons (30 mL) raisins, diced apples, or dried cranberries

Serves 2 to 3 people for breakfast.

Letter from a Patient

Before starting THE EATING ALIVE PROGRAM, everything I ate gave me gas and a lot of pain. I also had a choking problem and severe PMS symptoms (bloating, tenderness, mood swings, and sore ribs). After starting THE EATING ALIVE PROGRAM, these problems subsided.

And losing twelve pounds was a bonus. My new eating habits, having the mercury removed from my teeth, and my exercise regimen have made me feel like a new person.

Frances Galea
North Vancouver, BC

PART III

DETAILS! DETAILS! DETAILS!

CHAPTER 1

Mercury:
The Missing Piece

"...The primary symptoms of mercury-poisoning are vague psychic ones. Short-term memory deteriorates. You will find it difficult to concentrate on tasks which require attention and thinking. It is easier to execute tasks that are well known rather than to learn something new. You avoid social contacts which demand that you get out of your introvert behaviour. You lose your temper easily and switch between different moods for no particular reason.

"Little by little, a more physical kind of exhaustion is added to the condition. More and more effort is required to initiate activities and [you] sometimes break things due to inability to co-ordinate your movements with your visual impressions (ataxia). Occasional headaches, minor involuntary muscle spasms or ticks within groups of muscles can also appear. Hands and feet become easily cold, attacks of dizziness or vertigo can occur, and periodically you may find it difficult to focus your eyes and to see clearly. Joint and muscle pains, stiffness, lumbago and similar symptoms often appear at an early stage. They can be caused or increased by low availability of the trace element selenium.

"Nervous heart, sometimes accompanied by a weak pulse, sometimes by a hard pulse, creates a feeling of anxiety. You don't sleep well, you wake up stiff, and never feel thoroughly rested. As a whole, you need more sleep than before, and you are constantly tired.

"Some individuals develop pronounced intestinal and stomach disturbances. Bloating is common and diarrhea can alternate with constipation. From 50 to 200 micrograms mercury from amalgam daily passes the gastrointestinal tract. There is usually irritation where mercury first interacts with tissues. The upper respiratory tract easily becomes chronically inflamed and symptoms in mouth appear. The gums bleed when you brush your teeth, red and white irritations (lichen, leukoplakia) arise, blisters and sensitivity to certain nutritives develop, your teeth ache, the whole jaw can become more or less inflamed, and some persons develop sinusitis. Metal taste in your mouth is a direct sign of metal-poisoning (mercury, copper). The more poisoned you are, the more serious and chronic your problems become. The pituitary gland will be affected, which often leads to frequent urination. When the thyroid gland is affected, secondary effects on metabolism can appear. Both glands accumulate mercury. Neurological symptoms such as numbness, hypersensitivity, and paralysis exacerbate. It is often hard to determine if the cause is in the nervous or circulatory systems... ."

Swedish Association of Dental Mercury Patients,
Nov. 1993 (Booklet)

I went to Toronto several years ago for a book promotion. During the flight, I began talking to the person sitting next to me. His name was Michael Lyons; he was a medical doctor who had been working as a researcher with John Cline, an MD in Nanaimo, British Columbia (BC). One of the patients whose condition Cline claimed to have improved was a patient of mine with chronic fatigue.

I remembered this patient well. He was a big, burly guy who looked like he could wrestle grizzly bears for sport—not your typical chronic fatigue type. He was part-owner of an oyster farm that required a lot of heavy physical labour, which he had been unable to do for five years when I first saw him. He then followed my treatment program and within a few months, after taking a yeast-killer, he had reported that his energy was back up, and he had returned to work on the oyster farm.

I had considered him cured, but apparently his fatigue relapsed after several months, and he went to see Drs. John Cline and Michael Lyons. They recommended that he have his mercury-amalgam fillings replaced, which he did. After he had a number of **DMPS chelations**, he regained his energy.

DMPS is short for 2,3-Dimercaptopropane-1-Sulfonic acid. It is a sulfur compound that was developed in the former Soviet Union in the 1950s. In 1978, Heyl, a pharmaceutical company in Berlin, Germany, began manufacturing and distributing DMPS.

DMPS circulates in the blood and chelates—binds—metals into very stable and non-toxic molecules that can be excreted primarily by the kidneys within 12 hours. It binds strongly to mercury, arsenic, antimony, bisthmuth, lead, cadmium, cobalt, copper, and silver. DMPS binds weakly with gold, iron, manganese, molybdenum, thallium, tungsten, and zinc. It doesn't bind to calcium or magnesium.

DMPS can be given orally in capsule form or mixed in an acidic drink (such as orange juice) or it can be injected intravenously or intermuscularly. Heyl, a manufacturer of DMPS, states that oral administration is used for both acute and chronic metal poisoning, while IV administration is used primarily in acute metal poisoning when an oral treatment cannot be administered.

The "DMPS challenge," followed by a urine test for metals, is at this point the most accurate way to monitor mercury levels in the body—short of an autopsy. Before doing the DMPS challenge, a urine sample is collected from the patient. DMPS is then taken orally or injected intravenously. A second urine sample is collected over a period of two hours, six hours, or 24 hours after the DMPS is administered. The urine samples are sent to a lab, which measures the amounts and types of metals found in the urine. What consistently shows up is that there are *small amounts of metals* (usually within the reference range) in the urine sample taken *before* the DMPS is administered, and *greater amounts of some metals* in the urine collected *after* the DMPS, usually far above the reference range.

Of all the metals found in the urine after the DMPS challenge, mercury is the one that is usually detected the most frequently and in the highest quantities. Other metals, such as arsenic, however, are sometimes found in higher quantities than mercury. The DMPS challenges are usually repeated and mercury, lead, arsenic, aluminum, and cadmium often continue to be excreted in large quantities—presumably from the kidneys and liver. The signs and symptoms of health problems don't usually improve until the mercury levels in the body are reduced to within normal reference ranges.

By using DMPS chelations in their practice, Drs. John Cline and Michael Lyons saw improvements in more than 400 patients—most of them with stubborn chronic "mystery" illnesses such as chronic fatigue, fibromyalgia, various types of arthritis, and so on.

The insights that Dr. Lyons shared with me made me wonder whether metal toxicity might also be the missing piece for other patients of mine who weren't achieving complete or long-lasting results.

Soon after I returned home to my practice, I saw a patient that I had been treating for several years—with no improvement. She was suffering from chronic, unexplained diarrhea, severe allergies, and frequent urination that forced her to go to the washroom every 15 minutes, night and day. Years without adequate sleep had left her unable to work as an art teacher. She scraped out a meagre living selling her art in a local park—when she was able to make her way there.

Her knees were gradually giving out under her, probably due to an autoimmune connective disease; the best that medical specialists could do was give her stronger knee braces. By this time, she was using a cane and had a difficult time making it up stairs. It was hard to imagine her carrying her paintings to a park via bus each weekend.

I knew she had a yeast overgrowth in her intestine, but whenever she would start taking a yeast-killer, she would immediately get worse—especially the bladder symptoms. If she took antibiotics for the bladder, her diarrhea would worsen because the yeast would flare up again. Anyway, in spite of numerous attempts, she was unable to kill the yeast, and had no improvement in her complaints over a long period of time. She began to talk about her life becoming too great a struggle, and that maybe it was time to end it.

I told her what I had learned on my plane ride with Michael Lyons. She agreed to try an IV DMPS challenge with a local physician who did chelation treatments. At this time, I wasn't aware that DMPS could be taken orally. Because DMPS is such a strong extractor of mercury, she first had her old silver-amalgam fillings—which are approximately 50 percent mercury—replaced, so that the chelation wouldn't pull any metals from the fillings. (Later I learned that the DMPS does not pull mercury out of the fillings, so DMPS can be used even with people who have dental amalgams.) The removal of her fillings was done safely by a dentist with advanced training in mercury-amalgam removal.

A urine sample was collected before the DMPS. A second urine sample was collected over the 24 hours *following the DMPS*. A week later, the results came in.

- The first urine sample, taken before the DMPS was administered, didn't show the presence of any metals beyond the reference range.
- The urine sample collected over the 24 hours *following* the DMPS injection showed **25 micrograms (mcg) of mercury**; the reference range is 0 to 3 mcg. Cadmium measured 2.5 mcg; its reference range is 2 mcg or less (see Table 1).

(Note: All urine samples were analyzed by Doctor's Data, Inc., West Chicago, Illinois, www.doctorsdata.com.)

ELEMENTS REGARDED AS TOXIC

Elements	Result (µg/g creatinine)	per gram Creatinine Reference Range* (µg/g creatinine)	Within Ref. Range	Elevated	Very Elevated
Aluminum	8.9	0–35	• • •		
Antimony	.8	0–5	• •		
Arsenic	100	0–100	• • • • • • • •		
Beryllium	<dl	0–.5			
Bismuth	.4	0–30	•		
Cadmium	2.5	0–2	• • • • • • • • •	• •	
Lead	2.2	0–15	• •		
Mercury	25	0–3	• • • • • • • • •	• • • • • • • • • •	• • • • •
Nickel	7.3	0–12	• • • • • •		
Platinum	.8	0–2	• • • •		
Thallium	.6	0–14	•		
Thorium	.4	0–12	•		
Tin	1.4	0–6	• • •		
Tungsten	.8	0–23	•		
Uranium	.3	0–1	• • • •		

OTHER TESTS

	Result (mg/dl)	Reference Range* (mg/dl)	2 SD Low	1 SD Low	Mean	1 SD High	2 SD High
Creatinine	23.1	60–160	• • •	• • • •	• • • •	•	

Methodology: Analyzed by Induction Coupled Plasma Mass Spectrometry (ICP-MS). Creatinine by Jaffe Method. "dl" =detection limit.
*No safe levels established

Comments:
   (Post provocative challenge).

Table 1

This patient had DMPS chelations done once a month for four months. Following the fourth chelation, she was asked to collect her urine over a two-hour period. Her urine test results showed that the mercury level had dropped to 12— approximately *half the level* of the first chelation—but it was still above the reference range (see Table 2).

Subsequent chelations removed more mercury from her system. She tried the yeast-killer again. This time, she made it through the process without any major aggravation. Her bowels started working more consistently, and her hypersensitivities dropped off considerably. Her frequency of urinating every 15 minutes decreased to every two hours. And as she began to get more sleep, she was able to get a job teaching art at night school—a remarkable change in someone who had been struggling for so long without any improvement. She is not

ELEMENTS REGARDED AS TOXIC

Elements	per gram Creatinine Result (µg/g creatinine)	Reference Range* (µg/g creatinine)	Per 24-hour Result (µg/24-hour)	Reference Range* (µg/24-hour)		Elevated	Very Elevated
Aluminum	32	0–35	23	0–37	• • •		
Antimony	<dl	0–5	<dl	0–7			
Arsenic	100	0–100	72	0–140	• •		
Beryllium	<dl	0–.5	<dl	0–.6			
Bismuth	<dl	0–30	<dl	0–30			
Cadmium	1.7	0–2	1.2	0–3	• •		
Lead	1.3	0–15	.9	0–20	•		
Mercury	12	0–3	8.2	0–5	• • • • •	• • •	• •
Nickel	11	0–12	7.9	0–20	• •		
Platinum	<dl	0–2	<dl	0–2			
Thallium	.1	0–14	.1	0–14	•		
Thorium	<dl	0–12	<dl	0–13			
Tin	<dl	0–6	<dl	0–11			
Tungsten	<dl	0–23	<dl	0–22			
Uranium	<dl	0–1	<dl	0–2			

OTHER TESTS

	Result (g/24-hours)	Reference Range* (g/24-hours)	2 SD Low	1 SD Low	Mean	1 SD High	2 SD High
Creatinine	.708	.9–1.6	•	• • • •	• • •	• •	

Methodology: Analyzed by Induction Coupled Plasma Mass Spectrometry (ICP-MS). Creatinine by Jaffe Method. "dl" =detection limit. *No safe levels established

Comments:
  (Post provocative challenge.) high 24 hour volume

Table 2

"cured" in the sense that her knee damage is permanent—so she still needs a cane—and she is still much more sensitive to chemicals than the average person, but she is able to work creatively. She probably has more mercury in her body to deal with.

I had known for a long time that the main improvements in chronic health problems were found after patients finished taking a yeast-killer; but I had also known that some people had extreme difficulty during the yeast die-off period. After seeing the results with this patient, I began to realize that the metals played a significant role in the chronicity of her yeast problem.

Another one of my patients had stubborn chronic health problems that weren't responding to treatment. She had approximately ten mercury-amalgam fillings replaced, and had a DMPS chelation, followed by a 24-hour urine sample. The results showed no significant amounts of metals in her urine (see Table 3).

ELEMENTS REGARDED AS TOXIC

Elements	Result (µg/g creatinine)	Reference Range* (µg/g creatinine)	Result (µg/24-hour)	Reference Range* (µg/24-hour)		Elevated	Very Elevated
Aluminum	<dl	0–35	<dl	0–37			
Antimony	.2	0–5	.3	0–7	•		
Arsenic	28	0–100	31	0–140	•		
Beryllium	<dl	0–.5	<dl	0–.6			
Bismuth	.4	0–30	.4	0–30	•		
Cadmium	1.2	0–2	1.3	0–3	•	• •	
Lead	6.1	0–15	6.8	0–20	•	•	
Mercury	3.7	0–3	4	0–5	•	• •	•
Nickel	3	0–12	3.3	0–20	•		
Platinum	.1	0–2	.1	0–2	•		
Thallium	.3	0–14	.4	0–14	•		
Thorium	.1	0–12	.2	0–13	•		
Tin	2.5	0–6	2.8	0–11	•		
Tungsten	<dl	0–23	<dl	0–22			
Uranium	0	0–1	0	0–2	•		

OTHER TESTS

	Result (g/24-hours)	Reference Range* (g/24-hours)	2 SD Low	1 SD Low	Mean	1 SD High	2 SD High
Creatinine	1.11	.9–1.6		• • • •			

Methodology: Analyzed by Induction Coupled Plasma Mass Spectrometry (ICP-MS). Creatinine by Jaffe Method. "dl" =detection limit.
*No safe levels established

Comments:
(Post provocative challenge.) high 24 hour volume

Table 3

　　I told her that she obviously hadn't accumulated any metals in her body from her fillings, and therefore she didn't need to do any more DMPS chelations. She responded vehemently *that I was out of my mind*—she had done her research and knew that anybody who had ten mercury fillings for many years must be filled with mercury. She insisted that another chelation be done in a month, and that I had better find a way to get those metals out of her, because I obviously wasn't doing my job!

　　I thought about the fact that DMPS was a sulfur compound, and that brought the realization that maybe her body was so deficient in sulfur that it was stealing the sulfur from the DMPS chelation—before it could bind the metals. With this in mind, we increased her intake of **whey protein powder**, which is a good source of cysteine—a sulfur-containing amino acid— and **Methyl-Sulfonyl-Methane (MSM)**, which is a naturally occurring sulfur compound that is used as a dietary supplement. In a month, she had another DMPS chelation, followed by a 24-hour urine sample (see Table 4).

ELEMENTS REGARDED AS TOXIC

Elements	Result (µg/g creatinine)	Reference Range* (µg/g creatinine)	Result (µg/24-hour)	Reference Range* (µg/24-hour)		Elevated	Very Elevated
Aluminum	6.9	0–35	6.8	0–37	•		
Antimony	.1	0–5	.1	0–7	•		
Arsenic	400	0–100	390	0–140	• • • • •	• •	•
Beryllium	<dl	0–.5	<dl	0–.6			
Bismuth	<dl	0–30	<dl	0–30			
Cadmium	.4	0–2	.4	0–3	•		
Lead	8	0–15	7.8	0–20	• •		
Mercury	7.7	0–3	7.5	0–5	• • • •	• •	•
Nickel	7.8	0–12	7.6	0–20	• •		
Platinum	<dl	0–2	<dl	0–2			
Thallium	<dl	0–14	<dl	0–14			
Thorium	<dl	0–12	<dl	0–13			
Tin	1.7	0–6	1.6	0–11	•		
Tungsten	.3	0–23	.3	0–22	•		
Uranium	<dl	0–1	<dl	0–2			

OTHER TESTS

	Result (g/24-hours)	Reference Range* (g/24-hours)	2 SD Low	1 SD Low	Mean	1 SD High	2 SD High
Creatinine	.974	.9–1.6	• •	• • •	• •		

Methodology: Analyzed by Induction Coupled Plasma Mass Spectrometry (ICP-MS). Creatinine by Jaffe Method.
"dl" =detection limit.
*No safe levels established

Comments:
(Post provocative challenge.)

Table 4

This time, arsenic and mercury showed up in her urine. She continued taking the whey and MSM, and repeated the chelation after another month. This time, the chelation was followed by a *two-hour* urine sample (see Table 5).

ELEMENTS REGARDED AS TOXIC

Elements	Result (µg/g creatinine)	per gram Creatinine Reference Range* (µg/g creatinine)	Within Ref. Range	Elevated	Very Elevated
Aluminum	7.8	0–35	• • •		
Antimony	.3	0–5	•		
Arsenic	30	0–100	• • • •		
Beryllium	<dl	0–.5			
Bismuth	<dl	0–30			
Cadmium	1.1	0–2	• • • • • •		
Lead	30	0–15	• • • • • • • • • •	• • • •	
Mercury	34	0–3	• • • • • • • • •	• • • • • • • • • • • • •	• • • • • •
Nickel	4.5	0–12	• • • • •		
Platinum	<dl	0–2			
Thallium	.2	0–14	•		
Thorium	<dl	0–12			
Tin	4	0–6	• • • • • • •		
Tungsten	0	0–23	•		
Uranium	<dl	0–1			

OTHER TESTS

	Result (mg/dl)	Reference Range* (mg/dl)	2 SD Low	1 SD Low	Mean	1 SD High	2 SD High
Creatinine	46.7	60–160	• •	• • •	• • • •	• •	

Methodology: Analyzed by Induction Coupled Plasma Mass Spectrometry (ICP-MS). Creatinine by Jaffe Method. "dl" =detection limit. *No safe levels established

Comments:
  (Post provocative challenge).

Table 5

Test results from two-hour urine samples tend to show much higher levels of metals than 24-hour urine tests because most of the DMPS is excreted within the first two to six hours following the chelation injection. And of course, a two-hour urine sample is much easier to collect than a 24-hour urine sample. Likely, a six-hour urine test would be the most accurate, but I didn't know this at the time.

The arsenic that had appeared previously in her urine had virtually disappeared, and the mercury—which had shown itself so reluctantly on the second chelation—now revealed itself brazenly. So the lady *did* have a hidden load of metals—particularly mercury. Not until her body was saturated with sulfur compounds could the chelation sulfur make it down to the Mother Lode of metal, deep within her body, and begin to push it out through the urine.

From this insight, I began to recommend sulfur supplements more frequently. Whey was the one I suggested most often—usually along with MSM—but I also recommended N-acetylcysteine for a few patients. In some stubborn cases, I recommended stabilized glutathione (Recancostat®).

Later, I read studies that showed that when cysteine binds to mercury, it resembles the structure of the amino acid methionine, and could be transported directly into the brain. Using the sulfur-containing amino acid methionine is apparently a good way to block the transfer of mercury into the brain and provide much-needed sulfur, as well. For this reason, the amino acid levels of the patient, particularly methionine levels, should be monitored.

I tell my patients that they should not take whey powder or MSM at the same time as having DMPS chelation, because the sulfurs (from the whey or MSM) may "trip" the mercury into the brain. I suggest that they take the nutritional sulfurs only on days when they don't take the chelation sulfur, or at opposite ends of the day, at least 12 hours apart—or better yet, use methionine.

Mineral levels—especially those of zinc—should also be monitored. DMPS won't create a zinc deficiency in a person with normal mineral levels. People with heavy metal toxicity, however, are likely to already have low zinc levels—which should be monitored regularly before, during, and after chelation, because DMPS could remove enough zinc to create a wide range of symptoms.

Other patients that I had previously considered "difficult"—those who weren't achieving complete or long-lasting results—consistently showed low sulfur levels when tested, which I now interpreted as a suspicion that they had high levels of metals in their bodies.

To find out what types and quantities of metals might be the problem, I recommended that they have their mercury fillings replaced so that they could have a DMPS challenge. I had suggested that patients have their fillings replaced by dentists specially trained and equipped for safe removal of mercury, but several patients said they would just go to their regular dentists because they were nice people who would be able to do a good job.

Three of my patients went to three different dentists who all said I was crazy for recommending removal of the patients' amalgams—these dentists insisted there was nothing wrong with mercury-amalgam fillings! After the patients said they would go elsewhere to have the work done, all three dentists reluctantly agreed to replace the fillings.

Because the dentists apparently didn't believe that any mercury toxicity was involved in removing these fillings, they didn't use a rubber dam. The patients swallowed bits and chunks of the debris, and inhaled tremendous quantities of mercury vapour during the removal process.

One of the patients threw up bile for a week afterward; another was virtually paralyzed for a week, from the waist down. The third patient's arthritis—which had been completely relieved on my program—began to flare up. This motivated me to re-emphasize the necessity of having mercury-amalgam fillings replaced *only by dentists aware of the toxicity of mercury fillings*, and who know how to minimize the absorption of mercury particles and mercury vapour.

The results of recommending extra sulfur before undergoing DMPS chelations quickly became apparent, as is shown here in the urine tests of a number of different patients (see Tables 6–10).

ELEMENTS REGARDED AS TOXIC

Elements	Result (µg/g creatinine)	Reference Range* (µg/g creatinine)	Within Ref. Range	Elevated	Very Elevated
Aluminum	<dl	0–35			
Antimony	.3	0–5	•		
Arsenic	89	0–100	• • • • • • •		
Beryllium	<dl	0–.5			
Bismuth	<dl	0–30			
Cadmium	.9	0–2	• • • • •		
Lead	12	0–15	• • • • • •		
Mercury	61	0–3	• • • • • •	• • • • • • • • • • •	• • • • •
Nickel	3.4	0–12	• • • •		
Platinum	<dl	0–2			
Thallium	.2	0–14	•		
Thorium	<dl	0–12			
Tin	14	0–6	• • • • • • • •		
Tungsten	<dl	0–23			
Uranium	<dl	0–1			

OTHER TESTS

	Result (mg/dl)	Reference Range* (mg/dl)	2 SD Low	1 SD Low	Mean	1 SD High	2 SD High
Creatinine	205	60–160			• • • • •	• • • •	• •

Methodology: Analyzed by Induction Coupled Plasma Mass Spectrometry (ICP-MS). Creatinine by Jaffe Method. "dl" =detection limit.
*No safe levels established

Comments:
(Post provocative challenge.) pH=8; results checked by repeat analysis

Table 6

ELEMENTS REGARDED AS TOXIC

Elements	Result (µg/g creatinine)	Reference Range* (µg/g creatinine)	Within Ref. Range	Elevated	Very Elevated
Aluminum	<dl	0–35			
Antimony	1	0–5	• •		
Arsenic	39	0–100	• • • •		
Beryllium	<dl	0–.5			
Bismuth	1.5	0–30	•		
Cadmium	2.6	0–2	• • • • • • • • •	• • • •	
Lead	30	0–15	• • • • • • • • •	• • • •	
Mercury	54	0–3	• • • • • • • •	• • • • • • • •	• • • • •
Nickel	7.2	0–12	• • • • •		
Platinum	.6	0–2	• • • •		
Thallium	.9	0–14	•		
Thorium	.6	0–12	•		
Tin	10	0–6	• • • • • • •	• • •	
Tungsten	.6	0–23	•		
Uranium	.5	0–1	• • • • •		

OTHER TESTS

	Result (mg/dl)	Reference Range* (mg/dl)	2 SD Low	1 SD Low	Mean	1 SD High	2 SD High
Creatinine	39.9	60–160	• •	• • • •	• • • •	•	

Methodology: Analyzed by Induction Coupled Plasma Mass Spectrometry (ICP-MS). Creatinine by Jaffe Method. "dl" =detection limit.
*No safe levels established

Comments:
(Post provocative challenge.) lead and mercury checked

Table 7

ELEMENTS REGARDED AS TOXIC

Elements	Result (µg/g creatinine)	Reference Range* (µg/g creatinine)	Within Ref. Range	Elevated	Very Elevated
Aluminum	<dl	0–35			
Antimony	.3	0–5	•		
Arsenic	160	0–100	• • • • • • • • •	• •	
Beryllium	<dl	0–.5			
Bismuth	.6	0–30	•		
Cadmium	1	0–2	• • • •		
Lead	23	0–15	• • • • • • • •	• •	
Mercury	120	0–3	• • • • • •	• • • • • • • • • • • • •	• • •
Nickel	3.8	0–12	• • •		
Platinum	<dl	0–2			
Thallium	.3	0–14	•		
Thorium	<dl	0–12			
Tin	15	0–6	• • • • • • • •	• • • •	
Tungsten	<dl	0–23			
Uranium	<dl	0–1			

OTHER TESTS

	Result (mg/dl)	Reference Range* (mg/dl)	2 SD Low	1 SD Low	Mean	1 SD High	2 SD High
Creatinine	121	60–160				• •	• •

Methodology: Analyzed by Induction Coupled Plasma Mass Spectrometry (ICP-MS). Creatinine by Jaffe Method.
"dl" =detection limit.
*No safe levels established

Comments:
(Post provocative challenge.) results checked by repeat analysis

Table 8

ELEMENTS REGARDED AS TOXIC

Elements	Result (µg/g creatinine)	Reference Range* (µg/g creatinine)	Within Ref. Range	Elevated	Very Elevated
Aluminum	12	0–35	• • •		
Antimony	.3	0–5	•		
Arsenic	230	0–100	• • • • • • • •	• • •	
Beryllium	<dl	0–.5			
Bismuth	<dl	0–30			
Cadmium	1.1	0–2	• • • • •		
Lead	35	0–15	• • • • • • • •	• • • • •	
Mercury	110	0–3	• • • • • • • • • •	• • • • • • • • • • • •	• • • •
Nickel	4.1	0–12	• • • •		
Platinum	<dl	0–2			
Thallium	.2	0–14	•		
Thorium	<dl	0–12			
Tin	7.1	0–6	• • • • • • • •	•	
Tungsten	.2	0–23	•		
Uranium	<dl	0–1			

OTHER TESTS

	Result (mg/dl)	Reference Range* (mg/dl)	2 SD Low	1 SD Low	Mean	1 SD High	2 SD High
Creatinine	55	60–160	• • • •	• • • •	• •		

Methodology: Analyzed by Induction Coupled Plasma Mass Spectrometry (ICP-MS). Creatinine by Jaffe Method.
"dl" =detection limit.
*No safe levels established

Comments:
(Post provocative challenge.)

Table 9

ELEMENTS REGARDED AS TOXIC

Elements	Result (µg/g creatinine)	per gram Creatinine Reference Range* (µg/g creatinine)	Within Ref. Range	Elevated	Very Elevated
Aluminum	<dl	0–35			
Antimony	.1	0–5	•		
Arsenic	300	0–100	• • • • • • •	• •	
Beryllium	<dl	0–.5			
Bismuth	<dl	0–30			
Cadmium	1.6	0–2	• • • • • •		
Lead	9.9	0–15	• • • • •		
Mercury	440	0–3	• • • • • •	• • • • • • • •	• • • •
Nickel	8.6	0–12	• • • • • •		
Platinum	<dl	0–2			
Thallium	<dl	0–14	•		
Thorium	<dl	0–12			
Tin	7.6	0–6	• • • • • • •		
Tungsten	6.6	0–23	• •		
Uranium	<dl	0–1			

OTHER TESTS

	Result (mg/dl)	Reference Range* (mg/dl)	2 SD Low	1 SD Low	Mean	1 SD High	2 SD High
Creatinine	103	60–160			• • •		

Methodology: Analyzed by Induction Coupled Plasma Mass Spectrometry (ICP-MS). Creatinine by Jaffe Method. "dl" =detection limit.
*No safe levels established

Comments:
(Post provocative challenge.) Mercury checked

Table 10

Not only were all my "difficult" patients showing high levels of heavy metals in their bodies, mercury was showing as the most abundant and the most persistent metal. As more and more of my patients had DMPS treatments, it became clear that not only those with chronic health problems showed high levels of mercury; anyone who had ever had mercury fillings in his or her life was showing high levels of mercury—even if the individual had had them replaced years ago. I decided to get tested myself.

As a child, I lived up the coast of British Columbia where there was no road access. The dentist used to come by boat several times a year. If you were a good patient, he would give you a sucker and a pat on the head, and say, "I'll see you in six months." He'd appear six months later and, like magic, I'd always have another molar or two that needed filling. I was so happy that he could find those cavities so that I could get another sucker.

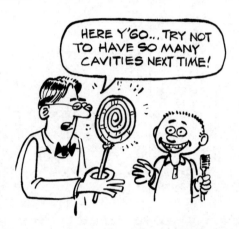

All my major molars had been filled with mercury amalgams in childhood. By my early 40s (ten years ago), the fillings were starting to break apart. Around this time, a patient came in who had been diagnosed with MS of the jaw. A look in her mouth revealed a large number of blackened old mercury-amalgam fillings. My passing comment was that perhaps she should consider having them replaced, because some research had implicated metal toxicity in MS. She had her mercury fillings replaced when she started on my program, and within a few months, her MS symptoms were gone.

Because my own fillings were in need of replacement, I asked my dentist to remove them, and replace them with non-mercury fillings. He thought that would be impossible, because the mercury was about the only thing holding my molars together. Without the support of the metal, the teeth would break apart. I insisted, and he reluctantly said he'd try to replace them with composite fillings, with which he hadn't had much experience.

These white plastic fillings cracked within a few years, so I went to a dentist who specialized in composite fillings. When he drilled out the failed composites, he found that the previous dentist had left large amounts of mercury underneath as a foundation—no doubt thinking he was doing me a favour. These mercury leftovers were removed, and new white composites were put in their place. I've had no trouble with them for ten years, other than an initial sensitivity to hot and cold temperatures, which eventually passed.

So the MS patient and I had had our amalgam fillings replaced with non-mercury fillings ten years ago, and I never thought any more of it. I didn't have enough proof of the benefits of removing mercury-amalgam fillings to recommend that other patients do the same. Anyway, in addition to having my mercury fillings replaced, I'd also taken a number of oral supplements like cilantro, chlorella, and pectin—which, at that time, were believed to remove metals from the body. I thought that over this many years, whatever metals might have accumulated in the past would now be gone—but decided I should do a DMPS challenge, just to make sure.

Because the urine sample taken *before* the DMPS injections had not shown significant metals in the first six patients, I had long since stopped recommending it for my patients. I did, however, collect a urine sample over the 24 hours following my first DMPS. My results are shown in Table 11.

You can see that all of the metals are within the reference range except for one—mercury. Removing my mercury fillings years ago obviously hadn't removed all the mercury from my body. While I didn't have any major symptoms to attribute to my mercury levels, this was probably because I followed my own dietary recommendations quite rigidly; I know from experience that if I stray from THE EATING ALIVE PROGRAM at all, I soon feel unwell.

Another of my patients, a 76-year old woman, had 12 DMPS chelations over a 12-month period. The two-hour urine results following her first, sixth, and 12th chelations—indicating a decline in mercury levels—are shown in Tables 12 to 14.

ELEMENTS REGARDED AS TOXIC

Elements	per gram Creatinine Result (µg/g creatinine)	Reference Range* (µg/g creatinine)	Per 24-hour Result (µg/24-hour)	Reference Range* (µg/24-hour)		Elevated	Very Elevated
Aluminum	<dl	0–35	5.6	0–37	•		
Antimony	.3	0–5	.6	0–7	•		
Arsenic	19	0–100	40	0–140	•		
Beryllium	<dl	0–.5	<dl	0–.6			
Bismuth	<dl	0–30	<dl	0–30			
Cadmium	.6	0–2	1.2	0–3	• •		
Lead	1.1	0–15	2.2	0–20	•		
Mercury	9.6	0–3	20	0–5	• • • • •	• • • •	• • • • • •
Nickel	5	0–12	10	0–20	• • •		
Platinum	<dl	0–2	<dl	0–2			
Thallium	.2	0–14	.3	0–14	•		
Thorium	<dl	0–12	<dl	0–13			
Tin	2	0–6	4.2	0–11	• •		
Tungsten	<dl	0–23	.1	0–22	•		
Uranium	<dl	0–1	<dl	0–2			

OTHER TESTS

	Result (g/24-hours)	Reference Range* (g/24-hours)	2 SD Low	1 SD Low	Mean	1 SD High	2 SD High
Creatinine	2.08	1.1–2.8			• • •		

Methodology: Analyzed by Induction Coupled Plasma Mass Spectrometry (ICP-MS). Creatinine by Jaffe Method.
"dl" =detection limit.
*No safe levels established

Comments:
(Post provocative challenge.) Initial pH=8.0

Table 11

ELEMENTS REGARDED AS TOXIC

Elements	per gram Creatinine Result (µg/g creatinine)	Reference Range* (µg/g creatinine)	Within Ref. Range	Elevated	Very Elevated
Aluminum	34	0–35	• • • • • • • • •		
Antimony	1.7	0–5	• • • • •		
Arsenic	66	0–100	• • • • • •		
Beryllium	<dl	0–.5			
Bismuth	2.5	0–30	•		
Cadmium	3	0–2	• • • • • • • • •	• • •	
Lead	37	0–15	• • • • • • • • •	• • • •	
Mercury	110	0–3	• • • • • • • •	• • • • • • • • •	• • • • •
Nickel	1.9	0–12	• •		
Platinum	.6	0–2	• • •		
Thallium	1.7	0–14	•		
Thorium	1.6	0–12	•		
Tin	2.8	0–6	• • • • • •		
Tungsten	3.4	0–23	• •		
Uranium	<dl	0–1			

OTHER TESTS

	Result (mg/dl)	Reference Range* (mg/dl)	2 SD Low	1 SD Low	Mean	1 SD High	2 SD High
Creatinine	17.7	60–160	• • •	• • •	• • • •	• •	

Methodology: Analyzed by Induction Coupled Plasma Mass Spectrometry (ICP-MS). Creatinine by Jaffe Method.
"dl" =detection limit.
*No safe levels established

Comments:
(Post provocative challenge.)

Table 12

ELEMENTS REGARDED AS TOXIC

Elements	Result (µg/g creatinine)	Reference Range* (µg/g creatinine)	Within Ref. Range	Elevated	Very Elevated
Aluminum	<dl	0–35			
Antimony	<dl	0–5			
Arsenic	130	0–100			
Beryllium	<dl	0–.5			
Bismuth	<dl	0–30			
Cadmium	1.8	0–2			
Lead	31	0–15			
Mercury	57	0–3			
Nickel	20	0–12			
Platinum	<dl	0–2			
Thallium	<dl	0–14			
Thorium	<dl	0–12			
Tin	2.7	0–6			
Tungsten	<dl	0–23			
Uranium	<dl	0–1			

per gram Creatinine

OTHER TESTS

	Result (mg/dl)	Reference Range* (mg/dl)	2 SD Low	1 SD Low	Mean	1 SD High	2 SD High
Creatinine	30.3	60–160					

Methodology: Analyzed by Induction Coupled Plasma Mass Spectrometry (ICP-MS). Creatinine by Jaffe Method. "dl" =detection limit.
*No safe levels established

Comments:
(Post provocative challenge.)

Table 13

ELEMENTS REGARDED AS TOXIC

Elements	Result (µg/g creatinine)	Reference Range* (µg/g creatinine)	Within Ref. Range	Elevated	Very Elevated
Aluminum	<dl	0–35			
Antimony	.1	0–5			
Arsenic	79	0–100			
Beryllium	<dl	0–.5			
Bismuth	<dl	0–30			
Cadmium	1.1	0–2			
Lead	21	0–15			
Mercury	27	0–3			
Nickel	2.7	0–12			
Platinum	<dl	0–2			
Thallium	.2	0–14			
Thorium	<dl	0–12			
Tin	2	0–6			
Tungsten	<dl	0–23			
Uranium	<dl	0–1			

per gram Creatinine

OTHER TESTS

	Result (mg/dl)	Reference Range* (mg/dl)	2 SD Low	1 SD Low	Mean	1 SD High	2 SD High
Creatinine	42.9	60–160					

Methodology: Analyzed by Induction Coupled Plasma Mass Spectrometry (ICP-MS). Creatinine by Jaffe Method. "dl" =detection limit.
*No safe levels established

Comments:
(Post provocative challenge.)

Table 14

One of my patients had been diagnosed at the age of 16 as paranoid schizophrenic, and branded as "retarded." She had been institutionalized at times, and had been on various psychiatric medications for the last 40 years or so. She followed my treatment program; by the time she finished her yeast-killer, she'd also had her mercury fillings replaced and had had six DMPS chelations. (Two of her urine test results are shown in Tables 15 and 16.)

ELEMENTS REGARDED AS TOXIC

Elements	per gram Creatinine Result (µg/g creatinine)	Reference Range* (µg/g creatinine)	Within Ref. Range	Elevated	Very Elevated
Aluminum	<dl	0–35			
Antimony	.7	0–5	• •		
Arsenic	71	0–100	• • • • • •		
Beryllium	<dl	0–.5			
Bismuth	<dl	0–30			
Cadmium	1.6	0–2	• • • • • • • •		
Lead	28	0–15	• • • • • • • • •	• • •	
Mercury	96	0–3	• • • • • • • • •	• • • • • • • • • •	• • • • • •
Nickel	3.9	0–12	• • •		
Platinum	<dl	0–2			
Thallium	.3	0–14	•		
Thorium	<dl	0–12			
Tin	8.4	0–6	• • • • • • • • •		
Tungsten	.3	0–23	•		
Uranium	<dl	0–1			

OTHER TESTS

	Result (mg/dl)	Reference Range* (mg/dl)	2 SD Low	1 SD Low	Mean	1 SD High	2 SD High
Creatinine	54	60–160	•	• • • • • • •	•		

Methodology: Analyzed by Induction Coupled Plasma Mass Spectrometry (ICP-MS). Creatinine by Jaffe Method. "dl" =detection limit.
*No safe levels established

Comments:
(Post provocative challenge.)

Table 15

ELEMENTS REGARDED AS TOXIC

Elements	Result (µg/g creatinine)	per gram Creatinine Reference Range* (µg/g creatinine)	Within Ref. Range	Elevated	Very Elevated
Aluminum	<dl	0–35			
Antimony	.7	0–5	• •		
Arsenic	73	0–100	• • • • • •		
Beryllium	<dl	0–.5			
Bismuth	.2	0–30	•		
Cadmium	1.5	0–2	• • • • • •		
Lead	19	0–15	• • • • • • • • •	•	
Mercury	11	0–3	• • • • • • • •	• • • • • • • •	• • • • • •
Nickel	1.1	0–12	•		
Platinum	<dl	0–2			
Thallium	.1	0–14	•		
Thorium	<dl	0–12			
Tin	4.7	0–6	• • • • • • •		
Tungsten	.2	0–23	•		
Uranium	<dl	0–1			

OTHER TESTS

	Result (mg/dl)	Reference Range* (mg/dl)	2 SD Low	1 SD Low	Mean	1 SD High	2 SD High
Creatinine	75.6	60–160		• • • • •	• •		

Methodology: Analyzed by Induction Coupled Plasma Mass Spectrometry (ICP-MS). Creatinine by Jaffe Method. "dl" =detection limit. *No safe levels established

Comments: (Post provocative challenge.)

Table 16

How did she feel? She was clearheaded, bright, and stable— as long as she stayed on her dietary program. She wanted to start a business, but a 40-year record of mental illness doesn't make you a prime candidate for a bank loan. (You can read her letter at the end of this chapter.)

Although I learned later that removing the amalgam fillings wasn't immediately necessary, at this point I was still encouraging my patients to have their amalgam fillings replaced in preparation for the DMPS removal of their accumulated mercury. Meanwhile, I continued to review the research on toxic metals.

During the same time all this was happening, I received several phone calls from very irate dentists. They were basically calling me a psychopath for telling their patients to have their

harmless mercury fillings removed when there was no scientific
justification for doing so. These irate dentists insisted:

- that mercury amalgams had been used for 160 years
  with no scientific proof of any side-effects;
- that you get more mercury from eating a can of tuna;
- that they had personally used them for decades and
  had no symptoms; and
- that they'd had blood and hair tests done regularly
  that had never shown any sign of mercury in their
  systems.

One of them even called me a *quack,* although I couldn't see
how that could apply. The word quack comes from *quecksilber,*
the German word for quicksilver—which is slang for mercury.

Mercury has anti-bacterial properties. Some of the most
famous physicians of a few hundred years ago used mercury
for treating their patients. One of these medical doctors was
Benjamin Rush, one of the signers of the *Declaration of
Independence,* who was later the first Treasurer of the US Mint.

It is believed that Mozart was treated with mercury for
syphilis—it's uncertain whether his death was due to the
mercury medicine he was taking or to the syphilis itself.

Mercuric chloride was long used as a disinfectant until it was
finally banned due to its severe toxicity. Mercurous chloride,
otherwise known as "Calomel," was widely used as a purgative
and an anti-fungal until it, too, was banned. Mercurous chloride
was also used in teething powders in the 1940s. "Pink
disease"—which consisted of irritability; insomnia; rash;
sensitivity to light; and cold, painful, red, and swollen
extremities—disappeared after mercurous chloride-containing
teething powders were discontinued in 1953.[2] When I was a
child, "Mercurochrome"—a mercury-based antiseptic—would
immediately be applied to my cuts and abrasions.

Throughout history, as the toxicity of mercury became
apparent, it was banned. *Those who continued to use mercury in
spite of its known poisonous side-effects were called quacks.*

So, it seemed ironic for a dentist who was using mercury in
his daily practice to call *me* a quack for telling patients *not* to
use mercury.

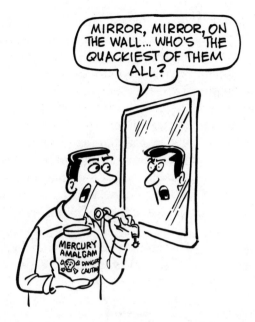

Obviously there was a giant discrepancy between these dentists' training and experience and what I was seeing in my practice. I told them I would put all the research I could find on mercury toxicity into this book, so they could better see the rationale for removing mercury fillings.

Mercury is the only element that is liquid at room temperature. This property, along with its metallic silvery appearance, gave it the name "liquid silver" or "quicksilver"—or in Latin, *Hydrargyrum* (water silver)—which was shortened to **Hg** to create its chemical abbreviation.

In ancient Roman mythology, each of the gods and goddesses was associated with a planet and a metal. Mercury (Mercurius), the god of Trade and Travel, was portrayed as having wings on his heels. He was associated with the *planet* Mercury, because of its quickness—it orbits the sun faster than any other planet—and the *metal* mercury, which runs so quickly.

Mercury has a strong attraction to sulfur; thus its main source is cinnabar ore—mercury sulphide—distinguished by its bright yellowish-red colour. Cinnabar ore is found only in low-temperature hot springs or volcanic areas, particularly in Spain. Two thousand years ago, slaves working in the Roman cinnabar mines were reported to quickly experience fatigue, shortness of breath, and digestive pain, soon followed by moodiness, tremors, and wasting.

The term "mad as a hatter" refers to the fact that felt hats were stiffened with mercury for shaping, with the result that years of exposure to mercury was observed to make old hatters moody, emotionally unstable, and somewhat confused. In *Alice in Wonderland*, by Lewis Carroll, the Mad Hatter exhibited the behavioural and neurological effects of exposure to mercury.

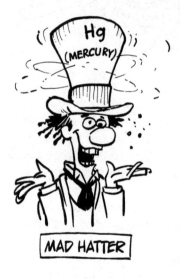

MAD HATTER

Alice in Wonderland was written in the mid-1860s—showing it was common knowledge that hatters were slowly being driven mad by mercury toxicity—*but mercury wasn't banned in the US hat-making industry until 1941; apparently the mercury was needed for the war industry.*

Gold had long been used in dentistry as a filler of dental cavities, but its main drawback was its expense, which made it more difficult for people with lower incomes to afford. Most people simply had the problem-tooth extracted. Perhaps this is why people in old photos never seemed to smile; they didn't want to show the gaps in their mouths.

While there were cheaper metals than gold, the main problem in using them to fill cavities was getting dissimilar metals to bond together, without using heat. Mercury is unique; at room temperature, it has the ability to bind dissimilar metals together.

This principle was first put to use in 1819 in England by Bell, and was fine-tuned in 1826 in Paris by Taveau, a dentist who found that mixing a variety of metals together with mercury allowed the metals to amalgamate into a paste, without heating. When this paste was inserted into the tooth cavity, it would harden into a tough, durable material. Thus was born the first silver amalgam filling.

Although it was called "silver" amalgam, only 35 percent was silver, and 50 percent was mercury. The rest of the compound consisted of zinc and copper. The early amalgam fillings tended to expand—thus cracking the tooth—but later, tin was added to solve this problem.

Amalgam fillings were introduced to North America in 1833 by the French brothers Crawcour, but the predominant dental association of the day—the **American Society of Dental Surgeons**—which had long used gold for fillings, banned the use of amalgam fillings in 1840 because of the known toxicity of mercury. Any member of the American Society of Dental Surgeons who was caught using mercury-amalgam fillings would be charged with malpractice. In 1848, the Society suspended 11 of its New York members for using mercury-amalgam fillings.[3]

Some dentists, however, must have surreptitiously experimented with these banned fillings, and found them extremely convenient to use and considerably cheaper than gold. The **American Dental Association (ADA)** was formed in 1859; it permitted members to use mercury-amalgam fillings. In 1984, the ADA continued to justify the use of amalgams by claiming that **"when mercury is combined with the metals used in dental amalgam, its toxic properties are made harmless,"**[4] though little proof of this bold statement has been offered.

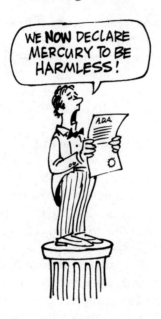

On this premise, the North American and European dental associations have been allowing dentists to insert mercury into the mouths of children and adults—not without controversy, however, as shown by an article on mercury fillings in the *Chicago Medical Journal*, in 1873. It stated: **"Neither Asiatic cholera, nor smallpox, nor any malarious disease, is doing half the mischief in the world that is done by this poisoning."** Little attention was paid to this type of statement because there was no scientific evidence to back it up.

In 1926, Alfred Stock of Germany—one of the world's leading chemists and a contributor to chemical nomenclature—published *The Dangers of Mercury Fumes*, which showed that the vapours from mercury fillings were more absorbable than the metal itself. Stock did an extensive series of experiments on mercury and its effects on people. He found that while some people could work in a room where they were exposed to 3 micrograms of mercury vapour per cubic metre of air for years without problems, he had become ill after a few hours of exposure to mercury vapour from his parquet floor, which gave off only 0.1 to 0.3 micrograms of mercury per cubic metre of air.

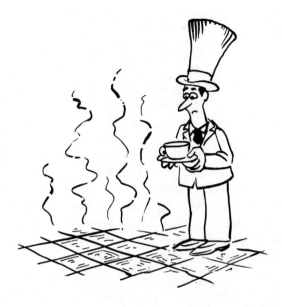

Stock personally inhaled air containing large quantities of mercury through his mouth, without experiencing any side-effects. However, if he inhaled just a few litres of air containing only small quantities of mercury—ten times less—*through his nose*, he soon suffered from dizziness, headaches, and nasal catarrh (inflammation of the mucous membranes).

In an attempt to determine how such small quantities of mercury could cause dramatic poisoning symptoms, he did studies on dogs and terminal cancer patients, exposing them to mercury vapours via the nose and doing autopsies after their deaths. The mercury was found to have accumulated to the greatest extent in the pituitary gland and the olfactory bulb portions of the brain—indicating a direct pathway of absorption of mercury vapours from the nose to the brain, via the nerves of smell.

Stock suffered from chronic mercury poisoning. He worked in a laboratory that had mercury-containing analytical devices; he therefore had a high level of exposure to mercury vapours. However, he concluded that this high intermittent exposure was not as detrimental as the lower levels he inhaled constantly from his amalgam fillings. It was only after he moved to a "mercury-clean" lab and had his mercury fillings replaced that his health improved.[5]

He proposed that there is a state of mercury toxicity that can occur from chronic exposure to even very low levels of mercury, and this results in predominantly mental symptoms. This became known as **"micro-mercurialism,"** a phrase coined by Russian researcher Trachktenberg. Symptoms include nervous irritability; excitability; moodiness; unpredictable outbursts of anger; concentration problems; inability to do intellectual work; shyness; introversion; lack of self-confidence; and depression.[6]

In 1937, Stock stated: **"In spite of my extreme hypersensitivity to mercury vapour, I don't have a general hypersensitivity to mercury as shown by the skin test."** This shows that the most common allergy test—skin-patch testing—isn't a reliable indicator for sensitivity to mercury.

In a 1928 German medical journal, Professor Fleischmann described cases in which a number of people with amalgam-related illnesses had recovered after removal of amalgam fillings.[7]

This research in Germany on the negative health effects of dental amalgams was leading toward the banning of mercury fillings in the late 1930s. The advent of World War II, however, suddenly and dramatically increased their use. The poor dental health of most North American military recruits resulted in the first mass use of mercury fillings by military dentists. After the war, dentists used amalgams to fill the dental cavities of the North American civilian population. Over 100 million mercury fillings are now inserted into North American teeth per year. In fact, it's difficult to find an adult *without* them. Let's take a closer look at the research to see if increasing the use of mercury amalgams was an appropriate thing to do.

When I began writing this chapter, I had about 40 articles that I felt were pretty convincing for showing that mercury fillings were a big health problem—but when I found out about **Bernard Windham**, the number of available research articles immediately increased more than ten-fold.

Bernard Windham is a chemical engineer in Tallahassee, Florida, whose health took a big turn for the better when he removed mercury from his body years ago. Aware of the routine statement used by defenders of mercury amalgam that "there's no scientific research," Bernie has made it a hobby to compile mercury research that he finds. His article, **Facts about Mercury and Dental Amalgam**, cites over 600 references condensed into more than 450 numbered groups. In addition, he has written several smaller articles.

With his gracious permission, I've used information from Bernard Windham's articles, and have cited references from them. These are represented by index numbers that are underlined and in **bold type**; this is an example of how they look: **1**. Each of these index numbers correlates with one or more reference numbers from Bernard Windham's articles, which are listed at the back of the book, under Bernard Windham's References. Please note that all other references cited throughout the book are marked with normal superscripts; this is how *those* index numbers will look: [1]. The references are located at the back of the book, under References.

Because much of the material in Bernie's articles may be too scientific and detailed for the average reader, I'll clarify some of the most important concepts.

Elemental—also known as inorganic—mercury is the form of mercury with which many people are familiar because it is the "liquid silver" that used to be found in thermometers. Elemental mercury—which was used in the hat, mirror, and thermometer industries and is still used in mercury-amalgam fillings—is poorly absorbed by the body. It can, however, be converted into two forms that are much more absorbable and highly toxic: **methylmercury** and **mercury vapour**.

METHYLMERCURY

When elemental mercury is methylated by algae and bacteria in the ocean, methylmercury is created. It works its way up the food chain into fish, shellfish, and sea mammals, although methylmercury only accumulates to dangerous levels in large, old fish or fish that live in waters polluted with mercury.[8]

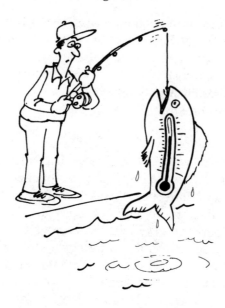

The bacteria and yeast in your mouth and intestine can also methylate elemental mercury into methylmercury,[1] which is readily absorbed through the gastrointestinal (GI) tract. Because the liver and kidneys are filters of the GI tract, they will be heavily exposed to methylmercury. Mercury can cause destruction of the stomach and intestinal lining, thereby altering permeability and adversely affecting bacterial populations, creating leaky gut syndrome and accumulation of Helicobacter pylori.[2] Helicobacter pylori is a bacteria found in the stomach in many people. If this bacteria gets under the stomach lining, the immune system's attack against it causes the damage associated with ulcers.

Methylmercury can also damage and weaken the immune system.[3] And Swedish professor Claes Ramel found that methylmercury is dramatically more destructive to DNA than any known carcinogenic chemical. (DNA is deoxyribonucleic acid; it's where your genetic information is stored.)

When methylmercury toxicity involves nerve symptoms, they tend to create difficulty in movement of limbs, and visual and hearing problems.

Methylmercury readily crosses both the blood-brain barrier and the placental barrier. When methylmercury passes into the placenta, it causes neurological damage to the fetus, such as cerebral palsy, seizures, and mental retardation.[9]

Of course, the standard rebuttal from dentists would be that people must have acquired methylmercury from eating too many cans of tuna.

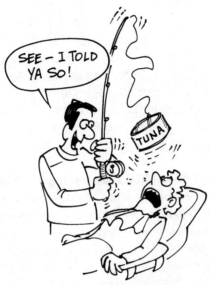

While large, long-lived fish have been known to accumulate high levels of methylmercury, the **tuna sold in cans** are usually smaller, shorter-lived albacore tuna whose levels of **methylmercury average 0.17 parts per million (ppm), far below the 1 ppm considered unsafe** by the Food and Drug Administration (FDA).[10] Studies show that **eating ocean fish increases the person's intake of selenium,**[11] and the **selenium from fish has been shown to reduce the toxicity of methylmercury from fish.**[12]

In another study, pregnant rats were exposed to two types of mercury: methylmercury—found in fish—and elemental mercury—found in dental amalgams. The rats' offspring were tested on reaching adulthood.

"The results show that, at the doses used, methylmercury alone did not affect the animals, while metallic mercury

caused a hyperactive behaviour and a slower learning.... . Extended selenium supplementation of the food prior to mating and throughout pregnancy counteracted the negative effects on behaviour caused by metallic methylmercury coexposure but not to metallic mercury only, indicating that selenium has an effect primarily on methylmercury." [13]

So nature has built a defence against mercury. We can eat small, short-lived ocean fish safely because nature has included a healthy dose of selenium in their make-up; selenium has protective properties against the methylmercury that these fish have accumulated. That pretty much refutes the notion that you'll get more mercury problems from a can of tuna than from mercury-amalgam fillings.

Studies have also found that the mercury showing in the urine after DMPS chelation is from amalgam fillings, not fish. In 1992, tests were done on **490 women** with **hormonal and infertility problems**. Only five had any history of occupational exposure to mercury, and their fish consumption was minimal.

On initial urine testing, 90 percent of mercury levels were below 5 micrograms. After DMPS chelation, a two-hour urine sample showed **all of them excreting mercury, lead, cadmium, copper, and arsenic—with mercury being the most predominant.** Urine mercury levels were over 100 micrograms in 25 percent of the women, and some were over 500 micrograms—an extremely high level.

Those women who showed high urine mercury after DMPS did a chewing gum saliva test. The women who had the most mercury-amalgam fillings also had the highest amounts of mercury in their saliva; the level was very high in women with ten or more amalgam fillings. **The conclusion is that bodily exposures to heavy metals play an important role in fertility disorders.** [14]

MERCURY VAPOUR

The average amalgam filling weighs 1 gram; about 50 percent of that amalgam is mercury. Thus, a filling contains approximately 0.5 grams (500,000 micrograms) of inorganic mercury. The dental associations generally consider the mercury in amalgams to be non-toxic. However, the vapour pressure of mercury causes it to continuously give off mercury vapour, which *is* toxic. As much as 50 percent (250,000 micrograms) of the mercury in a filling has been found to have vapourized within ten years, and 80 percent (400,000 micrograms) by 20 years.[4]

For people with mercury-amalgam fillings, the greatest source of systemic mercury intake is the mercury vapour coming from their amalgams.[5] The daily systemic intake from mercury vapour for a person with amalgam fillings is between 3 and 70 micrograms of mercury, with the average being at least 7 micrograms per day. [6] Most people with amalgams have daily exposure levels exceeding guideline levels set by government health organizations.[7]

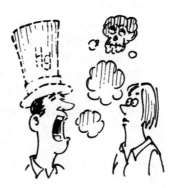

European studies have used saliva testing to measure mercury levels. It has been found that, on average, those with ten or more mercury fillings were exposed to more than ten times the mercury than those with no fillings.[8]

In another study, the DMPS challenge—three 100 mg DMPS capsules by mouth—was administered to college student volunteers with and without mercury-amalgam fillings. The results indicated that two-thirds of the mercury excreted in the urine of students with dental amalgams originated from the mercury vapour released from their amalgams.[15]

Some of the factors that increase the release of mercury vapours from amalgam fillings are: chewing (food or gum), bruxism (grinding of the teeth), hot foods and drinks, the acidity of foods and beverages, the presence of other metals in the mouth, and the brushing, drilling, and polishing of teeth.[16] For example, chewing gum or drinking hot liquids can produce ten to 100 times the normal levels of mercury exposure from amalgams.[2]

Polishing mercury-amalgam fillings increases the exposure to mercury vapour, for both the patient and the dental hygienist.[10] The use of high speed drills in the removal or replacement of amalgams increases the levels of mercury vapour and breathable particles; dental masks filter out only about 40 percent of these particles, and little of the mercury vapour.[11]

Mercury vapour that is swallowed in saliva may react with the hydrochloric acid (HCl) of the stomach, creating mercuric chloride—which, as mentioned earlier, was used in medicine for its antibacterial properties. Mercuric chloride can kill off your beneficial intestinal bacteria, allowing yeast and parasites to thrive. Also, by combining with the HCl of the stomach, there is less HCl available for the digestion of food, leading to heartburn, bloating, indigestion, and other digestive problems.[17]

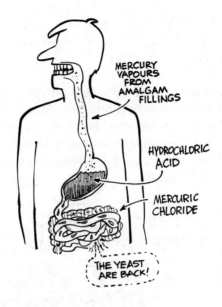

Some of the effects of mercury build-up in the mouth are gingivitis, oral lesions, burning mouth, mouth pain and discomfort, metal taste, chronic inflammation, lichen planus, autoimmune response, and cancer of the mouth.[12]

Mercury vapour readily crosses cell membranes and enters the blood from both the oral mucosa and the lungs.[18] Studies show that at least 80 percent of mercury vapour that reaches the lungs is absorbed and enters the blood.[13] Once in the bloodstream, mercury vapour binds to the hemoglobin of the red blood cells, thus reducing their oxygen-carrying capacity.[14] The red blood cells then deliver the mercury throughout the body, where it readily enters cells and accumulates in different organs.

Because the half-life of mercury vapour in the blood is ten seconds,[15] it will only show on blood tests if there is leakage of large amounts of mercury into the blood. Because hair grows from the blood supplied to it, hair tests will only show mercury if the blood has continually high levels of mercury over an extended period. Thus, the results of typical urine, blood, and hair tests are not accurate indicators of total mercury body burden.

Mercury inhibits the immune system, which can result in increased viral, bacterial, and fungal infections,[16] and increased bacterial resistance to antibiotics.[17]

Like methylmercury, mercury vapour readily crosses the blood-brain barrier into the central nervous system, especially the brain. Mercury vapour sometimes damages the blood-brain barrier on the way through,[18] allowing other toxins to enter, as well.[19] Once inside the blood-brain barrier, mercury is converted to a form that can't readily escape.

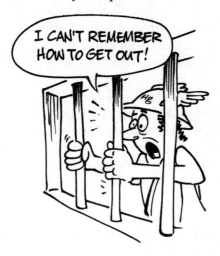

Mercury accumulates preferentially in the pituitary gland, hypothalamus, and occipital cortex of the brain, in direct proportion to the size and number of amalgam surfaces a person has.[20] Mercury has an effect on the functions of these areas. The pituitary gland plays a large role in hormonal balance—it is the master gland of the body because it influences other glands such as the adrenals, thyroid, and gonads. The hypothalamus is the major brain centre for regulation of internal body functions, and the occipital cortex is mainly involved in vision.

Patients who have diseases with memory-related symptoms have been found to have very high levels of mercury in areas of the brain associated with memory, such as the cerebral cortex and the hippocampus.[21]

The half-life of mercury in the brain is over 20 years, and chronic low levels of intake cause mercury to gradually accumulate in the tissues of the body.[22]

Mercury in the presence of other metals in the mouth undergoes galvanic action—the production of electrical currents flowing from one metal to a dissimilar metal—which increases the release of mercury vapours.[23] Therefore, **the claim by the ADA that "when mercury is combined with the metals used in dental amalgam, its toxic properties are made harmless" is actually incorrect. Dissimilar metals increase electrical activity which, in turn, releases more mercury vapour from fillings, dramatically increasing its toxicity.**

Corrosion induced by galvanic action deposits mercury into the gums, leaving an average deposit of 200 parts per million (ppm) near an amalgam filling.[24] The discharge of mercury vapour from amalgam fillings increases greatly if gold is used nearby, because of the galvanic action generated between dissimilar metals.[25] A gold cap on an amalgam filling could deposit 1,000 ppm of mercury in the nearby gum tissue,[26] while fish containing 1 ppm would be considered toxic and banned. So if cannibals lived among us, they would undoubtedly get mercury poisoning.

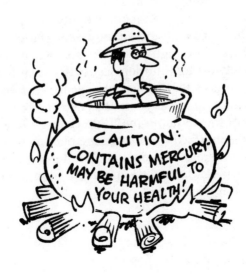

Newer amalgam fillings were developed. More copper was added to make the fillings less corrosive and less prone to fractures. They have, however, been found to be unstable when subjected to wear, polishing, chewing, and brushing; droplets of mercury form on the surface of the amalgams.[27] These high-copper amalgams can release up to 50 times more mercury and copper than conventional amalgams.[28] In the 1930s, German chemist Alfred Stock had already warned against the use of high amounts of copper in amalgams.

Nickel, such as is used in braces and crowns, is also a dissimilar metal that can generate galvanic action in proximity to amalgam fillings, and can therefore increase the release of mercury vapours. **Health Canada** has stated that **"new amalgam fillings should not be placed in contact with existing metal devices in the mouth, such as braces."** [19]

My personal experience was that after the installation of braces on my already amalgam-laden teeth, when I was about 12 years old, the lumbar area of my back (the kidney area) always felt cold. I used to lay with this part of my back directly on the heating vent in the floor, especially in the winter. Because it felt more comfortable there than being outside, I spent a lot of my time reading in this position.

By the end of grade 5, I had read virtually every book in the elementary school library—including the encyclopedias—so I was skipped ahead into high school. Incredibly shy, I wasn't emotionally ready for this sudden academic advance, although when I had my braces removed several years later, both the kidney sensitivity and my shyness lessened.

While some of these symptoms could be considered psychosomatic—due to the embarrassment of a "metalmouth" pubescent boy—there is a strong likelihood that the galvanic effect between the braces and the amalgam fillings increased the mercury load on my kidneys.

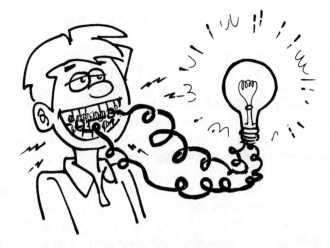

When the braces were removed, it was also found that most of my teeth had developed cavities at the gum line, which makes it even more likely that galvanic currents were at work.

The **Canadian Dental Association**'s position is, **"Galvanic effect, apart from its potential to contribute to heavy metal body burden, has not been demonstrated to be harmful... ."** [20]
So the dental association knows that galvanic action from dissimilar metals in your mouth could increase the amount of heavy metal in your body, but so what? They say, **"Scientific studies have not verified that dental amalgam is causing illness in the general population."** [21]

Let's take a look at some scientific studies to see if they agree that heavy metal body-burden is not harmful. Our first stop is at the **Karolinska Institute** in Sweden. The Karolinska Institute is Sweden's only medical university, with a budget of over two billion dollars per year, much of which comes from royalties on dynamite; it is devoted to academic research on health care. The Karolinska Institute is also where **Nobel Prizes** in Physiology and Medicine are issued.
Standard hair, urine, and blood tests for detecting mercury might be unreliable at assessing the total amount of mercury collected in your body during your life. But after you're dead, an autopsy should provide an accurate measure of how much

metal has accumulated in you, and where it's located in your body.

Autopsy studies done at the Karolinska Institute found that, on average, people with a history of mercury amalgams had three times more mercury in the brain and nine times more mercury in the kidneys than those with no history of mercury fillings.[22] Other autopsy studies have found high levels of mercury in dental workers—with levels in the pituitary and thyroid glands over ten times higher than in "controls," and levels in the kidney cortex seven times higher than in controls.[29]

Patrick Störtebecker, MD, PhD, neurologist at Karolinska Institute, wrote *Mercury Poisoning From Dental Amalgam—a Hazard to Human Brain*,[23] in which he points out that the teeth are only two inches from the brain. He shows that there are a number of ways that mercury, viruses, bacteria, and bacterial toxins can travel that short distance.

He revives Alfred Stock's insights of 50 years prior, in which he showed that mercury vapours can travel along the nerves of smell into the olfactory bulbs and the pituitary gland of the brain, accumulating there in large quantities.

Störtebecker also points out that the trigeminal nerves (the large sensory nerves of the face) are also capable of transporting toxins, viruses, and metals to the brain stem.

The veins and lymph tissue of the lower jaw drain substances from the lower teeth down the throat where they can easily react with the thyroid and thymus glands.

The upper teeth are drained into the cranio-vertebral venous system that runs throughout the brain and spinal column, and joins in with the venous system of the genital-urinary system. There are no valves in the cranio-vertebral system of veins, so any bacteria, toxin, or metal that enters from the upper teeth can travel freely throughout the delicate brain and into the spinal nerves.

Research using rats showed that the females were much more susceptible to mercury toxicity than the males. Studies of dental professionals agree with these findings; dental assistants and female dental workers generally showed higher mercury levels than male dentists.[30]

The DMPS challenge was used to study dental personnel who were occupationally exposed to mercury. The test group included ten dental technicians (all females), five dentists (one female and four males), and 13 non-dental personnel (five females and eight males).The urinary excretion of mercury was 88 times greater after DMPS administration than before administration for the dental technicians, 49 times greater for the dentists, and 35 times greater for the non-dental personnel.[24]

Dental staff have also been found to have:

- more eye and skin problems,[31]
- increased menstrual disturbances,[32]
- reduced fertility,[33]
- increased miscarriage rate,[34] and
- increased risk of ill health.[35]

Other studies have shown increased risk of lung, brain, kidney, and central nervous system cancers among dental workers.[36] Poor health in dental workers has been directly linked to their length of time on the job.[37]

Dentists were found to score significantly worse than a comparable control group on neurobehavioural tests of:

- motor speed, visual scanning, and visuo-motor coordination,[38]
- concentration, verbal memory, and visual memory,[39] and
- emotional/mood tests.[40]

Test performances were found to be proportional to exposure/body levels of mercury,[41] and even low levels of mercury exposure were correlated with significant adverse neurobehavioural symptoms, such as anger.

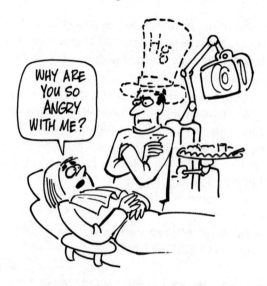

Older dentists, on average, have mercury levels that are about four times higher than those in controls,[42] although some have had levels up to 80 times higher.[43] Most studies of dentists have found increased irritability and tension,[44] high rates of drug dependency and psychological disability,[45] and higher suicide rates.[46]

The emotional and mood symptoms of mercury toxicity may be due to its effect on brain neurotransmitters. A study by Robert Siblerud at the University of Colorado found that people with mercury fillings had 45 percent more health symptoms—including emotional health problems, such as anger, irritability, less happiness, less peace of mind, and depression—than those without amalgams.[25]

Another of his studies showed that women who have mercury fillings are two-and-half times more likely to smoke. Siblerud states:

"one might postulate that, if the amalgam mercury reduces the function of neurotransmitters [such as serotonin and dopamine] **and results in anxiety, and if nicotine increases neurotransmitter functioning, people with amalgams would perhaps smoke more to relieve their anxious feelings."**

Some of the many symptoms associated with low serotonin are emotional instability, depression, anxiety, low self-esteem, memory weakness, obsessive-compulsive disorders, appetite disorders, insomnia, and suicidal tendencies. The presence of mercury toxicity explains why so many people need short-term serotonin enhancers, such as alcohol, to get through a week with any kind of self-esteem—or prescription serotonin recyclers such as Prozac, Paxil, Zoloft, Effexor, or Luvox to get through a day without depression—and sleeping pills, to get to sleep at night.

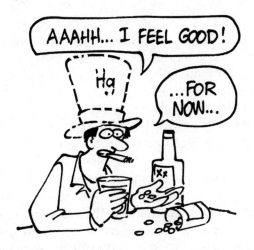

Symptoms of mercury vapour toxicity thus are primarily neurological and psychiatric:

"Common symptoms include depression, irritability, exaggerated response to stimulation (erethism), excessive shyness, insomnia, emotional instability, forgetfulness, confusion, and vasomotor disturbances such as excessive perspiration and uncontrolled blushing. Tremors are also common in individuals exposed to mercury vapor. These are exaggerated when a task is required but are minimal when the patient is at rest or asleep. A fine trembling of fingers, eyelids, lips, and tongue may be interrupted intermittently by coarse shaking movements. Both the erethism and the tremors are reversible." [26]

Erethism is:
"a peculiar form of psychic disturbance characterized by
self-consciousness, timidity, embarrassment with insufficient
reason, anxiety, indecision, lack of concentration, depression,
resentment of criticism, irritability or excitability; these
appear to cause a complete change of personality. Other
symptoms may include headache, fatigue, and weakness;
either drowsiness or insomnia also are characteristic
complaints and in more advanced cases, there may be
hallucinations, memory loss... ." [27]

In 1990, Siblerud also showed that those with amalgam
fillings had significantly higher blood pressure, lower heart
rate, and lower blood hemoglobin levels, causing anemia and
symptoms of chest pain, fatigue, low stamina, and rapid
heartbeat.[28] Numerous other studies, including one at Harvard,
have shown that while inorganic mercury—such as from
amalgam fillings—causes high blood pressure, organic
methylmercury from fish doesn't.[29]

Swedish researcher Mats Hanson stated in 1983:
"The majority of people might have sufficient resistance to
Hg [mercury] to have amalgam without becoming seriously
ill. However, mercury kills cells which are not renewed,
especially nerve cells. These cells are the ones we will need
later in life as a reserve. No dentist can guarantee that the
patient will not come to harm." [30]

The Canadian Dental Association has an information package
titled "Dental Amalgam Patient Information Sheet," which
refers to an article published in the *Journal of the American Dental
Association*.[31] The article estimates that approximately 3 percent
of the general population is sensitive to mercury—which means
allergic. If the population of Canada is 30 million people and 3
percent are allergic to mercury, that would mean approximately
900,000 Canadians would be allergic to mercury. In the US, it
would be ten times as many—about 9,000,000—who would be
allergic to the mercury in their fillings.

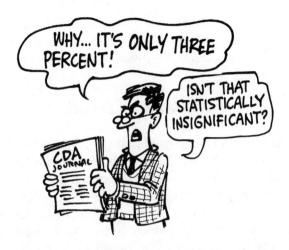

Do these people know that they're allergic to their mercury fillings? Mats Hanson continues:

"Allergy to mercury is often not testable on the skin. A patch test might show nothing at the application site but eczema can flare up at another part of the body. Immune reactions in the blood are the first reactions after exposure to mercury. A person can be extremely sensitive to inhaled Hg without showing a positive skin reaction. If the Hg comes to the skin from the circulation severe dermatitis can occur. Acrodynia—pink disease—was common when Hg-containing baby powders were used. Inner allergies of autoimmune type are not visible from the outside. They occur when proteins bind Hg (or other metals). The immune system will then not recognize the protein and react. Many manifestations of Hg poisoning have obvious immunological components. It is also known that autoimmune diseases can be elicited by mercury, i.e., myasthenia gravis and immune reactions towards kidney tissue are known. Since Hg can bind to thousands of different proteins and each individual has an unique immune system, the many and variable manifestations of mercury poisoning are not surprising." [32]

Because allergies to mercury could come from exposure to small quantities of mercury, and regular skin-patch allergy-testing has been shown to be unreliable, there are at least 900,000 Canadians out there for whom the cause of their health problems has been completely overlooked!

WHAT ARE ALLERGIES?

Because having allergies means that your immune system is reacting to something, let's start with a brief introduction to some of your key immune system characters.

When a "foreigner" (whether alive or dead) is spotted in your body by your largest, most rugged white blood cells—called **macrophages**—they immediately attack and destroy this alien. The macrophages then rip off a piece of it and wear it like a trophy.

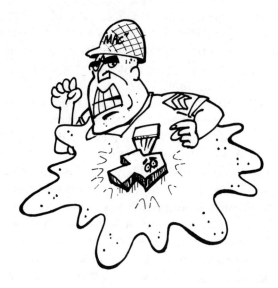

The piece they rip off is now called an **antigen**—another name for an enemy whose mugshot has been identified, and that must be attacked and killed if detected anywhere in the body.

In case this "foreigner" is just the scout of an offensive against you, your body immediately begins the production of mini-macrophages—called **neutrophils**—to back up your macrophages.

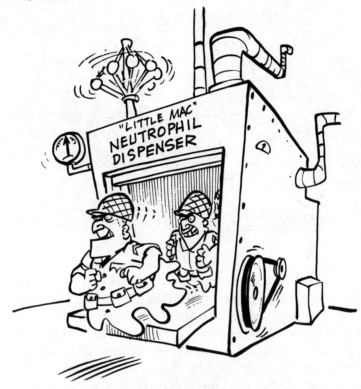

The macrophage will show this new antigen to smaller, naïve white blood cells—called **B** and **T lymphocytes.** They become sensitized to this antigen, and spend the rest of their lives searching out this alien so they can quickly destroy it.

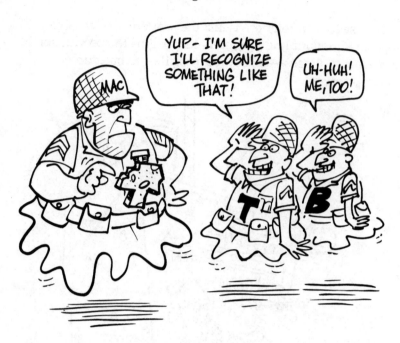

Your newly sensitized B lymphocytes make small
"harpoons"—called **antibodies**—that are designed to attack
that specific enemy. Seventy percent of the antibodies made
daily by your body are **IgA antibodies**, which patrol your
membranes, such as those in the upper respiratory tract and
digestive system—where the invaders are most likely to try
to force entry. Even if an invader were to get into your body
through these membranes, it is sure to be severely damaged
by the deadly double-pronged IgA antibody.

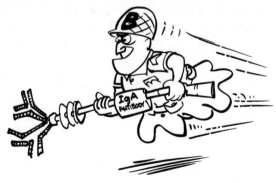

Backing up IgA is the much bigger **IgM antibody**—"Big Momma"—a large five-pronged antibody that rumbles around in the blood vessels, destroying any invader that dares enter.

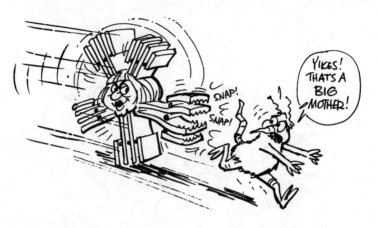

IgG antibody is a smaller, more dexterous antibody that is able to slip into the nooks and crannies of your body—such as the lymph system—to root out would-be invaders.

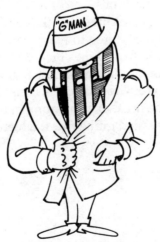

IgE antibody is only made in small amounts. Most IgE antibodies are bound to mast cells (in the tissues) or basophils (in the blood). They are like the protruding horns on a mine— when detonated by contact with a Bad Guy, they cause the mast cells or basophils to spray histamine and other inflammatory chemicals. This begins what is called an **immediate-type hypersensitivity allergy reaction**. The common test for this type of allergic reaction is done with skin-patch testing.

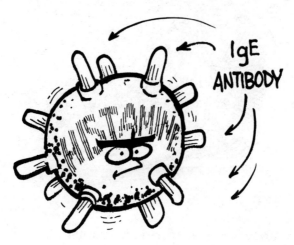

While the B cells are busy building antibodies for the expected invasion, the T cells—most of which are **helper T cells**—are preparing **cytokines**, which are high-tech secretions crucial for the immune system to win a war against a major adversary. The helper T cytokines include three types of **inteferon**, as well as **lymphotoxin** and a wide range of **interleukins**. The **cytotoxic "killer" T cells** secrete **perforin** to punch holes in the invader's membrane, through which they then pour enzymes called **granzymes**, which react to blow up the enemy.

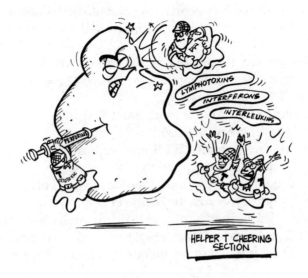

Thus your immune system has an array of defensive armaments that few invaders could withstand. In fact, your helper T cells are so effective at activating your immune system, **suppressor T cells** have to be made to prevent your immune system from totally destroying *you* along with the invaders.

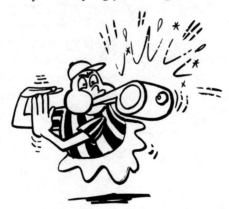

SUPPRESSOR T CELL

After the war has been won, the T and B lymphocytes continue to circulate in the form of **memory cells**, so that if the same invader should reappear, then your protective soldiers can be quickly armed with the right weapons to destroy this foe.

In a 1984 study, a 21-year-old dental patient with six amalgam fillings had his lymphocytes tested; **47 percent were found to be T lymphocytes.**
- After **removal of his six amalgam fillings,** the **T lymphocytes increased to 73 percent.**
- When four **new amalgam fillings were added,** the **T lymphocytes dropped to 55 percent.**
- When the fillings were finally **replaced with gold,** the **T lymphocytes rose to 72 percent.**[33]

This study clearly shows that your T cells—the controllers and coordinators of your immune system—can be dramatically affected by exposure to various metals installed in your mouth.

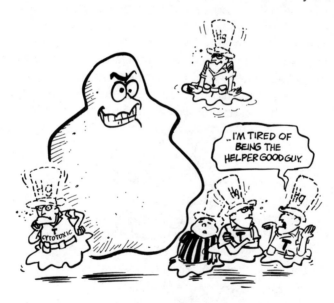

BACK TO SWEDEN

Let's return to Sweden, where **a new, more accurate way of testing allergies to metals has been developed; this new test has also given insight into how to reverse these allergies.**

While the skin-patch test is the most common allergy test for immediate-type hypersensitivity reactions, the Swedes felt that a test using **T memory cells** would give a broader and more accurate insight into immune reactions involving metals. Since using T memory cells as the tester involves **delayed-type hypersensitivity reactions**—which are common in autoimmune diseases—this test might also shed light on some of the mysterious autoimmune diseases that have become so prevalent in modern society. The test for metals that evolved from the research at Danderyd Hospital and the Karolinska Institute in Sweden became known as **MELISA**®, short for **ME**mory **L**ymphocyte **I**mmuno **S**timulation **A**ssay.[34] Let's take a look at a few studies that have used MELISA® testing to investigate metal allergies.

MELISA® testing for metal sensitivity was done on over 3,000 patients; the most common sensitizer identified was nickel, and females responded more frequently to it than males. Regardless of the patient's gender, the next most common metal found was mercury, followed by gold, cadmium, and palladium.

The effects of amalgam replacement on health was studied in 105 patients complaining of chronic fatigue syndrome. Eighty-six of the patients had their metal fillings replaced.

- 78 percent of them reported significant health improvement.
- 20 percent were unchanged.
- 2 percent reported a worsening of symptoms.

MELISA® testing of these patients showed that removing the amalgam fillings decreased reaction to all metals except nickel.[35] The conclusion from this study is that **an allergy to nickel is caused by nickel-containing jewellery that penetrates the skin, such as earrings. Other metal allergies were due to dental metals. Removal of the dental metals decreased the metal allergies, which eliminated the fatigue in most patients.**

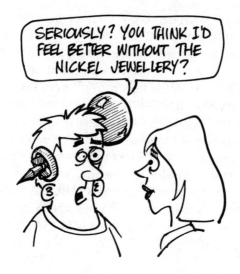

In another study, 72 individuals with **chronic fatigue syndrome** were divided into three groups.

- 22 with chronic fatigue with autoimmune thyroiditis (hormonal)
- 22 with chronic fatigue without autoimmunity
- 28 with chronic fatigue without hormonal problems

The study also included 13 healthy control subjects. The conclusion was: **"that fatigue, regardless of the underlying disease, is primarily associated with hypersensitivity to inorganic mercury and nickel."** Some of the patients had their amalgam fillings replaced with non-metal fillings. A six-month follow-up showed **"considerably alleviated fatigue and disappearance of many symptoms encountered previously. In parallel, lymphocyte responses to metals decreased as well."** [36]

MELISA® testing was done on 18 patients with mercury-amalgam fillings and a diagnosis of **lichen planus** of the mouth. There were also two control groups: 20 subjects with amalgam fillings, but no mouth disease, and 12 subjects with no amalgam fillings or mouth disease.

The patients with lichen planus showed significantly greater reactions to inorganic mercury with MELISA® testing, compared to the control groups. They also reacted to phenylmercury, which is used in root canals to kill bacteria. Removal of the amalgam fillings reversed the lichen planus.[37]

Magnetic resonance imaging (MRI) and MELISA® testing were done on 34 patients with central nervous system and systemic symptoms suggestive of toxicity from dental amalgams. The MRIs showed damage (called lesions) in 81 percent of the patients—primarily degeneration of the basal ganglia of the brain, which involves fine-tuning of movement. Damage to this part of the brain stem is also seen in Parkinson's disease. The MELISA® testing showed metal allergies in 88 percent of the patients, mainly reactions to **mercuric chloride**, suggesting **"that immunological mechanisms may play an important role in the development of the lesions."** [38]

As mentioned earlier, mercuric chloride is made when inorganic mercury from fillings is carried by saliva to the stomach, where it reacts with the chlorine of hydrochloric acid.

Is it the immune system's reaction against this mercury that causes Parkinson's disease? A 1989 study done in Singapore showed that high mercury levels were found in 54 people with Parkinson's disease.[39] Of course, further studies would be necessary for confirmation, but what if you have Parkinson's-like symptoms now? Do you have time to wait for more studies—or do you act now? What could be done to remove the immune reactions against mercury? **REMOVE THE MERCURY!**

A Japanese study, using a lymphocyte test similar to MELISA® testing, found that 34 out of 40 **psoriasis** patients showed reactions to one or more dental metals. All 40 were sensitive to house dust mites, as well. Within three months of removing dental metals and using mite-free bed linen, 83 percent of the patients showed improvement—67 percent of them markedly.[40]

MS patients can show reactions to mercury, cadmium, palladium, lead, or nickel. People with **Sjögren's syndrome** often react to gold and palladium.[41]

While nickel, mercury, cadmium, palladium, and gold were the source of most metal allergies, MELISA® testing done on 650 patients also showed three other substances to be problematic: **phenylmercury, thimerosal**, and **titanium dioxide**. [42] Phenylmercury, used as a bacterial killer in root canals, showed up in 14 percent of the patients. Of course, the phenylmercury must be leaking out of the root canal for the immune system to be attacking it.

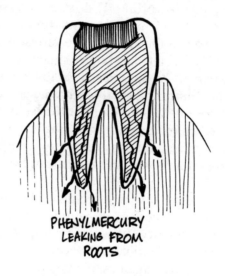

PHENYLMERCURY
LEAKING FROM
ROOTS

Thimerosal is a mercury compound that has been used as an antibacterial preservative in a number of products such as eye wash, contact lens disinfectant, and vaccines. Thimerosal showed up as an allergen in 7 percent of the patients. The third reactant, titanium dioxide, showed in 3 percent of the patients. Titanium dioxide is used as a white colouring agent in many dental products, including toothpaste, and is used in some pain-relief medications, as well. Since sodium lauryl sulphate is used in toothpaste, too—it increases the permeability of the membranes—the titanium dioxide will be more readily absorbed. For 3 percent of the population, this could be a significant health hazard.

So 3 percent of the population is allergic to titanium dioxide, · which is the same percentage that the North American dental associations admit is allergic to mercury. We've already calculated that would be about 900,000 people in Canada, and 9,000,000 in the USA.

But just how fixed is this 3 percent? We've already seen that in people with severe neurological disease, like Parkinson's, it could be that over 80 percent are allergic to mercury, so let's look at more studies.

A group of dental students taking a course involving work with amalgam had their urine tested before and after the course. The average urine level of mercury increased 500 percent during the course.[47] Allergy testing of another group of dental students showed that **of those with ten or more fillings at least five years old, 44 percent tested allergic to mercury.**[48] Other studies had similar results.[49]

Here are the obvious conclusions.
- The more metal you're exposed to, the more metal you're likely to have inside you, and the more likely you'll be allergic to it.
- The more allergic you are to metals, the sicker you're likely to be.

Even though MELISA® testing is relatively new, and only a few disease scenarios have been tested, the one important lesson that already jumps out is: *the less metal you have in you, the better*. Rather than running around trying to get MELISA® testing done, why not just bypass the test, and go straight to the one step that has been shown to reduce the reactions anyway? **GET THE METAL OUT!**

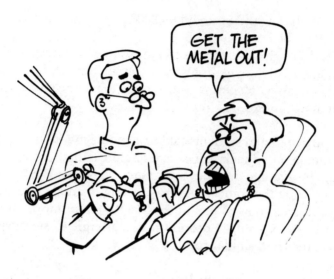

Mercury fillings were invented in Paris in 1826. By the 1840s—when mercury fillings were being introduced into North America—the first-ever case of MS was being recorded (coincidentally?) in Paris. Some MS patients have been found to have much higher levels of mercury in their cerebrospinal fluid.[50] One study found that MS patients had levels of mercury body-burden up to 300 percent higher than in controls.[51]

Numerous studies have shown that removal of mercury-amalgam fillings has led to improvement of MS.[52] In one large German study, replacing the mercury fillings in MS patients gave a recovery rate of 16 percent, while total tooth extraction resulted in an 85 percent recovery rate.[53]

How can removing the teeth of MS patients achieve results that are five times better than the results achieved by simply replacing the fillings? Let's go back to Patrick Störtebecker, neurologist from the Karolinska Institute, and his book *Mercury Poisoning from Dental Amalgam*. Störtebecker states that:

"Multiple Sclerosis (MS) is the denomination of a disorder of the nervous system, characterized by the occurrence of scattered or disseminated lesions (plaques) in the brain and spinal cord... ."

"Post-mortem examinations have revealed that the 'plaques' always are located around the venous blood-vessles [sic]... and moreover in the initial stage always surrounded by a circular 'zone' of white blood corpuscles, round cells, and plasma cells. A finding that provides real evidence of an inflammatory process of infectious origin!"

"As all the 'plaques' are situated within the territory of the valve-less cranio-vertebral venous system, this venous system itself constitutes the only possible pathway for transport of the causative noxa [noxious substances]. Any other explanation is not possible." [43]

Störtebecker believes that the brain lesions of MS result from infections in the upper teeth that have spread their toxins via the veins to the brain, while spinal cord lesions of MS are caused by toxins from infections in the genito-urinary system.

Mercury-amalgam fillings don't escape without blame in MS, however, as Störtebecker has this to say, "...mercury may enhance the symptoms of multiple sclerosis...by causing vascular damage to the brain and the spinal cord... ."

Störtebecker goes on to show that not only MS but also brain tumours are more common in the countries where the "civilized" diet is eaten. He states:

"People of the Western industrialized countries have a high degree of dental caries, and mostly they have undergone conservative dental treatment, with several root-fillings protected by amalgam, as well as by golden crowns.

"Many of the conservatively treated teeth harbour chronic infections, with all possibilities existing for spread of microbial carcinogens to the brain.

"In more rural and primitive districts of the world, on the other side, we encounter people, who either have escaped a conservative dental care including root-fillings, or have got the aching teeth extracted!" [44]

From these insights, we can see that removing the teeth from MS patients may have given such positive results because latent bacterial infections were also removed.

Numerous other studies have shown that people who have had their mercury-amalgam fillings replaced experienced significant improvement in their health problems, such as the following.

- **allergies**[54]
- **ALS**[55]
- **Alzheimer Disease**[56]
- **anger**[57]
- **anxiety/confusion**[58]
- **arthritis**[59]
- **asthma**[60]
- **blood conditions**[61]
- **cancer/leukemia**[62]
- **chemical sensitivities**[63]
- **Crohn's disease**[64]
- **depression**[65]
- **dizziness/vertigo**[66]
- **eczema**[67]
- **epilepsy**[68]
- **eye inflammation**[69]
- **fatigue**[70]
- **fibromyalgia/muscle/joint pain**[71]
- **hair loss**[72]
- **headaches/migraines**[73]
- **heart problems**[74]
- **immune/autoimmune problems**[75]
- **infertility**[76]
- **insomnia**[77]
- **infections**[78]
- **lupus**[79]
- **memory disorders**[80]
- **mouth lesions (pre-cancerous)**[81]
- **nerve conditions**[82]
- **Parkinson's/tremors**[83]
- **periodontal diseases**[84]

- PMS[85]
- psoriasis and skin conditions[86]
- schizophrenia[87]
- sinusitis[88]
- stomach problems[89]
- tinnitus[90]
- urinary/prostate problems[91]
- vision disturbances[92]

While all of the above studies have shown major improvement in the specific conditions listed, after removal of amalgam fillings, it is possible to find many studies that say that there are *no* health problems that can be attributed to mercury-amalgam fillings. How do you reconcile these different insights?

Picture a birthday party with ten children in a large orchard. Put blindfolds on them, give them each a stick, and tell them there might be a *piñata* somewhere in the orchard. After a long period of many swings, most of the children would give up, saying there isn't any *piñata*. If one child happened to hit the *piñata* once, he or she would know better where to swing, and would soon hit it frequently. If each of the children were interviewed, nine of them might say there is no *piñata*, while one child would know for certain that there was one.

Such is the history of research on mercury. Some researchers found the mercury and zeroed in on it quickly. Researchers like Stock in Germany, Vimy in Canada, and Siblerud in the USA have done many studies proving the health hazards of mercury, while others have found nothing. Quoting those who found nothing is pointless—those who found health problems have discovered the truth.

The mercury *piñata* was finally broken open when the accumulated research resulted in Sweden's banning the use of mercury in 1994; it is to be completely phased out in industry and dentistry by the year 2000.[45] Some of the other European countries are well along the way to discontinuing the use of mercury amalgams. The rest of the world still uses mercury because they've listened to too many of the researchers who had false-negative results.

The rest of the world must eventually ban mercury, as well. The following information is from **www.talkinternational.com**. It represents a summary of the findings from studies that examined the health effects of replacing mercury amalgams with non-mercury dental fillings. It comprises evaluations of **1,569 patients from six different sources.**

- 762 Patient Adverse Reactions Reports submitted to the FDA (USA)
- 519 patients in Sweden from Dr. Mats Hanson
- 100 patients in Denmark from Dr. Henrik Lichtenberg
- 80 patients in Canada from Dr. Pierre Larose
- 86 patients in Colorado from Dr. Robert Siblerud
- 22 patients from Dr. A. V. Zamm

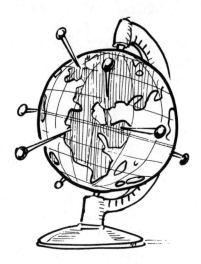

While the math in this report is a little shaky, the numbers still give an idea of which types of symptoms might improve following replacement of mercury fillings. These would likely correspond to the 3 percent of North Americans—or was it 44 percent?—who might have a sensitivity to mercury. Note that almost half of the 1,569 patients complained of fatigue, and 86 percent of them reported improvement after replacement of mercury fillings—not too different from the 78 percent improvement reported on the MELISA® allergy test studies.

Selected Health Symptom Analysis of 1569 Patients who Eliminated Dental Fillings Containing Mercury

% of total symptoms reported	Condition	Reported number	Number improved	% improved
14%	Allergy	221	196	89%
5%	Anxiety	86	80	93%
5%	Bad temper	81	68	89%
6%	Bloating	88	70	88%
6%	Blood pressure problems	99	53	54%
5%	Chest pains	79	69	87%
22%	Depression	347	315	91%
22%	Dizziness	343	301	88%
45%	Fatigue	705	603	86%
15%	Gastrointestinal problems	231	192	83%
8%	Gum problems (OLP)	129	121	94%
34%	Headaches	531	460	87%
10%	Heartbeat, irregular	159	139	87%
6%	Heartbeat, rapid	115	68	70%
12%	Insomnia	187	146	78%
8%	Irritability	132	19	90%
17%	Lack of concentration	270	216	80%
6%	Lack of energy	91	88	97%
17%	Memory loss	265	193	73%
17%	Metallic taste	260	247	95%
3%	Migraines	45	39	87%
7%	Multiple sclerosis	113	86	76%
8%	Muscle tremor	126	104	83%
10%	Nervousness	158	131	83%
8%	Numbness anywhere	118	97	82%
20%	Skin problems	310	251	81%
9%	Sore throat	149	128	86%

Selected Health Symptom Analysis of 1569 Patients who Eliminated Dental Fillings Containing Mercury

% of total symptoms reported	Condition	Reported number	Number improved	% improved
4%	Thyroid problems	56	44	79%
12%	Ulcers & sores in mouth	189	162	86%
7%	Urinary tract problems	115	87	76%
29%	Vision problems	462	289	63%

A large-scale Swedish study has shown that virtually all patients who had their amalgam fillings replaced due to health problems reported significant, long-lasting improvements in health. The length of the study was 17 years.[93]

Caution must be used when removing amalgam fillings because more mercury will be spilled into the body. This spilling can be reduced by up to 90 percent if the dentist uses a rubber dam, high-velocity evacuation, water spray, outside air supply (to be breathed in through the nose), and an aspirator tip.[94]

Studies show that after the removal of dental amalgams, mercury levels in the blood and urine are typically increased for a few days. However, these levels decrease significantly within two weeks, and are often reduced from the original levels by 80 percent or more, within a few months. [95] Does this mean that the mercury has been removed from the body, or is it now bound to the sulfur in the organs?

If you're going to remove your mercury fillings, what do you replace them with? Gold has been used for centuries and works well for most people, but MELISA® testing has shown that gold can also be an allergen to some people. Also, because pure gold is very soft, other metals are added to it as hardeners, especially palladium. Some "gold" fillings have over 75 percent palladium. Since palladium can also be methylated by your bacteria and therefore made very toxic, this is not the ideal choice.

Porcelain is made by fusing feldspar and silica with finely ground glass at high temperatures to form an extremely hard filling. Most porcelain crowns use metals like nickel for reinforcing; nickel has been shown to release from these fillings into the body. Nickel is even more allergenic than mercury and, like mercury, is very toxic to the nervous system and—also like mercury—is very prone to inducing autoimmune reactions.

These problems with metals have led researchers to search for non-metallic fillings; about 50 years ago, composite fillings were produced. These plastic resins ("plastic" refers to flexibility, not the plastic material we generally think of) were inserted into the cavity, and chemical reactions would quickly harden them. When these composite fillings were used in the large back teeth—the molars—where the greatest strain of chewing takes place, they would shift, thereby allowing bacteria to get underneath them. These failures caused many dentists to discontinue their use. Also, these fillings made the teeth very sensitive to hot and cold temperatures.

In 1975, composite resins were produced that would not harden until exposed to an ultraviolet (UV) light, which gave the dentist more control over the filling. The UV-sensitive materials were soon replaced by white light-sensitive materials, but there was still difficulty in bonding these composites to the large teeth that are subject to tremendous chewing pressure. Japanese research solved this problem in the early 1970s with "acid etching" of the teeth, allowing a much better bond and seal between the teeth and the composite filling, thereby making them feasible in molars.

For larger cavities in molars, however, it has been found that mixing glass particles with composite resins to form ceramic has produced a filling virtually as tough as the original enamel, with less sensitivity to hot and cold than the composites. Studies have shown that ceramic fillings are virtually as wear-resistant as gold.[46] The state-of-the-art in ceramic dentistry at this point is the Cerec method, which uses computer-cutting of

the ceramic to get a perfect fit. The Cerec fillings are much less
prone to fracture than other ceramics.[47] These studies refute the
idea that there aren't strong alternatives to mercury-amalgam
fillings.

Since not everyone with mercury-related health problems
gets better just from having amalgam fillings replaced, the
process of chelation can help remove some of the accumulated
metal burden. Studies that used DMPS chelation to remove
accumulated body mercury after amalgam replacement
reported that over 80 percent of patients with chronic health
problems showed significant improvement.[96] Because DMPS
chelation doesn't penetrate the blood-brain barrier very
effectively, the mercury showing in the urine after a DMPS
chelation is primarily being flushed out of the kidneys, liver,
and GI tract.

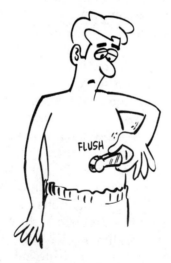

FLUSH

Since the mercury is being pushed out through the kidneys
after DMPS chelation, it's important to monitor kidney
function, and not do the chelation too frequently.
    DMPS has proven to flush large quantities of stored metals—
mainly mercury—out of the organs and into the urine. It
verifies the Swedish autopsy studies that showed that virtually
everyone who has had mercury fillings has accumulated

mercury, primarily in their kidneys, brain, and liver. Removing the fillings does not remove this accumulated mercury. In fact, if the dentist is not properly trained in the safe removal of amalgam fillings, this procedure may add considerably more mercury to the body.

It will take one to three years of chelation to remove the accumulated metals from the body. I have discontinued recommending IV DMPS for my patients. **I find that a smaller dose of DMPS, taken orally, is tolerated better, and is cheaper for the patient.**

DMSA (2,3-Dimercaptosuccinic acid) is another sulfur chelation substance that is taken orally. It is even cheaper than DMPS, and was once thought to be capable of penetrating the blood-brain barrier to remove metals—this may not hold true, however.

DMSA has been shown to increase urinary elimination of mercury by 163 percent.[48] The usual precautions must be taken if the person is sulfur-allergic—and, if gas or bloating, headaches, anxiety, or irritability appear, then the DMSA must be reduced or stopped. **I must add this CAUTION: Those with central nervous system disorders, such as MS or autism, should use extreme caution with DMSA.**[49]

Some doctors are also using **alpha lipoic acid** to assist the chelation sulfurs in removing mercury from the body.

Because of the potential dangers of stirring up mercury, chelation should only be done under the guidance of a licensed practitioner.

In addition, **because some minerals—particularly zinc— are also drawn out by the chelation, it is recommended that minerals be supplemented.** A common symptom of zinc deficiency is feeling spacey or having poor concentration. Because zinc is important for hundreds of enzymes in the body, a weakened immune system and weakened digestion can soon follow. This is why I recommend taking oral DMPS or DMSA for only a few days at a time, to allow zinc levels to increase. If zinc supplementation is used, it should be taken approximately 12 hours away from the chelation.

While the dental associations have long denied the connections between their use of metals and the declining health of their patients, all they have to do is look at the *Material Safety Data Sheet* issued by the manufacturers of amalgam fillings. It states:

"Inhalation of mercury vapor over a long period may cause mercurialism, which is characterized by fine tremors and erethism. Tremors may affect the hands first, but may also become evident in the face, arms and legs. Erethism may be manifested by abnormal shyness, blushing, self consciousness, depression or despondency, resentment of criticism, irritability or excitability, headache, fatigue, and insomnia.

"In severe cases, hallucinations, loss of memory and mental deterioration may occur. Concentrations as low as 0.03 mg/m3 have induced psychiatric symptoms in humans... . Other effects may include salivation, gingivitis, stomatitis, loosening of the teeth, blue lines on the gums, diarrhea, chronic pneumonitis, and mild anemia... . Intrauterine exposure may result in tremors and involuntary movements in infants. Mercury is excreted in breast milk. Paternal reproductive effects and effects on fertility have been reported in male rats following repeated inhalation exposures." (Caulk Company)

If you take into account the dozens of other symptoms listed in the previous pages, you'll see the full extent of the mercury problem. In fact, they cover all the chronic diseases of young and old in "civilized" countries.

In 1987, a Swedish National Department of Health, Mercury Amalgam Review Panel concluded that, "from a toxicological point of view, mercury is too toxic to be used as a filling material." [97]

In 1987, the Federal Department of Health in Germany issued an advisory warning against the use of dental amalgam in pregnant women,[98] and, other than the US, most major countries have similar or more extensive warnings or bans.

On December 16, 1990, the TV program *60 Minutes* televised the most heavily viewed story of that show's history, titled, *"Is There Poison In Your Mouth?"* which exposed the potential dangers of amalgam fillings.[50]

Yet, even back in 1992, the Swedish Medical Research Council still stated the following.

- "Mercury released from dental amalgams does not, according to available data, contribute to systemic disease or systemic toxicological effects.
- "No significant effects on the immune system have been demonstrated with the amounts of mercury which may be released from dental amalgam fillings... .
- "Available data do not justify discontinuing the use of silver-containing dental amalgam fillings or recommending their replacement." [51]

In 1994, the BBC did a show whose title dropped *the question* about mercury fillings; it was more bluntly titled, "The Poison in Your Mouth."

Also in 1994, mercury fillings were banned in Sweden for those under age 19, and a general ban was passed to end the use of mercury in industry and dentistry by the year 2000.

A World Health Organization Scientific Panel concluded, in 1995, that there is no safe level of mercury exposure.[99]

In 1995, a report from Health Canada concluded that any person with any number of amalgam fillings is exposed to levels of mercury that are above the guideline levels set by government health organizations.[100]

Finally, in 1998, the massive accumulation of scientific evidence indicting mercury as a health hazard came to fruition as the Swedish Council For Planning and Coordinating Research unanimously recommended to the government "...discontinuing the use of amalgam as a dental material." [101] As a result, **the Swedish government has banned the use of mercury-amalgam fillings**, while the rest of the dental world carries on business as usual.

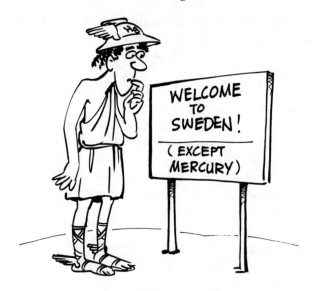

I know, I know—your dentist says there's no research proving that mercury fillings are a health concern. Maybe the problem is that he or she can't read Swedish. Ironically, even though my grandparents on my father's side were both Swedish, I can't read a word of Swedish either—and look at all the research I've managed to track down.

Perhaps it is possible that mercury only leaks out of Swedish amalgam fillings into Swedish brains, kidneys, and livers—and if so, then it obviously has been leaking into their brains, kidneys, and livers over the last 160 years. Perhaps if you don't have any Swedish blood in you, you will be okay with a mouth full of mercury amalgams. Just to be on the safe side, don't you think it would be safer to *not put any more of it into your mouth, and to remove what you can?*

The claim that there is no scientific data *to **not** allow the use of mercury in fillings* is just as weak today as it was in 1840. Because the toxicity of mercury was well known then, the onus should have been on the dentists to prove that mercury wasn't a problem **before** it was used. At the very least, every patient should have been informed about the potential toxicity of mercury, *if it did prove to leak* out of the filling, so that the patient could have the option to refuse to take the risk. If people had been informed of the potential toxicity, mercury fillings would not have become as prevalent as they are today.

In spite of all the international research showing the toxicity of mercury fillings—and in spite of all the studies showing how removal of dental amalgams has improved the health of over 20,000 people with a wide range of illnesses—the majority of dentists continue to use mercury amalgams without providing any warning to patients about their potential toxicity.

If a patient questions the safety of mercury fillings, the standard reply is, "There's nothing wrong with mercury fillings." End of debate—no explanation of the potential side-effects. These dentists are obviously not aware that the individual dentist may be personally liable for the health of that patient if the dentist's "safe" mercury fillings should be proven to leak mercury—as Swedish researchers have already proven, conclusively.

I get calls every now and again from angry dentists calling me a psychopath for advising patients to have their mercury fillings replaced when there's "no scientific proof for such idiocy." At first I was a little intimidated by these calls, but after reading the research again and realizing that the dentists phoning me were older individuals—older dentists have been shown to accumulate the most mercury in their brains—these wild statements were as ironic as being called "mad" by the Mad Hatter himself.

I've had several patients insist that their dentist *not* give them mercury fillings, yet when they got home and looked in the mirror, they found that mercury fillings had been placed in their teeth. Perhaps the Mad Hatter has a dark sense of humour.

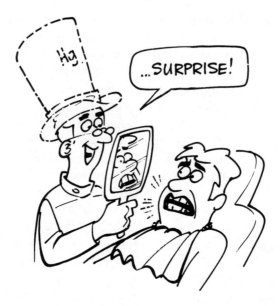

It also seems clear that dentists aren't aware that a crack has occurred in this madness, similar to what happened with the cigarette companies. For decades, the cigarette companies vigorously refuted any scientific research implicating cigarettes with health problems by saying:

- the research wasn't done properly;
- it wasn't interpreted properly; or
- it was insufficient to make any final conclusions.

When one of their insiders finally admitted they had been aware all along of the health problems of smoking—but had proceeded anyway because they were making big bucks—whatever controversy that had existed immediately ended; the public realized they had been duped. Smoking and its ill-health effects haven't stopped, but the confusion about it is over; the courts will write the ending to this sad story.

With the banning of mercury-amalgam fillings in Sweden, a similar chink has appeared in the dental associations' armour of 160 years of strident denial. It's the end of the controversy in Sweden, but unfortunately, not yet the end of the story in North America, as the inevitable politics have yet to be fully played out.

In Canada in 1998, the first of a number of class-action lawsuits was filed, based on informed consent and the use of mercury-amalgam fillings. In 2001, the Americans followed suit with four lawsuits already filed. Targets of these lawsuits include dentists who have failed to provide to patients their right to informed consent, and the American Dental Association.

The North American dental associations are carrying on *business as usual*—allowing the use of mercury amalgams. One professional who got into trouble for suggesting that mercury amalgams were health hazards is American dentist Hal Huggins. Huggins is the author of a number of books, including *It's All In Your Head,* which gives fair warning to the public of the dangers of mercury-amalgam fillings. His licence to practise dentistry in Colorado was suspended in 1996. The judge in the case even forbade patients from requesting removal of amalgams fillings based on mercury's toxicity.

This decision was eventually overruled, due to public outcry. A bill was introduced in the State Legislature that allows patients *to not have* mercury fillings, and assures that dentists can use mercury-free fillings without fear of retribution.

During one of Huggins' trials, the president of the American Dental Association, **"insisted that any dentist recommending the removal of amalgams for the sole purpose of eliminating the mercury vapors would be guilty of 'unethical' conduct."** [52]

Isn't this an ironic historical twist on the statements of the 1840s, when the predominant dental association of the day would charge any dentist *using mercury amalgam* with unethical conduct?!

Don't they realize that the Swedish researchers have proven conclusively that mercury *does* leak out of mercury fillings, and it *does* pose such a severe health risk that the authorities overcame the resistance and inertia inherent in bureaucracy, and banned the use of mercury fillings to protect the people of Sweden?

Do the dental associations of North America not trust the research of the Swedes, or do they not care about the health of North Americans? It has to be one or the other, doesn't it? Or is

there a greater fear—fear of financial liability? If dentists were
given freedom from lawsuits over mercury usage, would they
be more cooperative?

The ultimate liability, of course, lies with the health
departments of the countries that allow mercury to be used.
In Canada, Dr. Pierre Blais, an employee of Health Canada,
Medical Devices Bureau, wrote a report on mercury amalgams.
In a memo to his superiors, he stated that:
**"the potential hazards with the product (silver/mercury
fillings) are so transparently obvious that we (Government
of Canada) cannot even appear to ignore it without
attracting ridicule... ."** [53]

This was on August 31, **1976**. Since then, four other internal
Health Canada documents by medical scientists have also
warned of the dangers of amalgam.
- Chawla and Karov, July 10, 1991
- Karov, May 5, 1993
- Sinclair, July 15, 1994
- Richardson, August 18, 1995

Health Canada officials ignored all of them.

In 1985, instead of warning the public of the known dangers
of amalgam fillings, Health Canada apparently made an
arrangement with the Canadian Dental Association and the
Dental Industry Association of Canada, to exempt dental
restorative materials—including amalgam—from review.[54]
As a result, the scientific studies that might prove mercury
amalgam to be toxic—or not—needn't be done.

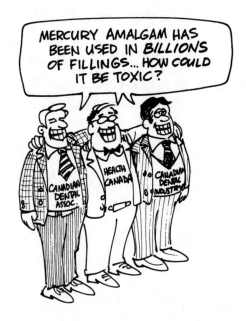

A giant proportion of the health problems in civilized societies has obviously been directly caused by—or at least been affected by—the slow but steady accumulation of mercury throughout the bodies of hundreds of millions of people. The full extent of this is impossible to fathom, but surely the whole concept of pathology as it is now taught will have to be revised, to put much less emphasis on individual diseases and more concern for the underlying cause.

Governments are spending billions of dollars annually on people's "health care," for medical and pharmaceutical disease-treatment that might only mask the symptoms of the deeper problems with metals. Not only is this a waste of billions of dollars, the overprescribing of medications will only worsen people's health in the long run.

It seems that the Swedish Health Department is the only one in the world that puts the health of its citizens above its own political interests. Who knows *if and when* the rest of the health departments in the world will follow.

In the meantime, I will continue to recommend that my patients avoid having mercury fillings put into their mouths, and to have their existing mercury fillings replaced, as their budgets permit. It's a real shame that some of the sickest patients have the most mercury fillings—they are the least able to afford their removal and replacement.

At this point, I thought this chapter on the mercury link to chronic disease was closed. The research on mercury was done, and the material was written—but when you start digging up dirt, it seems you keep finding more dirt. The mercury trail leads us into another chapter, focused more on the health of children, but overlapping into the health of the elderly.

Author's Note, April 2004

I have stated that Sweden banned the use of mercury in 1994 and planned to completely phase out its use in industry and dentistry by the year 2000. This, however, has not happened to date. Sweden actually *began* the process in 1994 but numerous committees appointed to study the issue have delayed the banning of mercury use.

Letter from a Patient

The very qualities that give a healthy human being the opportunity for a full and worthwhile life have, I believe, worked against me since late childhood. I was born June 10, 1943, in Vancouver, British Columbia, Canada, into an average, middle-class Protestant family. My intelligent, caring, responsible parents gave me and my two sisters the best of what they knew. They have always been hard-working, generous, and friendly people, who taught us good values to live by. We learned respectfulness, independence, and responsibility from them.

I was born with a good IQ, as well as other good qualities that could have given me a great opportunity for a successful life: naturally curious, determined, and friendly, with a healthy courage, and a passionate desire to strive for excellence in life. They are qualities that do not always make a person popular, therefore, difficulties would have followed me at the best of situations in life, I believe.

So what happened to my life? My story is a long and painful one, with myriad symptoms plaguing my life for nearly 48 years. My perception, memory, and intuition was precariously disrupted and distorted, and my emotional world was thrown about by depression, paranoia, anger, hostility, despair, and suicidal desires—while a mess of physical symptoms, from a poor immune system, also made my life, many times, a lonely and hellish trip.

All this drove me, at different times in my life, without rhyme or reason, into a strange psychotic world. It was not until I read Dr. Jonn Matsen's book, *Eating Alive,* in 1992, while working at Nature Works Natural Foods, in the town of Ganges on Salt Spring island, that I first learned of his clinic in North Vancouver: the North Shore Naturopathic Clinic. Eventually, seven years later, after my last total psychotic crash, I finally began to find the answers to a lifetime of misery.

As a teenager, I was considered a hypochondriac and a neurotic. At 31, when I had my first long-term psychotic crash, which lasted about four years, I was classified as a paranoid schizophrenic.

In late childhood, I was plagued with night panics, unreal fears, and loud ringing in the ears, which is still with me today. In my early teens, I began to suffer from extreme self-consciousness that would come and go; paranoia around my family and friends began to torment me, with a strange comfort when I was around strangers, sometimes. I had a fear of public places (agoraphobia), claustrophobia, nervousness, and fatigue; my teenage years and twenties were miserable, much of the time.

But a great desire for learning, I believe, took, what many times could have been a totally disastrous life, and continued it on the road to an answer. I have been through over 45 jobs in my life, as well as a two-and-a-half-year start at a navy career, where I became a sonar operator at 19, and worked on an Oceanographic Research base in Shelbourne, Nova Scotia. Eventually I trained new recruits from the Fleet Sonar School in Key West, Florida. I was plagued with one short bout of psychosis while in the navy, but was allowed to remain in the services, if I returned to my base. Which I did, as I surely did not want to leave the navy on the grounds of a mental problem.

I did finally leave the navy early to enter the Registered Nurses training program at the Vancouver General Hospital, in Vancouver, BC. But I left the nursing program after 14 months, as I was accepted at the University of British Columbia in the Pre-Med program, in September 1966—the real dream of my life. But I became depressed and paranoid by the end of my first university term, and had to drop out—with terrible emotional pain over the loss of my dream. I managed to eventually move on.

Because I was very good in bookkeeping, typing, and shorthand in high school, I eventually got a bookkeeping job in 1967. By 1970, I was a senior bookkeeper, and started the Certified General Accountant's course at UBC at night school, while working full-time. I only managed two years of the course before my life started unravelling again.

In December 1974, while working as a junior accountant at a large cedar mill in Langley, BC, I finally crashed into four years of severe psychosis, which took me out of my accounting job and into a psychiatric ward for a couple weeks, and then into my parents' home, where they looked after me as long as they were able, which was about a year.

Trouble came, and into a prison remand section I went in May 1976, in a terrible psychotic state. After two weeks, my family, lawyer, and forensic psychiatrist had me transferred into Riverview mental hospital. After six months of psychiatric treatment, and a five month trial for arson, I went on to a forensic ward, from which I was not finally released until October 1978.

These were horrible years, which nearly did me in. Four years of drug treatment—with Valium, then shock treatments, and finally anti-psychotic drugs—put a deeper shadow over my so-called illness, I believe, than had the original symptoms.

From the time I was released from the forensic hospital in October 1978, until my final serious psychotic crash in October 1998, which lasted four months, I had one minor collapse in the winter of 1984, with a mess of symptoms throughout the next nine years. Then came a more serious collapse in August of 1993, which lasted nearly two years, until the spring of 1995.

It was after the four months of psychosis, starting in October 1998, that I finally made an appointment to see Dr. Jonn Matsen at the end of January 1999. After being a patient of Dr. Matsen's for ten months, I found that all of my symptoms were starting to diminish, though they had not gone away totally. Dr. Matsen told me in November 1999 that I needed to go and get all the remaining mercury fillings out of my mouth, of which I had five or six.

I only had eight teeth of my own left. As a child I had soft teeth, and had many fillings before I was 25. At 25 I had all of my top teeth removed because they were soft and misshapen; I also had an accident in high school while playing grass hockey.

After having my fillings changed, I have had DMPS IV shots every month since the end of January 2000. My whole world has changed. The mental, emotional, and physical symptoms have nearly all disappeared. The mercury and other heavy metals in my body are considerably lower now, and hopefully after a few more months, they will finally all be removed from my body.

The paranoia, anger, hostility, depression, psychosis, immune system problems, personality problems, and extreme self-consciousness have disappeared, as have a mass of other symptoms. I am left, at 57, with a sense of peace I have hardly ever known as an adult. But I am also left with a very different kind of anger: an anger over a terrible injustice that can tear a person's life to shreds for so long, for which no one is held responsible in our system.

Carolynn J. Brown
Salt Spring Island, BC

CHAPTER 2

Vaccines: Unanswered Questions

"The inherent danger of all vaccination procedures should be a deterrent to their unnecessary or unjustifiable use. Vaccination is far too often employed, especially in the developing countries...and should not be used as an excuse from applying the well tried standard methods for the prevention of infectious disease. Most important is to realize the potential dangers of mass immunization. In such an operation time does not permit an inquiry into the suitability of each individual subject for vaccination."

Sir Graham Wilson
London School of Hygiene and Tropical Medicine

In the last several years, I've seen the following: in any adults who have their mercury fillings replaced, and who show sulfur deficiency when I test them, the DMPS chelation-challenge urine test will show mercury as the most predominant heavy metal in their bodies. From this I presume that mercury depletes sulfur because mercury *binds* to sulfur, decreasing the amount available to the body.

355

So whenever sulfur deficiency shows up on the preliminary test, I immediately suspect mercury is present in the patient's body. While everyone who has followed up with the DMPS chelation urine test has shown positive for mercury, I've never recommended the DMPS test for children because DMPS might be too strong for kids.

Does mercury leak from children's amalgam fillings as it does from adults' fillings?

In 1994, a study was done on 81 children *with* amalgam fillings and 86 children *without* amalgam fillings; the children ranged in age from three to 15. A direct correlation between the number of dental amalgams and the concentration of mercury in the urine was found. Urine from children with amalgams averaged 0.66 micrograms of mercury, while those without amalgams averaged 0.16 micrograms of mercury. No correlation was found with consumption of fish or mercury-thermometer accidents.[55] Since this scientific study shows that mercury *does* leak from the amalgams of children, one must assume that the mercury *will* affect the health of these children, as it has been proven to do in adults. Not according to the Canadian Dental Association. They say, **"Scientific studies have not verified that dental amalgam is causing illness in the general population."** [56]

When children show sulfur deficiency, my immediate suspicion is that mercury might be involved in their chronic health problem. Without the DMPS test, however, I have no way to verify that, as I could with an adult.

If children have amalgam fillings, I recommend that they have them replaced, because the mere existence of mercury-amalgam fillings is proof enough that mercury is likely accumulating in their bodies. But what are you to think when sulfur-testing arouses your **suspicions for mercury, but their history tells you that they have never had amalgam fillings? If sulfur deficiency is indeed the indicator for mercury, where could the mercury be coming from?**

On looking through Bernard Windham's main collection of research on mercury, it didn't take long to come up with a possible explanation.

Soon after the placement of mercury-amalgam fillings in a pregnant woman's teeth, mercury moves from her blood through the placenta, and appears in the amniotic fluid, and in the blood, liver, and especially the pituitary gland of the fetus.[102] Exposure of the mother to mercury vapour was found to cause an accumulation of mercury in the fetus that was ten times more than if the mother was exposed to an equivalent dose of inorganic mercury.[103] Developmental behavioural effects have been found even at low levels of exposure to mercury vapour.[104]

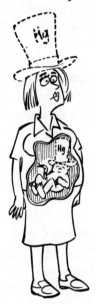

- Mercury can reduce the ability of the mother's blood to transport essential nutrients to the fetus, including oxygen, glucose, amino acids, zinc, magnesium, and vitamin B_{12}.[105]

- Mercury can depress the fetal enzyme isocitric dehydrogenase, interfere with iodine uptake, and cause hypothyroidism.[106]

- Mercury can cause learning deficiencies and impairment, and reduction in IQ,[107] as well as birth defects.[108]

- Mercury has an effect on the fetal nervous system at levels far below that considered toxic in adults, and background levels of mercury in mothers correlate significantly with incidence of birth defects and still births.[109]

- Mercury can accumulate in the fetus and in breast milk at much higher levels than in the mother's tissues.[110] Dental amalgams are the main source of the mercury found in breast milk,[111] and milk further increases the bioavailability of mercury.[112]

- There is a significant correlation between the number of amalgam fillings a mother has and both the level of mercury in her fetus and older infants, [113] and the level of mercury in her breast milk.[114] For example, milk from mothers with seven or more fillings was found to have mercury levels approximately ten times that of the breast milk of amalgam-free mothers.[115]

- Studies have found that exposure to toxic metals, including mercury, has major effects on classroom behaviour and learning ability. High levels of exposure to toxic metals have also been found in patients with mental illness, and those involved in criminal behaviour.[116]

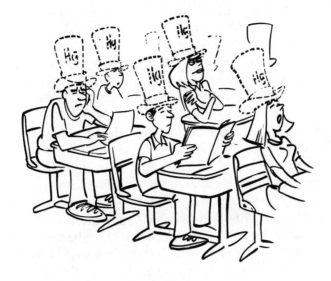

The research shows clearly that a mother's mercury level can have an effect *on her developing fetus* that is greater than the effect mercury has *on her*. While fish is known to be a source of mercury for the mother, studies of mothers and their children in the Republic of Seychelles—where 85 percent of the population consumes ocean fish daily—showed no adverse effects on the development of the children up to age 66 months.[57] Shellfish found in coastal waterways, however, are more likely to be contaminated with mercury and cadmium.[117] In Florida wildlife studies, mercury was found to be present at levels that feminized males, and that had adverse effects on female reproductive systems. Similar effects have also been documented in humans.[118]

The transfer of mercury from mother to fetus is widely recognized now. In some countries, putting mercury fillings in women who are pregnant *has been banned*. This is not going to entirely solve the problem because most women don't know they're pregnant until a few weeks along in their pregnancy; it's possible for them to have dental work done without realizing they are pregnant.

Also, while acute exposure to mercury vapour is increased during placement of *new* mercury fillings, chronic exposure to mercury from *old* fillings will still be ongoing. Plus—as the DMPS chelation tests and autopsies have so clearly shown—the accumulated total-body-burden of mercury must be considered. Banning placement of mercury fillings in pregnant women is only the first step toward the inevitable *complete ban* on mercury fillings that is 160 years overdue.

I was content with this research—which showed that mercury can pass from mother to child via the placenta and mother's milk—to explain the fact that sulfur deficiency was showing when testing children with chronic diseases that weren't responding to my treatment.

Then a child patient of mine tested sulfur-deficient, which made me suspicious of mercury, **but that child had never had any mercury fillings and neither had the mother! How could a positive test for sulfur deficiency indicate that the child carried mercury, if the child hadn't been exposed to mercury amalgam?**

My first reaction was that sulfur deficiency wasn't as reliable an indicator of mercury as I had first thought—until Bernard Windham came through with a batch of research that gives another explanation about how mercury can affect children. That research showed that mercury—in the form of **thimerosal**—had been injected directly into babies, children, and adults. Thimerosal is a substance that for years has been used to increase the shelf-life of vaccines. Let's take a closer look at the history of vaccines, and the research that's been done, to see if there's any connection between health problems and vaccinations.

VACCINES

Smallpox (*Variola major*) was a disease that killed several hundred to a thousand people per year in England in the 1700s, except in parts of western England, where dairy workers appeared to have found a way to develop resistance to smallpox. A farmer named Benjamin Jesty noticed that cowmilkers who had contracted the viral disease cowpox

(*Variola vaccinae*) did not get very sick, and at the same time, seemed to acquire immunity against the more deadly smallpox disease. In 1774, Jesty inoculated his wife and two sons with pus from a cowpox pustule using a darning needle; they did not develop smallpox, while other people did.

Doctor Edward Jenner heard about this. He inoculated an eight-year-old boy named James Phipps—and later, his own son, as well—with cowpox. Even though he later injected them with smallpox, no symptoms appeared. This apparent ability of cowpox vaccination to give protection against smallpox was quickly accepted as a major breakthrough in preventing this deadly disease. This resulted in the first mass vaccinations with live cowpox virus. These vaccines became compulsory in England in 1853, and have been spread around the world by enthusiastic government health departments ever since.

Paul Ehrlich later proposed a theory that vaccinations resulted in the production of specific antibodies for that disease, which would protect the person against the organism that caused that disease.

LEGAL ENFORCEMENT OF
UNPROVEN VACCINES ON THE NAÏVE MASSES

Mandatory smallpox vaccinations in Holland and Switzerland were eliminated in 1904, due to suspicions about their benefits. In the same year in the USA, "the Land of Freedom," a remarkable case was being played out in the Supreme Court. A law enforcing vaccinations and revaccinations against smallpox had been passed in Cambridge, Massachusetts. A man named Jacobson refused to be revaccinated; he claimed that he and his son had bad reactions to previous smallpox vaccinations. He felt that vaccination could cause injury or even death, and that he should be exempted from having further vaccinations. The Court ruled that:

"It was the duty of the constituted authorities to keep in view the welfare, comfort, and safety of the many, and not permit the interests of the many to be subordinated to the wishes or convenience of the few." [58]

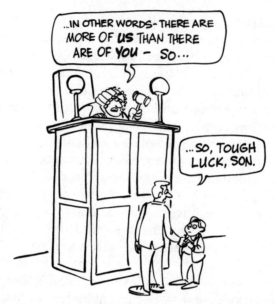

Thus the Court ruled that the government had the right to force vaccinations on people, and also that **doctors had the ability to predetermine who would have bad reactions to a vaccine; therefore, the ultimate authority lay with doctors,** not with Jacobson. Did Jacobson and his son have another smallpox vaccination forced upon them? Did they suffer dire consequences from it? The answers seem to have been lost in time. However, this shift of power away from the individual to the government and the medical profession was an omen, as mass vaccinations were only beginning.

After the smallpox vaccine came vaccines for **tetanus** and **diphtheria**, both of which seemed to help in limiting these deadly childhood diseases. **Pertussis** vaccination was created to stimulate the body to make specific antibodies against the pertussis bacteria in the late 1930s; it was combined with the diphtheria and tetanus vaccines to become the **DPT shot.**

Pertussis, or **whooping cough,** is a highly contagious bacterial infection of the upper respiratory system that causes the most pronounced symptoms in young children. The pertussis bacteria produces several toxins; one is sometimes called **histamine sensitizing factor (HSF)**, which makes the person much more allergic. For example, the child might start out with a mild cough for several weeks, but by late in the second or third week, the bacterial toxins can irritate the membranes of the lungs into producing tremendous quantities of mucous, especially at night, so that the child is choking, gagging, and coughing it up. This severe coughing can last for two to three weeks, although full recovery can take months.

Secondary infections accompanying pertussis can be severe—and if the pertussis toxins penetrate the blood-brain barrier, they can cause convulsions, brain injury, and death. In 1934, in the US, 265,000 cases of whooping cough were reported, with 7,500 deaths. Obviously, pertussis is a disease we want to prevent children from contracting.

At first, pertussis vaccine was administered to the children of wealthier, more educated parents, but by the late 1950s, it began to be used on a mass basis in all the industrialized countries. While each state in the US controls its own vaccination program (many of them with mandatory laws), under the Carter administration in the 1970s, the federal government pushed for total vaccination in the population, and eventually achieved a DPT vaccination rate of over 95 percent in many geographical areas.

ARE VACCINES DANGEROUS?

A 1997 conference on "Living and Learning with Autism," with Paul Shattock and Dawn Savery of the Autism Research Unit, University of Sunderland, UK, had this to say:
"The suggestion that autism and other disorders with serious and lifelong implications could be caused by vaccinations has been in circulation for many years. There are few rational texts on the topic and most literature can be placed in one of two categories. Some authors adopt what appears to be a fanatical anti-vaccine stance and so overstate their case that even the valid points become unbelievable. On the other hand, orthodox medical

literature exhibits such complacency and lack of
willingness to accept that any problems could exist that it
too becomes devalued."

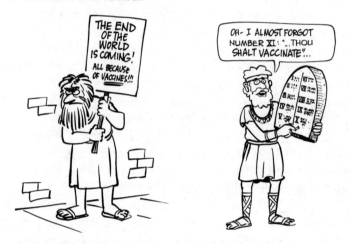

In the 1970s, while US politicians were gloating about
achieving almost universal vaccination rates on young children,
parents of thousands of them were left grieving over their dead
or brain-damaged children. They formed a group called **DPT
(Dissatisfied Parents Together)** in 1982, which grew into the
National Vaccine Information Center in Vienna, Virginia—
dedicated to preventing vaccination death and injury, through
public education.

One of the founders was Barbara Loe Fisher; her oldest son
had a severe reaction after his fourth DPT shot, which left him
with multiple learning disabilities and attention deficit disorder.
She is co-author, with Harris Coulter, of *A Shot in the Dark*,[59] a
well-referenced exposé of the political and medical cover-ups of
the side-effects of pertussis vaccinations.

While vaccine manufacturers and their medical and political
allies have long touted the benefits of vaccinations—ignoring
or downplaying their known side-effects—in 1986, the US
Congress, under pressure from concerned parents, passed the
National Childhood Vaccine Injury Act (Public Law 99-660).
The *Act* recognized that a significant number of recipients of
mandatory vaccines would be killed and injured each year.

The law requires doctors to warn parents of the potential dangers of vaccinations before administering a vaccine. Also, all bad reactions within 30 days after a vaccine—such as convulsions, shock, or paralysis—are to be recorded and reported by the person who administers the vaccine. This person is not to judge whether the reactions are from the vaccine, but to simply report the occurrence.

I'm sure most people who have had vaccinations can't recall hearing the potential side-effects of vaccinations explained to them, or having pertinent questions asked of them before the needle was stuck into their arm or their posterior. More ominous is that the vice president of the National Vaccine Information Center, Barbara Loe Fisher, stated:

"The will and intent of Congress in enacting the *National Vaccine Injury Act* of 1986 is being subverted. This subversion is resulting in an appalling underreporting of vaccine reactions and deaths by both private and public health physicians... ."

The National Vaccine Information Center has estimated that reported incidences of vaccine injury may be 10 percent, or lower, of the actual injuries sustained.

Underreporting of vaccine injury seems to prevail in England, as well, according to Sir Graham Wilson of the London School of Hygiene and Tropical Medicine. In his book, *The Hazards of Immunization*, he states that:

"...a large number of accidents—I suspect the majority—have never been reported in print, either through fear of compensation claims, or of giving a weapon to anti-vaccinationists... . I have come to the conclusion that no vaccine...has been free from complications or accidents." [60]

The US Department of Health and Human Services was ordered by Congress to develop and disseminate vaccine information, including adverse reactions and contraindications before December 22, 1988. The **National Vaccine Advisory Committee** was formed to do that. By March 1991, the information was yet to be published; the chair of the

subcommittee, Barbara Loe Fisher, reports her version
as to why:

**"Not only is there a lack of concern about the subject of
vaccine reactions on the part of some committee members,
but there is a deliberate attempt to deny the reality of
vaccine reactions, deaths, and injuries."**

On October 1, 1988, Congress established a tax on a number
of vaccines—from a few cents per polio vaccine, to several
dollars per DPT and MMR vaccine—to pay for deaths or
injuries from those mandatory vaccinations. What's the reality
behind this somewhat-secretive "insurance" against vaccine
injury?

The FDA reported that in the **three-year period** ending
December 31, 1993, there had been **31,000 reports of adverse
effects due to vaccinations, and 500 were deaths**. Of course, if
accusations of underreporting vaccine reactions are real, then
the true damage could be much higher than that. If, in a three-
year period, one child died from taking a vitamin or a herb, that
supplement would be banned immediately—and 500 deaths of
young children in three years would lead to a major
investigation to immediately halt this travesty.

Even if three of every four claims are dismissed as
unsubstantiated—often because the reactions didn't occur
within hours after the vaccination—money paid out in the four
years ending May 16, 1994, was more than $437 million for
death and injuries—mainly of the brain (such as **mental
retardation, paralysis, seizures, and learning disabilities**)—
with most of the suits involving pertussis vaccine. By February
28, 1998, compensation payments were $871 million, and a
billion-dollar surplus was being held against future claims.

Lawsuits against vaccines aren't confined to the US. In
October 1998, **the French government abandoned its
mandatory hepatitis B vaccination for school children after
more than 15,000 lawsuits were filed for brain damage and
autoimmune reactions, including arthritis, MS, and lupus**.

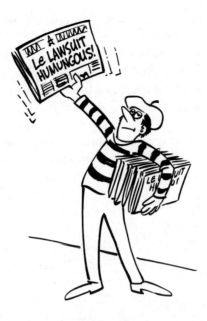

Hepatitis B is a vaccine that, like pertussis, commonly **contains thimerosal**, the mercury preservative.

The US government Vaccine Adverse Event Reporting System reported that **in 1996, 872 children under the age of 14** suffered severe adverse **reactions to hepatitis B vaccine; 48** of these reactions **were fatal**.[61]

In the 1980s, the mystery of **Sudden Infant Death Syndrome (SIDS)** was reported in the media, with increasing numbers of children suddenly dying in their sleep without apparent reason.

Some research implicated the addition of flame-retardant chemicals to mattresses as possible suspects. **Phosphorus, antimony,** and **arsenic** added to mattresses were found to be consumed by the fungus *Scopulariopsis brevicaulis,* that then gave off the heavier-than-air gases **phosphine, stibine,** and **arsine**— which, when breathed by a sleeping baby, can have fatal effects.

From this insight, New Zealander T. J. Sprott invented a mattress cover called **BabeSafe®**, which blocked the exposure of the sleeping baby to the gaseous emissions, and virtually ended crib death for those using it. In Japan, the much-safer boron was used as a fire-inhibitor.[62]

The rash of baby deaths had also caught the attention of Australian research scientist Viera Scheibner. Her insight was to design a monitor that could tell when a sleeping baby was in distress so that help could be brought to bear before the child passed away in his or her sleep. In 1985, she met an electronics engineer named Leif Karlsson. Together they developed a monitor called **Cotwatch**. Sensors detected the sleeping baby's breathing patterns and recorded them. Any delay in breathing would activate an alarm so that the parent or attendant could rush to wake the child before death ensued.

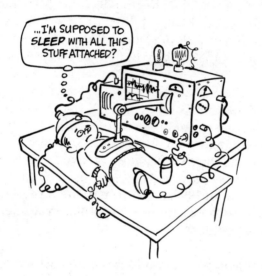

Note: The Cotwatch sensors are actually under the mattress; nothing is attached to the baby.

It was found that when a child was under stress, he or she would exhibit a shallow breathing pattern using only about 5 percent of normal air volume. If the child were developing a cold, low-volume breathing would occur a night or two before the actual cold symptoms would manifest. By picking up this early-stage breathing response—which would normally be overlooked by the parents or attendant—Cotwatch was able to sound the alarm so that the baby could be immediately picked up and treated. One of the key insights seen with the Cotwatch system was that: **"all vaccine recipients whose breathing was recorded with the microprocessor Cotwatch showed reactions to vaccine injections."** [63]

While there were individual differences in the amplitude of stressed-breathing reactions from vaccinations, the reactions reoccurred for a number of days afterward, with the 16th day often being a key crisis point—after which the baby either recovered or worsened, possibly suffering brain injury or death. This apparent link between vaccinations and SIDS was a surprise to Dr. Scheibner; it led her to review 30,000 pages of medical literature on vaccinations. From this research arose her book, *Vaccination: 100 Years of Orthodox Research Shows that Vaccines Represent a Medical Assault on the Immune System.*[64]

In this book, she shows, in great detail, how researchers have long suspected the link between vaccinations and the subsequent death or injury of the child—although this has been greatly ignored because the politics of medicine continued to urge parents to vaccinate their children. She believes that both the polio epidemic of the 1950s, and the increases of *Hemophillus* influenza in more recent times, are likely caused from a weakening of the immune system by the DPT vaccine. Her conclusion, based on her monitoring experiences and her research, is: **"vaccination is the single most prevalent and most preventable cause of infant deaths."**

Australian microbiologist Glen Dettman gives a possible explanation: large amounts of an antigen will cause a massive release of adrenal hormones, and the amount of brain endorphins could be as much as 1,000 times greater than the number normally released. He states:

"The endorphins will suppress respiration and cardiac function. Thus if a child with malnutrition, or an immune problem, is given a load of antigen larger than it can handle—and this antigen may be an immunisation— endorphins may result in respiratory or cardiac failure and death." [65]

This wouldn't be a surprise to the flying doctor, A. Kalokerinos, whose vaccination experiences came from flying

into the Outback of Australia, where he would inoculate the
Aboriginal children. On returning later, he would sometimes
find that half of the children had died since the previous
vaccinations. As he said in his book, *Every Second Child*:

**"A health team would sweep into an area, line up all the
Aboriginal babies and infants and immunize them. There
would be no examination, no taking of case histories, no
checking on dietary deficiencies. Most infants would have
colds. No wonder they died. Some would die within
hours.... . Others would suffer immunological insults and
die later from 'pneumonia,' 'gastroenteritis,' or
'malnutrition.' "** [66]

Let's take a look at the research to see if there is anything
to back up these Australian observations on the hazards of
vaccination. Two cases of SIDS were reported in the *Journal of
the American Medical Association* (*JAMA*) in 1933 as occurring in
two infants within hours of receiving pertussis vaccination.[67]
Another two cases were reported in 1946, by Werne and
Garrow, after identical twins died following their second
pertussis shot.[68]

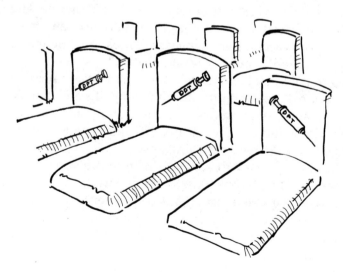

Bernier and associates reported in the *Journal of Pediatrics* in 1982, that a number of infant deaths in Tennessee were unusual, but the fact that they died after DPT vaccinations wasn't in itself proof that the vaccinations were the cause.[69]

Torch, in 1982—commenting on a large number of random Sudden Infant Deaths—stated:

"DPT vaccination may be a generally unrecognized major cause of sudden infant and early childhood death, and that the risks of immunization may outweigh its potential benefits. A need for re-evaluation and possible modification of current vaccination procedure is indicated by this study." [70]

In 1983, Baraff and associates, reporting on their investigation of 145 Sudden Infant Deaths in LA, mentioned suspicion of a link between DPT and SIDS.[71]

The *American Journal of Epidemiology*, in 1992, showed that **children die within three days of a DPT vaccine** *at a rate eight times greater than normal.*[72]

While suspicions of a direct link between pertussis vaccine and SIDS met with more criticism than acceptance in the US, and mandatory vaccinations have continued as the norm, the response in Western Europe was the opposite—most countries abandoned mandatory pertussis vaccinations in the 1970s.

After Germany stopped mandatory pertussis vaccinations, the incidence of whooping cough again climbed to high levels, but *the death rate* from whooping cough was at the lowest level ever recorded.

In Sweden, where pertussis vaccinations were virtually eliminated in the 1970s—partly because the population refused them—it has been seen that pertussis occurs in cycles, every three to four years, yet there have been virtually no deaths from it. Sweden banned the use of amalgam fillings in pregnant women 20 years later; in 1997, Sweden reported its first decline in SIDS in decades. **Could these reductions in exposure to mercury have contributed to that decline?**

In Japan, in 1975, two babies died after DPT shots. As a result, the Japanese delayed giving DPT shots to all infants until they were 24 months of age, which drastically reduced the number of bad reactions—and virtually ended SIDS. The incidence of whooping cough, however, did increase in Japan.

The Japanese developed a purer pertussis vaccine with the hope of reducing vaccination reactions. This was tested on a Swedish population that had long refused the regular pertussis vaccination. One version of the **new Japanese vaccine was only 69 percent effective** at preventing pertussis, while the other was even less effective, at **54 percent.**

More ominous, **11 Swedish babies contracted invasive bacterial infections after receiving the new pertussis vaccine, and four died.** The Swedish government withdrew from further study, preferring to go without any pertussis vaccine rather than risk further young lives to this new vaccine, which wasn't particularly successful at preventing pertussis—and possibly made the body **more** susceptible to other bacterial infections.

Storsaeter and associates stated in their evaluation of the new pertussis vaccine, **"The hypothesis of an immunosuppressive effect of the vaccines, which would explain the deaths…could not be refuted by the data."** [73]

You can see that there have long been connections linking pertussis vaccine to infants dying in their sleep, but let's go further, to see if vaccines have been linked to other diseases.

In 1992, the *Journal of Infectious Diseases* reported that after DPT shots, children in Oman were significantly more likely to contract **paralytic polio** than children who were not vaccinated with DPT.[74]

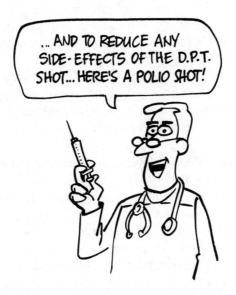

The *Journal of the American Medical Association*, in 1994, reported that children receiving pertussis vaccinations were five times more likely to get **asthma**.[75]

In 1997, a New Zealand study, which was reported in *Epidemiology*, showed a 23 percent incidence of **asthma** in children who had received DPT and polio vaccines, while those who were not immunized did not develop asthma.[76]

Two other studies reported serious reactions to DPT vaccinations; in one study, the number was as high as *one in every 200 children*, while the other study reported that *one in every 600 children* had severe reactions, including **grand mal epilepsy** and **encephalopathy**.[77]

In New Zealand, J. B. Classen observed a 60 percent increase in **Type 1 juvenile diabetes** within several years of mass hepatitis B vaccine campaigns.[78]

Other negative side-effects seen with hepatitis B vaccines are: **demyelination of the central nervous system,**[79] **polyneuropathy,**[80] **thrombocytopenic purpura,**[81] **liver dysfunction,**[82] **transverse myelitis,**[83] **arthritis,**[84] and **Evan's syndrome.**[85]

MMR vaccine (for Measles, Mumps, Rubella) has also had some bad press. A study in 1992 concluded that there is an increased risk of **arthritis** associated with MMR vaccine.[86]

In 1995, a study in *Lancet* reported that those who received the measles vaccine were three times more likely to develop **Crohn's disease**, and more than twice as likely to develop **ulcerative colitis.**[87]

Another report three years later found that **autism** is a possible side-effect of the MMR vaccine.[88]

The MMR vaccine was banned in Japan in 1993, after a large number of children developed **non-viral meningitis** and **other adverse reactions**. One study showed that one in every 900 children experienced problems, which was more than 2,000 times higher than the expected rate of *one child in every 100,000 to 200,000*. Instead, today, in Japan, individual vaccines for measles, mumps, and rubella are used.[89]

Robert Mendelsohn, MD, professor at the University of Illinois, had this to say about vaccinations, in his article, "The Medical Time Bomb of Immunization Against Disease":

"There is growing suspicion that immunization against...childhood diseases may be responsible for the dramatic increase in auto-immune diseases since mass inoculations were introduced. These are fearful diseases such as cancer, leukaemia, rheumatoid arthritis, multiple sclerosis, Lou Gehrig's disease, lupus erythematosus, and the Guillain-Barre syndrome.... Have we traded mumps and measles for cancer and leukaemia?" [90]

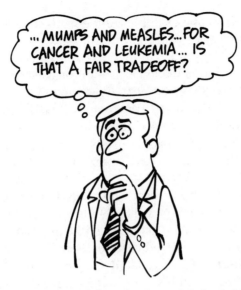

You can see why Barbara Loe Fisher and the other parents of brain-damaged children have been so frustrated. The politicians of Big Medicine constantly deny and belittle the side-effects of vaccines, while the researchers—in 3,000 studies—keep proving those politicians wrong. **What if, after 70 years of killing and brain-damaging babies and children world-wide, it was proven that vaccines didn't even do the job they were originally claimed to do—give long-lasting immunity against a dangerous disease?**

DO VACCINES ALWAYS WORK?

In February 1979, a report in *Pediatrics* showed that 12 years after DPT vaccination, up to **95 percent of the recipients were susceptible to pertussis** infections.[91]

The *Journal of Pediatrics* published an article in 1989 that showed that Nova Scotia **children vaccinated against pertussis were still susceptible** to the disease.[92]

In 1993, an epidemic of pertussis occurred in Cincinnati, Ohio, and **82 percent** of those who came down with it **had received regular doses of the vaccine**.[93]

Even more dramatic examples of ineffectiveness have been reported with measles vaccinations. Measles vaccines were made mandatory in the US in the 1960s, and an over-95 percent vaccination rate was achieved. Cases of measles dropped from 400,000 to 5,000 in the early 1980s. Just when it looked like measles would be completely eradicated, it began to resurface—although this time, in the vaccinated population.

In 1984, in Waltham, Massachusetts, **27 cases of measles** occurred at a high school where **over 98 percent of the students had been vaccinated.**[94]

The next year, Corpus Christi, Texas, had **157 cases of measles**, even though there was a **99 percent vaccination rate.**[95]

A year later, in 1986, it was the turn of Dane County, Wisconsin, with **235 reported cases of measles**, of which **only 6 percent had *not* been vaccinated.**[96]

In 1989, an Illinois high school had **69 cases of measles, in spite of a 99.7 percent vaccination rate.**[97]

So, a number of incidents have been reported where vaccinated populations still contracted the disease they were vaccinated against—and even though their blood contained antibodies against the disease.

Perhaps the whole premise that antibodies induced by vaccinations give protection is wrong to begin with—at least that's what Dr. Manwaring, Professor of Bacteriology and Experimental Pathology at Leland Stanford University, concluded:

"I believe that there is hardly an element of truth in a single one of the basic hypothesis [sic] embodied in this theory. My conviction that there was something radically wrong with it arose from a consideration of the almost universal failure of therapeutic methods based on it.... . Twelve years of study with immuno-physical tests have yielded a mass of experimental evidence contrary to, and irreconcilable with the Ehrlich theory, and have convinced me that his conception of the origin, nature, and physiological role of the specific 'antibodies' is erroneous." [98]

The possibility that billions of people on our planet have been vaccinated and perhaps had their health worsened, due to a faulty understanding of how our immune system works, is at first an incredulous thought—until we realize that it has happened before.

In 1911, Dr. Sidney Lange, a medical radiologist in Cincinnati, Ohio, reported that a woman whose previous two children had died of SIDS—then known as crib death—had a third child who was turning blue from difficulty with breathing. Suspecting an enlarged thymus gland was causing the breathing problems, he irradiated the thymus gland, and credited the radiation with saving the child's life.

For the next 40 years, it became the norm for many hospitals to x-ray the thymus glands of infants. If the thymus was more than half the width of the heart, as shown on x-ray, then the child was given a series of radiation treatments. This treatment was so enthusiastically embraced by radiologists that it was expanded to treat sore throats, chronic coughs, enlarged tonsils, and acne. Millions of children were exposed to extremely high doses of radiation.

By the late 1940s, studies were beginning to show that accumulated doses of radiation could cause adverse health effects, and thymus radiation was generally discontinued in the early 1950s. Studies done in the 1970s and 1980s show that those children whose thymuses were irradiated have an 80-fold increased risk of thyroid cancer and a two-fold higher risk of developing other cancers.[99]

Now it is known that the thymus gland is often enlarged in infancy because it is the controlling gland in the newly developing immune system. **Will studies one day show that vaccines have been an even bigger blunder? Will long-term studies ever be done?**

Yet the faithful still cling to their belief that vaccines are successful because of the tremendous results that smallpox vaccine achieved, beginning with Jenner's triumphant inoculations of James Phipps and his own son with cowpox, so many years ago.

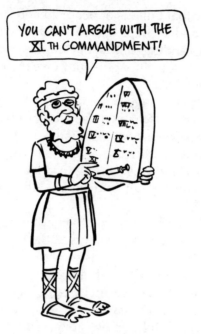

James Phipps was inoculated by Jenner 20 times, and died at the age of 20 from tuberculosis, as did Jenner's son, at age 21. Neither contracted smallpox, so in that sense, perhaps the vaccinations may have been a success; but the vaccines obviously didn't improve the young men's defences against tuberculosis. **Could it be possible that the smallpox vaccine actually weakened their immune defences against the tuberculosis bacteria?**

What would be the point of winning a battle against smallpox, yet losing the war against tuberculosis as a result? While proponents of mass vaccinations have spent no money on long-term studies—to verify that short-term gains might have been made at the expense of other health problems—most have spent even less time pondering the possibility that they might be doing more harm than good.

Ironically, Jenner's use of cowpox was soon shown *to not work* very well, because people still contracted smallpox after being vaccinated—so the theory arose that re-vaccinations were necessary to guarantee immunity.

We have all heard the claim that the smallpox vaccine has been so successful that the smallpox virus has been virtually chased off the planet—but did the smallpox vaccine play any role at all? Bubonic plague also virtually disappeared in the same time period, and no vaccine was used against it. Had bubonic plague just run its course as we, as a society, developed a natural "herd immunity," or is it because we have developed better sanitation, such as not pooping into our drinking water?

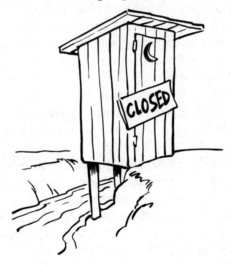

In the 1950s, the World Health Organization (WHO), the health branch of the United Nations, initiated a vaccination program to eradicate smallpox from the world—37 million doses were administered over 20 years. The *WHO Chronicle* reported in 1968, 1969, 1971, and 1975 that numerous countries that had been vaccinated still experienced deadly outbreaks of smallpox.[100]

In 1980, Dettman and Kalokerinos summed up their research on smallpox thus:

"...we claim that if the evidence is honestly evaluated that smallpox has actually been prolonged and that the so called protective vaccinations actually put the recipient at risk from...the disease itself." [101]

THIMEROSAL: MERCURY PRESERVATIVE IN VACCINES

In July of 1999, the US FDA requested that US manufacturers of vaccines plan to remove **thimerosal** from vaccines. Thimerosal is a mercury compound that has been used as a preservative in many medications—including some vaccines—for the last 70 years.

In November 1999, in the *Journal of the American Medical Association*, Halsey calculated that if all the vaccinations recommended by the American Academy of Pediatrics are given—and if they all contain thimerosal as a preservative—by the age of six months, the infant would have received 187 micrograms of ethylmercury, which exceeds the Environmental Protection Agency (EPA) guidelines for mercury.[102]

The **Pharmaceutical Research and Manufacturers of America (PhRMA)** noted in a statement that while there is currently:

> **"no clinical evidence that the use of thimerosal has caused adverse health consequences, there is general consensus that it would be preferable to eliminate thimerosal from vaccines whenever possible. The vaccine industry is working closely with FDA and other government agencies to meet this objective."** [103]

No adverse health effects from thimerosal!? How about this study published in 1994: thimerosal was injected into mice, which resulted in a swelling response that peaked after one hour, and lasted for more than 24 hours. The authors concluded:

> **"These results suggest that part of these hypersensitivity reactions against thimerosal observed among patients were possibly induced by the toxic effect of thimerosal. Therefore, thimerosal contained as a preservative in vaccine may augment the side-effects of the vaccination."** [104]

Let's see if this insight holds up in a human study. In an Italian study published in 1998, 670 children—between six months and 12 years of age—who had **dermatitis** and **eczema**, underwent skin-patch testing with **47 different substances; 282** children **(42 percent) were positive** to one or more of the substances tested, indicating an immediate-type hypersensitivity allergy to that substance. Of the 31 substances that showed positive, **nearly half the reactions were to one substance, and that was thimerosal.** The researchers' comments were:

> **"In our patients the high incidence of positivity to thimerosal may be related both to compulsory vaccinations and to exposure to antiseptics containing this substance... ."** [105]

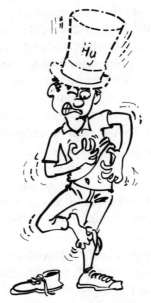

If over 20 percent of children with eczema or dermatitis were allergic to thimerosal on the immediate-type hypersensitivity testing (skin-patch testing), what would delayed-type hypersensitivity testing—such as MELISA® testing—show? Also, if skin allergy reactions to thimerosal are so common in children, and have been overlooked by the manufacturers, couldn't immune reactions involving much more serious problems have been overlooked, as well?

Because Dr. Scheibner's experiences with the Cotwatch detection system showed that all her test children reacted badly to all vaccines—even the ones that didn't contain mercury—there is no doubt that the negative reactions to vaccines involve more than just a reaction to mercury. **However, because mercury is one of the most toxic of substances—especially to a developing nervous system—couldn't mercury have been the main instigator of dramatic increases in allergic responses and decreased learning ability in children, especially in the last 40 years, when vaccines were pushed onto the naïve masses?**

Shouldn't research be done to find out the extent of the damage done to our children by mercury-laced vaccines? Not according to the joint statement issued by the **US Public Health Service** and the **American Academy of Pediatrics**: **"Infants and children who have received thimerosal-containing vaccines do not need to have blood, urine, or hair tested for mercury** because the concentrations of mercury would be quite low and **would not require treatment."** [106]

Is this because there wouldn't be any mercury found in the little toddlers, or is it because if mercury were found, the political embarrassment (and lawsuits) would be too much to bear? Of course, the small amounts of mercury from vaccines might not be all that easy to find. Conventional hair, blood, and urine tests haven't been reliable at detecting the level of mercury accumulating in our bodies from amalgam fillings. The only accurate way to determine the amounts of accumulated mercury is through autopsies—and compare the results of those who received vaccinations with those who didn't, as was done in Sweden, with amalgam fillings.

David Satcher, the former US Surgeon General, had this to say about the matter:

"The risk of devastating childhood diseases from failure to vaccinate far outweighs the minimal, if any, risk of exposure to cumulative levels of mercury in vaccines." [107]

Excuse me, Dr. Surgeon General, sir. You are saying that there has been minimal risk to children's health from the mercury-laced vaccines that have been forced on them for the last 70 years. **Could you show us the studies that have been done to back up this statement?** If you have none, then it must be asked if the government is more interested in the health of the vaccine industry than in the health of the millions of children who are entrusted to its care.

Perhaps you are too busy to do such onerous research, so let me help you out by showing a few reasons why you should reconsider. In a three-year period, at least 500 American children were killed by vaccinations that likely contained thimerosal, and many more became brain-damaged.

What killed them? What damaged them?

There have been dramatic increases in **dermatitis, asthma, allergies, eczema, autism, schizophrenia, psoriasis, vitiligo, diabetes, lupus, attention deficit disorder, hyperactivity, dyslexia, and behavioural disorders** in children over the last 50 years—the same period in which mandatory vaccines have been given *en masse*. **Why?**

Recently a teenage boy came in to see me with the results of his urine test after having a DMPS challenge. The results are shown in Table 17.

ELEMENTS REGARDED AS TOXIC

Elements	Result (µg/g creatinine)	per gram Creatinine Reference Range* (µg/g creatinine)	Within Ref. Range	Elevated	Very Elevated
Aluminum	<dl	0–35			
Antimony	<dl	0–5			
Arsenic	53	0–100	· · · ·		
Beryllium	<dl	0–.5			
Bismuth	<dl	0–30			
Cadmium	<dl	0–2			
Lead	<dl	0–15			
Mercury	43	0–3	· · · · · · · · · · ·	· · · · · · · ·	· · · · · · ·
Nickel	6.8	0–12	· · · · ·		
Platinum	<dl	0–2			
Thallium	.4	0–14	·		
Thorium	<dl	0–12			
Tin	<dl	0–6			
Tungsten	<dl	0–23			
Uranium	<dl	0–1			

OTHER TESTS

	Result (mg/dl)	Reference Range* (mg/dl)	2 SD Low 1 SD Low Mean 1 SD High 2 SD High
Creatinine	18.2	75–200	· · · | · · · | · · · | ·

Methodology: Analyzed by Induction Coupled Plasma Mass Spectrometry (ICP-MS). Creatinine by Jaffe Method. "dl" =detection limit. *No safe levels established

Comments:
(Post provocative challenge.)

Table 17

He is the first of my patients with **no history of mercury-amalgam fillings** to be tested for the presence of toxic metals, yet his test results show *high levels of mercury*. He came to see me because he had developed severe ulcerative colitis shortly after receiving a hepatitis B vaccination. It is likely that his high mercury levels are from the thimerosal used in that vaccine. However, his mother worked in a dental office while she was pregnant with him, so that may have also been a contributing factor.

During the last few weeks, I've also seen children in their early teens who have contracted juvenile diabetes, chronic fatigue, and attention deficit disorder (ADD) after receiving hepatitis B vaccinations, and juvenile rheumatoid arthritis after receiving a meningitis shot. Studies show that autism has also dramatically increased since the advent of hepatitis B vaccines.

Now, as of June 1, 2001, newborns in British Columbia, Canada, will be immunized with *mercury-free* hepatitis B vaccines. Existing stocks of mercury-containing hepatitis B vaccines, however, will still be administered to those over 20 years of age. My own experience of seeing patients who have developed immune diseases in their early teens—in addition to medical research on the subject—indicate this may not be a good idea. Injecting this old mercury-laden hepatitis B stock into anyone, of any age, may create another round of serious health problems.

Why are we injecting our children with hepatitis B vaccines anyway, since hepatitis B mainly occurs in IV drug users? Is it feasible to assume that all children are going to grow up doing IV drugs? If juvenile diabetes can be caused by a hepatitis B shot—presumably from the mercury (thimerosal) in the vaccination—**isn't it plausible that adult-onset diabetes could be caused by the mercury in flu shots? Have any studies been done?**

In her book, *Endangered Minds,* Dr. Jane M. Healy notes there has been a dramatic change in the mental functioning of students since the 1960s. She examines how "today's fast-paced media culture" has negatively affected children's levels of concentration and learning ability. Dr. Healy states:

> **"Today's students looked and acted differently, of course, and they talked about different things, but I became increasingly convinced that the changes went deeper than that—to the very ways in which they were absorbing and processing information."**

> **"Yes, attention spans are noticeably shorter. Yes, reading, writing, and oral language skills seem to be declining— even in the 'best' neighborhoods."** [108]

Overall scholastic ability has decreased, and Dr. Healy shows conclusively that teachers have lowered the difficulty of the exams to make it easier for students to pass.

However, while marks are down, shootings are up.

REPORT CARD

READING.........D
WRITING.........C
ARITHMETIC......C
HISTORY.........D
SCIENCE.........C
AGGRESSION......A
BULLYING........A
SHOOTING........A

Could this change in mental functioning be connected to the increase in mandatory vaccinations imposed on these children during the same time period? The **American Psychiatric Association's handbook** for diagnosing mental handicaps, *Diagnostic and Statistical Manual of Mental Disorders*, states that the following conditions can be caused by heavy metal toxicity:

"**pervasive development disorder, borderline intellectual functioning, mild to profound mental retardation, autistic disorder, academic skill disorder, passivity, dependency, low self-esteem, low frustration tolerance, aggressiveness, poor impulse control, self-stimulating behavior, and self-injurious behavior.**"

Most of this research was done on lead toxicity, but it also applies to cadmium toxicity—which is much more toxic than lead—and to mercury, which is even more toxic than cadmium. My recent experiences with DMPS chelation have shown that mercury is far more common in chronically ill adults than lead, cadmium, arsenic, or aluminum—and much slower to be eliminated from the body. **Does the same pattern hold true for children?**

Here's a bit of research on infants—which seems to have been overlooked by the government in an attempt to save the vaccine industry from its potentially embarrassing moment. Studies researching the reasons for the increase in infant reactive conditions seem to implicate earlier and higher usage of thimerosal-containing vaccines as a possible connection.[119] The incompletely formed blood-brain barriers of fetuses and young infants offer little protection against mercury, and thus the resulting damage is commonly neurological. Underweight infants who get the same dose of thimerosal as other infants have been found to be more vulnerable. Pregnant women who are RH negative commonly get RhoGAM shots; these carry a further 30 micrograms of mercury-containing thimerosal.

Studies have also shown that mercury has adverse effects on the cellular mineral levels of calcium, magnesium, zinc, and lithium,[120] and that mercury decreases levels of vitamins B_6 and B_{12}. Clinically, mercury seems to block the conversion of cobalamin (vitamin B_{12}) into methylcobalamin—the form of B_{12} that provides protection for the nerves—thus leaving the person much more vulnerable to nerve damage.

Mercury is mined from cinnabar ore in the form of mercury sulphide, which shows that mercury has a strong attraction to sulfur.

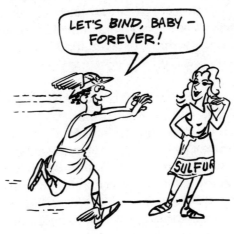

When it binds to sulfur in your body, mercury interferes with enzymes that require sulfur for proper function. This process can be responsible for the allergic, immune-reactive conditions that can result from vaccinations.[121]

Some of the sulfur-carrying enzymes that are inhibited by mercury are **xanthine oxidase** and **dipeptyl peptidase**—which play a key role in digestion of the **casein of milk** products[122]— and an enzyme that digests **gluten in grains**.

Studies involving a large sample of **autistic, schizophrenic, and manic patients** found that over 90 percent showed defective enzymes for the digestion of milk proteins[123] and wheat gluten[124]; these patients also had high levels of the **milk protein beta-casomorphine-7** in their blood and urine. Beta-casomorphine-7 is a morphine-like compound from dairy products that can cause nerve dysfunction,[125] increase histamine reactions, and induce skin reactions.[126] Similar reactions were seen to a gluten protein.[127]

The same studies showed that the poor digestion of dairy protein also led to immune reactions against various parts of dairy, such as high levels of IgA antibodies for casein, lactalbumin, and beta-lactoglobulin, and high IgG and IgM antibodies for casein.

Children who were tested for toxic exposures have also showed reactions to other toxic metals and organochlorine pollutants.[128] The effects of these substances on the immune and neurological systems can be factors in the increasing incidences of eczema, allergies, asthma, delayed food allergies, and other sensitivities.[129]

Studies have found that mercury increases the levels of suppressor T cells,[130] while other studies have shown a reduction in B cells,[131] leaving autistic patients with increased incidence of viruses, leaky gut, lymph node enlargement, and intestinal parasites. Ironically, vaccinations that are given to improve the immune system's reactions against a specific disease can have a devastating effect—derailing the immune system, and damaging the digestive and neurological systems at the same time.

All autistic children were found to have disrupted liver enzyme function. In fact, by the time you've finished this book, you'll relate most chronic diseases back to these key liver enzymes—and you'll know how to keep them working at their optimum.

What is the most important reason for finding out whether a child's vaccine-related health problem was caused by mercury? There is a possibility that improvement may come from removing the mercury. The MELISA® metal-allergy testing from Sweden found that **thimerosal** (the mercury preservative used in vaccines) showed as **an allergen in 7 percent of the people tested**. We have already calculated that if 3 percent of the population are allergic to mercury in dental amalgam fillings, that would mean that 900,000 Canadians or 9 million Americans are affected.

So "7 percent allergic to thimerosal from vaccines" would be more than double those numbers—perhaps 2 million Canadians or 20 million people in the US. **Do you then add these new numbers to the numbers of people already known to be allergic to mercury, to calculate that 10 percent of the population is allergic to mercury from fillings and vaccinations?**

Or, because children are the ones most exposed to thimerosal from vaccinations, should the 7 percent be calculated as a percentage of *children*, **rather than the general population?** (Remember: in that Italian study of children with eczema and dermatitis, over 20 percent have been shown to be allergic to thimerosal.) **Hasn't it already been calculated that 20 percent of children in parts of the US are learning-disabled, since the time that mandatory vaccinations have been injected into 95 percent of all American children?**

Because the vaccine is injected directly into the bloodstream, the spleen—the primary filter for the bloodstream (the liver being the primary filter for the gut)—could receive the brunt of the foreign antigens in the vaccine, including the thimerosal.

Your spleen is a hornet's nest of immune activity because your immune system's main components are here, *en masse,* "frisking the blood" for any aliens. As the blood enters your spleen, it passes into the white pulp area, where it's thoroughly exposed to numerous T cells and B cells, which begin targeting any potential invader.

As the blood leaves the white pulp area, it has to squeeze through the narrow penicillar arterioles. This squeezing bursts any weak, old, or infected red blood cells, spilling their contents. The red blood cell debris and any still-intact red blood cells enter the red pulp of the spleen through the venous sinusoid, where macrophages gobble up and digest any potential invaders.

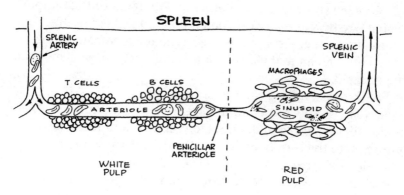

Anything foreign that enters your spleen is set upon by your immune system with a ferocity that can spill over into the rest of your body, where incredible damage can be done to you. Activation of the spleen's potent immune response by vaccine debris could be behind the dramatic increases in allergies, asthma, eczema, dermatitis, and autoimmune diseases, which are so common today.

Let's see what Israeli researchers say in the *Journal of Autoimmunity*, February 2000, under the title, **"Vaccination and Autoimmunity –'Vaccinosis': A Dangerous Liaison?"**

"The question of a connection between vaccination and autoimmune illness (or phenomena) is surrounded by controversy. A heated debate is going on regarding the causality between vaccines, such as measles and anti-hepatitis B virus (HBV), and multiple sclerosis (MS).

Brain antibodies as well as clinical symptoms have been found in patients vaccinated against those diseases. Other autoimmune illnesses have been associated with vaccinations. Tetanus toxoid, influenza vaccines, polio vaccine, and others have been related to phenomena ranging from autoantibodies production to full-blown illness (such as rheumatoid arthritis [RA]). Conflicting data exists regarding also the connection between autism and vaccination with measles vaccine." [109]

It goes on to state that only one controlled study—using dogs—has been done. So, for the last 70 years, in spite of the suspicions that vaccines probably create autoimmune diseases in a significant number of recipients, **no studies have been done to evaluate the risk!**

In other words, you have been one of the billion guinea pigs in an experiment in which the pharmaceutical companies, the medical profession, and the government health workers have made few observations on the long-term side-effects of vaccines. In fact, you can see from some of the previous quotes that they've gone out of their way to avoid such observations.

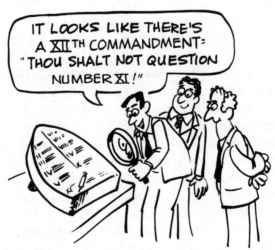

By the time you read this, mercury may have been quietly removed from most vaccines sold in the industrialized countries, and it will be business-as-usual for the vaccine industry. Of course, the formaldehyde, antibiotics, monosodium glutamate (MSG), sulfites, and aluminum will still be in the vaccines—and quite capable of inducing harsh reactions by your immune system.

On his Website, www.mercola.com, Dr. Joseph Mercola lists the following fillers found in vaccines (in addition to the viral and bacterial RNA or DNA): aluminum hydroxide; aluminum phosphate; ammonium sulfate; amphotericin B; animal tissues—pig blood, horse blood, rabbit brain, dog kidney, monkey kidney, chick embryo, chicken egg, duck egg; calf (bovine) serum; betapropiolactone; fetal bovine serum; formaldehyde; formalin; gelatin; glycerol; human diploid cells (originating from human aborted fetal tissue); hydrolized gelatin; monosodium glutamate (MSG); neomycin; neomycin sulfate; phenol red indicator; phenoxyethanol (antifreeze); potassium diphosphate; potassium monophosphate; polymyxin B; polysorbate 20; polysorbate 80; porcine (pig) pancreatic hydrolysate of casein; residual MRC5 proteins; sorbitol; sucrose; thimerosal (mercury); tri(n)butylphoshphate; VERO cells: a continuous line of monkey kidney cells; and washed red-blood cells from sheep.

Research on Alzheimer Disease has shown, on autopsy, high levels of aluminum and mercury in the brain—up to nine times that found in normal brains. Studies published in 1998 and 1999 assert that the mercury found in those with Alzheimer's is not from mercury fillings.[110]

Could the mercury and aluminum used in flu shots—so fervently pushed onto senior citizens—be responsible for the dramatic increase in Alzheimer Disease in the last decade? Equally important: if so, can these metals be removed?

The ADA says: "There is no scientifically valid evidence linking either autism or Alzheimer Disease with dental amalgam." However, Dr. Boyd E. Haley, a researcher at the University of Kentucky, disputes this claim. His research implicates mercury from dental amalgams and/or mercury-containing thimerosal from vaccines.[111]

Let's take a closer look at **autism**. It is a neurological disorder that affects the functioning of the brain. It usually begins during the first three years of life—coincidentally, the time of greatest exposure to vaccination—and boys are four times more likely to be affected than girls. It has been estimated that as many as one in 500 American children develop autism; there are more than 500,000 cases in the US alone. Symptoms and degree of the disorder are individually variable. Those with autism generally have difficulty with communication. In addition:

- **they may be overactive or very passive;**
- **they may throw tantrums without reason;**
- **they may be obsessed with an idea, activity, person, or object;**
- **they may be aggressive;**
- **they may have difficulty with changes in routine;**
- **they may exhibit repeated body movements, like hand-flapping; and**
- **they may experience sensitivities in the five senses of sight, hearing, touch, smell, and taste.**[112]

Autism was first identified in the 1960s, in children of wealthier families. It was at first thought to be a result of their bad genes or of bad parenting skills—both of which were later disproved.

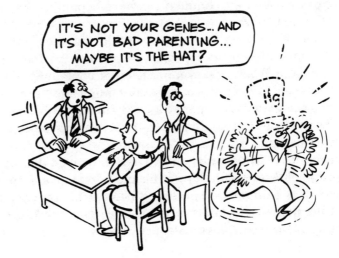

IT'S NOT YOUR GENES... AND IT'S NOT BAD PARENTING... MAYBE IT'S THE HAT?

Testing in the 1970s and 1980s subsequently found autism across the economic and racial spectrum. No cause is recognized by researchers at this point, and MMR vaccines have tentatively been ruled out by recent studies in Finland and the United Kingdom.[113]

The problem with these studies is that they are looking for "acute" reactions that occur within two to three weeks after the MMR vaccination. Autism is known to be a delayed-onset disease that may not present itself for months or years. Also, prescribing physicians are notorious for underreporting adverse reactions.

In the previous chapter, I had mentioned that many in search of the "mercury *piñata*" will swing blindly before any will ever get close to hitting it and finding the truth. The same holds true for vaccines. The following research is one of the first solid hits on the "vaccine *piñata*." A study using the latest biotechnology found that one of three patients with ulcerative colitis, and three of nine children with autism, were positive for measles virus from vaccine.[114] How many more hits on the "vaccine *piñata*" will be necessary to overrule the false-negative studies?

So the live viruses in the MMR vaccine have been shown to be involved in autism and ulcerative colitis, but what about the role of thimerosal used in DPT and hepatitis B vaccines? On the day of birth, babies are commonly given a hepatitis B vaccine, which contains 12 micrograms (mcg) of mercury. At four months of age, they are given DPT and HiB vaccines, which contain a total of 50 mcg of mercury. At six months, they are given hepatitis B and polio vaccines, which contain 62.5 mcg of mercury. At 15 months, vaccines containing another 50 mcg of mercury are given. Since the blood-brain barrier is not completely developed in infants, the brain and spinal cord take a tremendous beating.[115]

Because the Italian study shown earlier proved that 20 percent of children with dermatitis and eczema were found to be allergic to thimerosal, couldn't it be possible that autism and other neurological disorders in children might just be "eczema of the brain"—and also, an allergy to thimerosal?

The fact that DPT shots were first used by wealthy families—before mass vaccinations across the social spectrum occurred a decade later—may explain the initial observations in wealthier families. If thimerosal is part of the problem with autism, then you would expect to find mercury in autistics. Let's take a look.

A study done at the Edelson Center in Atlanta, Georgia, with 56 autistic patients from the ages of three to 12, determined that:

> **"All 56 (100%) of the children tested positively for the presence of one or more heavy metals (lead, mercury, tin, aluminum, or arsenic) above reference levels.... These tests clearly indicate that an overwhelming number of autistic patients have impaired liver detoxication processes and that their bodies are under toxic chemical and heavy metal stress."** [116]

In another study done by Edelson and Cantor, and published in *Toxicology and Industrial Health*, all 20 autistic children who were tested also showed abnormal liver detoxication. The authors propose that:

> **"Exposure to ordinary environmental chemicals like paints, plastics, glues, carpets, pastes, etc., to the healthy organism usually doesn't present any difficulty unless there is a massive exposure. To the individual with a dysfunctional liver detoxication system however, these ordinary chemical exposures can be devastating and we propose that lipophilic [fat-loving] chemicals are not properly metabolized. Thus, lipohilic compounds pass directly into the brain at a developmental juncture where the blood brain barrier cannot protect developing brain structures."** [117]

Where did these metals come from, that affected the liver so strongly? Amalgams? Vaccines? So many questions remain unanswered.

In her book, ***Turning Lead Into Gold***, Nancy Hallaway describes how her twin three-year-old boys were diagnosed with autistic tendencies, hyperactivity, and attention deficit disorder. Removal of heavy metals with chelation led to immediate and spectacular improvement in their symptoms.

Her final questions are:

> **"So why is no one testing for heavy metals in children that display these disorders? And when the incidence is rising so steadily and affecting the intelligence and mentality of these affected children, why aren't we looking at better, more effective methods of evaluating their body burden of metals?"** [118]

The **Cure Autism Now (CAN) Foundation**—another parents-of-damaged-children group—is presently polling scientists to investigate the links between childhood vaccinations and autism (www.cureautismnow.org). **How about MELISA® testing for metal allergies?**

As suspect as vaccinations have been in the developed world, an even greater "experiment" is going on in the Third World, as the WHO sets goals to vaccinate all the children of the world. Raymond Obomsawin is the author of **Universal Immunization: Medical Miracle or Masterful Mirage?** Obomsawin was born in the US, but was at one time, manager of CUSO, Canada's overseas international development agency, which gave millions of dollars to vaccinate Third World children. He says in his book:

> **"A minority of qualified scientists are now postulating that the full vaccine schedule as routinely employed in early childhood vaccination inevitably weakens the immunologic system of the child, leaving this system crippled in its ability to protect the child throughout life, and in turn opening the way for other infectious diseases due to immunologic dysfunction. It is also being postulated by such scientists that mass immunization is directly contributing to the now widespread escalation of various auto-immune, degenerative disease and allergic conditions."** [119]

Obomsawin's well-referenced book, which also shows the crucial roles that proper farming and nutrition play in sustaining human health, is available from:

www.eatingalive.com

Health Action Network Society (HANS)
#202-5262 Rumble Street
Burnaby, BC, Canada V5J 2B6
Tel: (604) 435-0512
Fax: (604) 435-1561

The Association of American Physicians and Surgeons
(AAPS), at its 57th annual meeting in St. Louis, in October 2000,
passed a resolution calling for a moratorium on all government-
mandated vaccines. Jane M. Orient, the Executive Director, said:

**"Our children face the possibility of death or serious long-
term adverse effects from mandated vaccines that aren't
necessary or that have very limited benefits."**

**"This is not a vote against vaccines. This resolution only
attempts to halt blanket vaccine mandates by government
agencies and school districts that give no consideration for
the rights of the parents or the individual medical
condition of the child."**

**"AAPS believes that parents, with the advice of their
doctors, should make decisions about their children's
medical care—not government bureaucrats. This
Resolution affirms that position."** [120]

On March 23, 2001, the law firm of Waters & Krauss LLP, of
Dallas, Texas, filed a lawsuit alleging that mercury poisoning
in many children has been caused by the use of thimerosal in
vaccines. This is probably the first of many legal actions to bring
justice to those who have been adversely affected by mercury.

I'll close this chapter with another quote from Raymond
Obomsawin's book. This statement was made by Thomas
McKeown, past chairman of the World Health Organization
(WHO) Advisory Group on Health Research Strategy:

**"All the countries that advanced rapidly achieved a
substantial improvement in nutrition, which led to
increased resistance. Indeed in some countries this was the**

only important direct influence. It is perhaps surprising that immunization appears to have contributed relatively little to the advances...the reduction in mortality occurred during a period when vaccine coverage was still low.

"To anyone who has traveled extensively in the rural areas of the Third World, the common causes of ill health may seem self-evident. Many children are visibly malnourished, sanitary conditions are primitive, drinking water is unclean, the food...is contaminated, and the number of people competing for the means of life is clearly excessive. Our conclusions concerning the determinants of health can be epitomized by the simple statement that people must have enough to eat and must not be poisoned." [121]

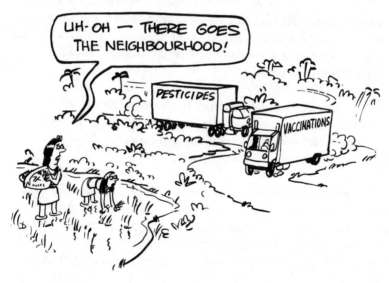

Thomas McKeown obviously has faith in physiology—put the nutrients in and keep the poisons out, and the body will run itself. From *Universal Immunization: Medical Miracle or Masterful Mirage?* it's clear that the $150 million that Canada spent, between 1986 and 1991, to vaccinate Third World children did little to help the health of these children—and probably contributed further to their poisoning.

Letter from a Patient

I am a 16-year-old patient of Dr. Matsen. I have known him since I was in grade four, at elementary school.

The circumstances through which I came to be acquainted with Dr Matsen were lucky for me. I don't like to think about how I might have turned out, had my family not explored the possibilities of Naturopathy.

My story begins when I was about nine years old. My twin sister and I were attending grade four at Gleneagles Elementary School. At that point, just after the summer of '94, I began to feel some peculiar symptoms, including fatigue, light-headedness, and immediate nausea after eating anything except certain sugary foods.

Until that time, my twin and I had always physically been the same; we were the same height, the same weight, and had the same eye and hair colour. We even lost our teeth at the same time. Because of this, my parents couldn't help wondering why all of a sudden, in grade four, I was behind my sister in my development. I was shorter, lighter, and skinnier than my sister, and her teeth were beginning to develop faster. Kids began to compare us, saying I was the "weak one" or "chicken legs," and *that* didn't help my self-esteem at all.

Seeing as my symptoms appeared to be worsening, my parents decided it was time to go to the doctor. I started to feel sick at just the thought of food, and my already-tiny appetite was getting smaller. We went to see some doctors over the course of several months, all of whom took ample blood samples that all came back negative for any sort of sickness that would cause my particular symptoms. The doctors seemed to think that because nothing showed on the tests, there was nothing to worry about.

We began to get a bit sceptical regarding their opinions, given the fact that I didn't look as if I was just going to "grow out of it." Heck, I wasn't even growing *at all!* Luckily, my parents—being open to new ways of doing things—started to look elsewhere for answers.

First they tried avoiding the foods that made me feel sick, but that didn't help much because most foods made me feel sick. I would have become malnourished before that had worked. Finally, on the advice of a good friend, my mom learned of Dr. Matsen, and booked an appointment for me as fast as she could.

I still remember the day when we went to see the friendly, knowledgeable Naturopath who would soon cure my ailments. He gave me various supplements and homeopathic medicines to take, and a strict diet of no sugar, no raw vegetables, no dairy, or any other things that would cause the yeast to grow.

The improvement was astounding. After just 12 hours, I had no nausea and felt like I could eat more. Finally! I was going to be better again! By the time I was off the treatment and totally cured, my appetite was bigger than most of my family members, and I was growing like a weed. I can happily say that nobody will call me chicken legs anymore.

Because of this amazing experience, I've been seeing Dr. Matsen over the years; he's kept my yeast at bay when needed, and successfully dealt with other problems that have cropped up, such as recurring earaches and minor skin problems. Most recently, he is in the process of dealing with the fatigue and minor circulation difficulties that have plagued me since childhood.

After discovering that the previous yeast problem wasn't causing my fatigue and cold limbs, Dr. Matsen decided to treat me for mercury toxicity. I thought, "mercury toxicity? How could I have mercury toxicity? I learned about the deadly effects mercury had on people who worked with it in the 1800s, but where would *I* get it from?" Well, according to Dr. Matsen's most recent research, mercury has been used as a preservative in some vaccinations and flu shots that all my peers and I have received since we were born.

Mercury is also in every amalgam filling that we've ever had (fortunately, I've never had a cavity); some of my friends and family have a lot of fillings. What's even worse is the fact that low levels of mercury won't show up on a blood test because it's stored in our tissues, not our blood. I was also horrified to see the pages and pages of symptoms and diseases that mercury toxicity causes, among which my symptoms were listed.

So now I'm currently on chelation treatment in capsule form, to remove the mercury. Yet again, I have already seen results after only a month of treatment. I feel less fatigue and for the first time, haven't had to wear socks and slippers to bed. My hands no longer get icy when I play the clarinet, and my feet heat up quickly when they're cold.

Thanks to Dr. Matsen, I've been able to live healthier—and therefore happier—through treatments I know to be safe and natural.

That's the good thing about his treatments: they're all natural. I especially appreciate how Dr. Matsen always takes care to explain exactly what is going on in my body—for example, the way his treatment would help my liver enzymes or leach out toxins, etc.

Not only does his treatment rise above that of regular doctors, but he also takes the time to inform his patients—using diagrams, etc.— about his treatments, so they *understand*. I've always enjoyed the results of his treatments and his humour, and the kindness extended to me in his clinic. I'm sure I will continue to rely on Dr. Matsen's expertise in the future and to recommend his all-natural treatments.

Fenella Brandvold
Lions Bay, BC

CHAPTER 3

The Liver Connection

"For some years past, reported deaths from 'heart failure' have become frequent and fashionable among reporting physicians, and perhaps the reports may have been true, but not the whole truth, for it is probable that, in nine cases out of ten, the heart failure was secondary and brought on by an ineffectual effort of the stomach or alimentary tract to cast off indigestible matter clogging the way...a mass of ptomaines to be seized...and thrown back into the general circulation, poisoning tissues wherever they go and defying the liver...to cast them out of the system. Congestion, inflammations, abscesses, and all the catalogue of pathological complications are liable to ensue. Most likely a large majority of chronic diseases take their origin from this cause." [122]

R. H. Dalton
Journal of the American Medical Association, 1893

Your brain, nerves, heart, joints, and DNA are delicate, and your gut is always toxic—so your liver evolved to filter and neutralize your gut toxins, to protect your more fragile parts.

Some toxins originate in the foods themselves. For example, if **benzoic acid** comes to your liver via the food you've eaten,

then your liver binds it with the amino acid **glycine** to form
hippuric acid, which is easily eliminated through your kidneys.

Some toxins come from the process of digestion. When
protein is being broken down, the nitrogen stripped off the
protein is turned into **ammonia**, which is extremely toxic to
nerve cells. Your liver will normally bind two ammonias with a
carbon dioxide to create **urea**, which is much less toxic and
more easily eliminated by your kidneys. People whose livers
can't filter and neutralize ammonia might see "pink elephants"
and "snakes" because the ammonia aggravates their sensitive
brain neurons.

The amino acid **methionine** is shipped from the gut to the
liver in a form called **homocysteine**, which is toxic—especially
to the heart. Your liver should reconvert homocysteine back to
methionine before releasing it into the general circulation, but
it needs adequate tools to do that, such as the **B vitamins—
B_{12}, B_6,** and **folic acid.**

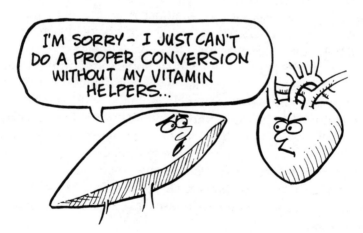

The toxins on which this chapter will focus, however, are the
ones actually **made by your liver.** These are the cause of most
**digestive problems; chronic fatigue; allergies; thyroid
problems; asthma; arthritis; autoimmune diseases; heart and
stroke attacks; and cancer.**

I can write this with confidence because I've seen these diseases reversed in some of my patients, as they regained their proper liver function. I've written my books with the purpose of trying to explain—as much to myself as to the readers—how working with diet and digestion could reverse such a diverse assortment of "mysterious" diseases.

My second book, *The Secrets to Great Health*, lists 575 medical research excerpts that show how **improper functioning of liver detoxification enzymes creates chronic disease**. Since I've had that book as my own reference for the past two years, and can now draw upon my more recent insight into heavy metals, **I'm going to fine-tune that statement even more, to say that one particular liver detoxification enzyme is at the root of most chronic disease.**

Before we get into the details about the ailments this liver enzyme can cause—and what you can do to fix it—let's take a refresher course on how your liver's detoxification enzymes normally work.

Every drop of your digestive juices and the nutrients contained in them are picked up by your **portal vein** and delivered to your liver—where any potential invader or toxin must be screened out, neutralized, and eliminated through the bile or kidneys. When the portal vein enters your liver, it splits off into millions of branches; each branch enters a **liver sinusoid**.

LIVER LOBULES

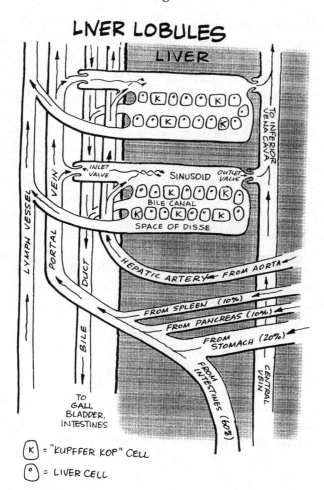

$\left(\text{K}\right)$ = "KUPFFER KOP" CELL

$\left(\circ\right)$ = LIVER CELL

The flow *into* the sinusoid is regulated by an **inlet valve**, while the flow *out* the other end of the sinusoid, into the central vein, is regulated by an **outlet valve**. Anything that passes through the outlet valve into the central vein is now truly *inside* the body, and free to travel throughout the circulation system.

The blood that is carried by your portal vein swirls into the sinusoid, where it is joined by a smaller amount of blood from the hepatic artery, which carries red blood cells with their supply of fresh oxygen, as well as hormones.

Lining your liver sinusoids are a large number of cells; 30 percent of them are macrophages, called the **Kupffer cells** (I call them Kupffer Kops). Their job is to gobble up any foreigners, such as bacteria, that are trying to sneak into your body via your gut and liver. They also break down any **immune complexes** that pass through your liver. So you can see that **30 percent of your liver's cells are macrophages of your immune system that can benefit from any treatment that helps immune function.**

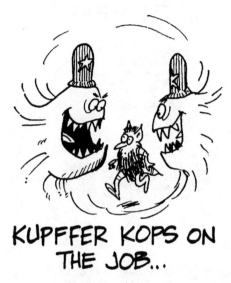

KUPFFER KOPS ON THE JOB...

The other 70 percent of the cells lining your millions of liver sinusoids are called **liver cells**. Their bland name totally understates how incredibly talented and versatile they are. The hundreds of jobs they do daily—including detoxification, breaking down hormones, regulating blood sugar and fat levels, as well as producing an endless number of products—should earn them a more appropriate name, like **Superhero Cells**. They are the balancers of your body, and when anything is out of balance—like blood sugar, hormones, energy, or emotions— you can suspect that these crucial liver cells might be at fault.

Complete failure of these liver cells to do their jobs will result in a rapid death, while partial failure of these cells will lead to loss of health, at the least. You'll learn in the next few chapters that guiding these crucial cells' function toward either health or disease is pretty much in your control.

With all the digestive goodies and baddies that enter your liver every minute of every day of your life, your liver cells' first priority is to neutralize any incoming toxins before they can do any harm. These vital cells are only as dexterous and strong as they are because of the **superhero enzymes** they contain.

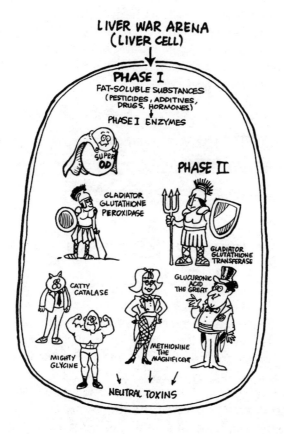

I have already mentioned that glycine can bind with benzoic acid to form hippuric acid so it can be eliminated by your kidneys—but there are also enzymes called **glucuronic acid, methionine, catalase, glutathione peroxidase,** and **glutathione transferase.** Together these are referred to as **Phase II enzymes.** Phase II enzymes can **conjugate**—which means neutralize—a wide range of toxins so that they can be easily eliminated through your kidneys or bile.

One crucial limiting factor with these Phase II enzymes is that they can only neutralize *water-soluble* toxins—which excludes fat-soluble toxins and fatty hormones. Fortunately, another group of liver detoxification enzymes can make a *fat-soluble* substance water-soluble, by attaching an **oxygen** to it. These enzymes are called **Phase I enzymes**. Together with Phase II enzymes, they provide a one-two punch in knocking out toxins. Phase I enzymes make it easier for Phase II enzymes to finally neutralize and eliminate fatty toxins such as **phenols**, which are extremely common in modern society—most man-made chemicals are phenols.

LIVER LOBULE

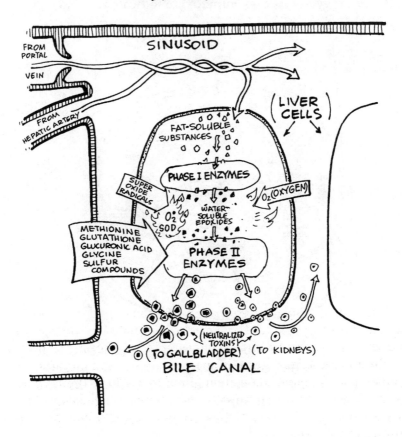

There is, however, a potentially fatal flaw in this system. The products created by your Phase I enzymes—water-soluble epoxides and peroxides—can be much more toxic, even cancer-causing, than the original fatty substances, if they're not quickly neutralized by the Phase II enzymes.

Let's go back to a liver cell in one of your liver's sinusoids and see what happens to fat-soluble toxins—such as **benzopyrene**. Benzopyrene might enter your body when you eat smoked or charbroiled food, or when you inhale smoke from cigarettes, cigars, smelters, or power plants. Ordinary oxygen molecules (O_2) have two oxygen atoms. When one oxygen atom is added to a fatty substance like benzopyrene—to make it more water-soluble for the Phase II enzymes—the leftover oxygen becomes a **superoxide radical**.

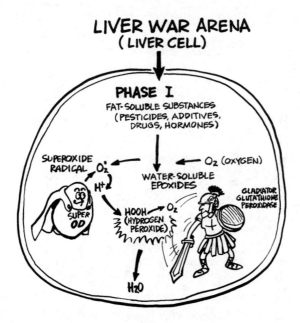

LIVER WAR ARENA
(LIVER CELL)

PHASE I
FAT-SOLUBLE SUBSTANCES
(PESTICIDES, ADDITIVES,
DRUGS, HORMONES)

SUPEROXIDE
RADICAL $O_2^{\cdot}$

← O_2 (OXYGEN)

WATER-SOLUBLE
EPOXIDES

H^+

SUPER
OD

HOOH → O_2
(HYDROGEN
PEROXIDE)

GLADIATOR
GLUTATHIONE
PEROXIDASE

H_2O

Having superoxide radicals ricocheting around in your liver cells could cause tremendous destruction to your own cell membranes. To get rid of them, your **superoxide dismutase (SOD) enzyme**—I call it **Super OD**—must immediately grab the superoxide radicals and bind them with hydrogen, to create hydrogen peroxide.

Less toxic than a superoxide radical, hydrogen peroxide
is still able to damage any membrane on contact, so another
enzyme—**glutathione peroxidase enzyme**—quickly comes to
the rescue. The name of an enzyme usually ends with the suffix
"ase," and begins with the name of the substance upon which it
acts. Peroxidase means an enzyme that works on peroxides.
Glutathione peroxidase, therefore, is an enzyme that uses
sulfur-containing glutathione to work on peroxides. With its
glutathione shield and selenium sword, glutathione peroxidase
deftly chops deadly hydrogen peroxide into water. End of
peroxide; end of problem. You live happily, healthfully ever-
after, thanks to glutathione peroxidase.

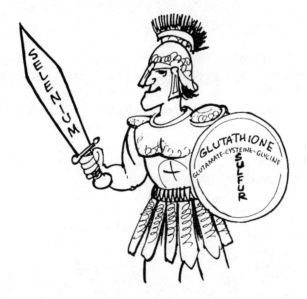

At least that's the way it's supposed to work in fairy tales
and physiology textbooks. The trouble starts when hydrogen
peroxide is being made by your Phase I liver enzymes faster
than the glutathione peroxidase in the Phase II enzymes can
chop it into water. As the hydrogen peroxide builds up in your
liver cells, your body will pour water-soluble antioxidants—like
vitamin C and bioflavonoids—into the liver cells, desperately
trying to neutralize the hydrogen peroxide, as a fireman might
try to douse a fire.

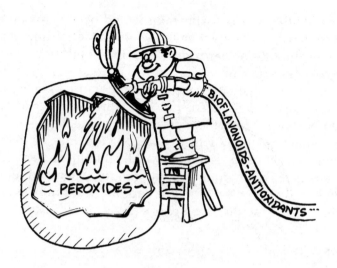

In the military hierarchy of your body, your liver is on the front line of the war against potential invaders. It therefore gets "first pick" of recruits. If your liver runs low on water-soluble antioxidants to neutralize hydrogen peroxide, it will strip them out of the areas ranked lower in priority, such as your connective tissue. This action can deplete your collagen so that ligaments, tendons, cartilage, intervertebral discs, joints, eyes, veins, arteries, gums, nails, etc., are weakened.

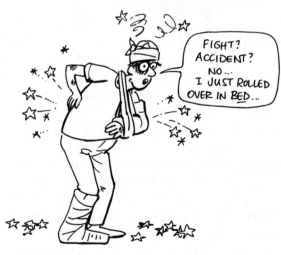

If your liver fails in this last-ditch attempt to neutralize hydrogen peroxide, then the hydrogen peroxide binds to cholesterol and fatty acids—collectively called **lipids**—to form **lipid peroxides**.

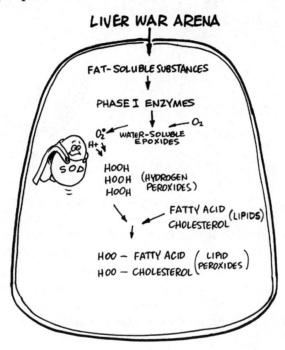

While hydrogen peroxide can't travel far without breaking up, lipid peroxides can travel long distances, and wreak havoc throughout your body—destroying cell membranes on contact. A cell membrane is made up of two layers of fatty acids linked together. Along the membrane are found many of the proteins—including enzymes—that are crucial for a cell to do its work.

Whenever a lipid peroxide contacts a membrane, it can release an OH group—a deadly **hydroxyl radical**—into the fats of the membrane. A hydroxyl radical set adrift in this sea of delicately linked fatty acids has the effect of a bowling ball knocking over bowling pins. And, the fats that get knocked over by this free radical can generate even *more* hydroxyl radicals—which can rip holes in nearby enzymes.

If those enzymes leak metal particles, such as iron or copper, any peroxides that the metal contacts can cause an explosive increase in free radicals. This can lead to a dramatic increase in damage to the membrane and the release of a number of gases, including pentane, ethane, octane, and butane.

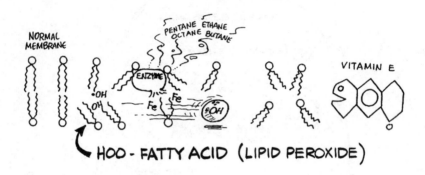

HOO - FATTY ACID (LIPID PEROXIDE)

Eventually the free radical will be gobbled up by vitamin E, which is stationed about every 1,000 fats along each membrane. Of course, 999 fats could have been destroyed before the vitamin E could nab the free radical.

The vitamin E will be knocked out of commission permanently if it can't get rid of the free radical it has so valiantly inhaled. Vitamin E needs help to pass the free radical out of the membrane into the cell, where it can be eliminated; a few of the fat-soluble bioflavonoids that assist vitamin E are alpha and beta carotene, and lycopene.

Inside the cell, vitamin C and its water-soluble bioflavonoid buddies—such as quercitin, hesperidin, and rutin—can pass the free radical on to glutathione for final elimination. So sulfur-carrying glutathione is critical to release the teams of vitamin C and vitamin E, so they can get on with their job of helping to eliminate free radicals.

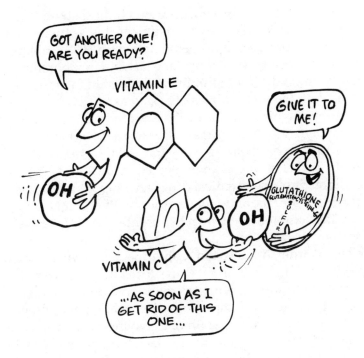

Of course, if you had an adequate supply of glutathione, perhaps glutathione peroxidase would have chopped the hydrogen peroxide into water in the first place, and lipid peroxides would not have formed.

The more unsaturated fats there are in a membrane, the more susceptible the membrane is to lipid peroxide damage. Because the membranes of the brain contain the largest number of unsaturated fats, lipid peroxidation is most likely to occur there. **Parkinson's disease** results from damage to the brain stem. Studies of people with Parkinson's have shown both increased lipid peroxidation and decreased activity of glutathione.

Tardive dyskinesia can occur from long-term use of pharmaceutical drugs called neuroleptics. Research has shown the damage to the basal ganglia to be due to lipid peroxidation, because as the liver makes the drug water-soluble, peroxides are produced.

Studies of patients with **schizophrenia** indicate the possibility of a brain injury early in life which was further aggravated by increased lipid peroxidation. In 1993, Phillips measured increased levels of pentane gas in schizophrenics' breath—a sure indicator of lipid peroxidation of membranes.

People with **Down Syndrome** have an extra "21st chromosome," which causes the liver to produce more hydrogen peroxide than normal; this causes glutathione enzymes to be overwhelmed. More than 50 years ago, Dr. Henry Turkel of Michigan pioneered medications—a combination of pharmaceutical drugs and supplements such as vitamins, minerals, and other nutrients—that dramatically reduced the symptoms of Down Syndrome; the FDA blocked its interstate distribution.

Dr. Jack Warner, of Fullerton, California, has further refined a supplement formula without drugs for Down Syndrome. The intent of the supplement is to reduce the production of hydrogen peroxide, and improve the breakdown of hydrogen peroxide by catalase and glutathione enzymes. It is claimed that using diet and supplements to block lipid peroxidation in Down Syndrome has shown astounding results in this genetic disorder.[123]

Studies of people with **Alzheimer Disease** have shown increased lipid peroxidation—combined with decreased glutathione activity—in the hippocampus area of the brain, which is responsible for short-term memory.

Subsequent to the brain and nervous system, the liver is the next part of the body with the most fatty membranes susceptible to damage from lipid peroxidation. Decreased glutathione levels (up to eight-fold less) have been found in both alcoholic and non-alcoholic **cirrhosis** of the liver, as well as in acute and chronic **hepatitis**.

When I wrote *The Secrets to Great Health,* I knew that at least one of the Phase II liver enzymes wasn't keeping up its job of neutralizing the toxins made by the Phase I enzymes. It's clearer to me now that increased lipid peroxidation activity goes hand-in-hand with decreased glutathione activity.

We'll soon take a closer look at why glutathione might be struggling to do its job, but first let's take a further look at what happens in the liver, when glutathione peroxidase enzyme fails to do its job of neutralizing hydrogen peroxide into harmless water.

PEROXIDES IN THE BILE CREATE DIGESTIVE TROUBLES

The build-up of lipid peroxides in the liver, due to failure of glutathione enzymes to neutralize them, can result in the spilling of peroxides directly into the central vein, where they could go directly to your brain and create lipid peroxide damage. Your liver partially closes the outlet valves, trying to protect your brain. This will create a back-pressure in the liver sinusoids, and contribute to the spilling of proteins and lipid peroxides through the bile canal into the bile that is being made by your liver.

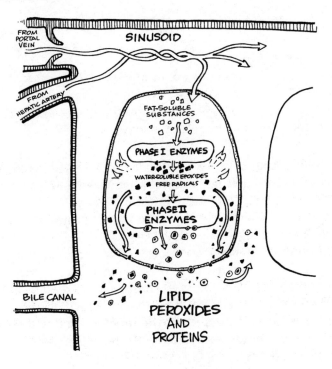

Spilling proteins into the bile could cause your bile to thicken, which will make it more prone to forming both bile sludge and gallstones; the peroxides could make your bile toxic. This toxic bile could irritate your bile ducts and, because your surplus bile is concentrated and stored in your gallbladder, it could also irritate your gallbladder.

Every time you eat—especially when you eat saturated fats, fried food, or spicy food—bile comes from your liver and gallbladder to aid digestion. It enters the small intestine just below your stomach, at the duodenum. Toxic bile can irritate your duodenum and your pancreatic duct—as well as disrupt your fat metabolism.

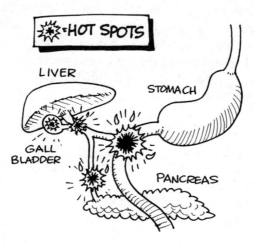

Now that your bile is toxic with peroxides, it will irritate this digestive musculature. Your esophagus, stomach, and duodenum—in fact, your entire intestinal tract, from mouth to rectum—all contain muscle fibres. An irritated muscle will first respond by spasming.

Muscle shortens when it spasms, and the shortening of your esophagus will pull your stomach up against the diaphragm, inhibiting the stomach's ability to churn and make digestive juices. Reduced production of digestive juices will lead to weaker digestion and sluggish bowel function, and will give the intestinal flora more opportunity to create gas and bloating in the lower abdomen.

As the stomach spasms up into the diaphragm, the valve at the top of the stomach can be forced open, and digestive juices can flow backward, up into the esophagus—and even up into the mouth—creating symptoms of nausea, heartburn, reflux, sore throat, burping, belching, pain below or under the sternum, or vomiting.

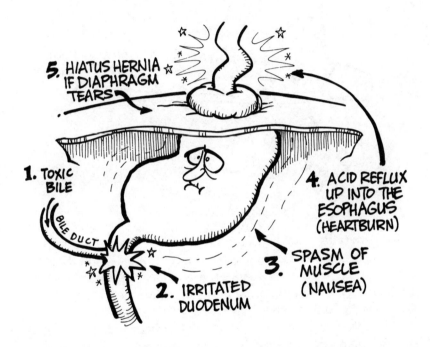

If the diaphragm should tear due to this relentless upward pressure, the stomach can literally pop up through the diaphragm into the chest cavity, pushing the lungs against the heart. This is called a **hiatus hernia**. It can cause symptoms of extreme discomfort under the chest—such as shortness of breath or heart symptoms—and/or accentuate the problems of acid reflux, so that lying down or bending over causes acid to escape upward.

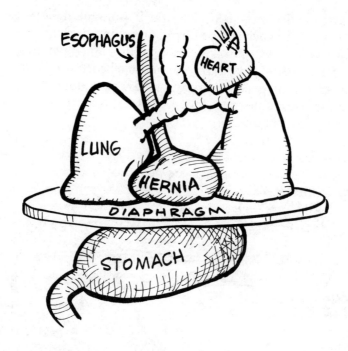

It's generally believed that more than half the population over the age of 60 has a hiatus hernia. It didn't start on their 60th birthday, but many years prior—when their livers' Phase I enzymes began making more peroxides than their Phase II enzymes could neutralize.

While there is no alarm system in your liver to tell you when it's producing more peroxides than it can handle, there certainly is one in your diaphragm—the nerves there will usually let you know that your stomach is protruding into your diaphragm.

The standard treatment for acid reflux is antacids, though there is nothing in these symptoms that says you are actually making too much acid. These symptoms are telling you that your stomach acid is flowing backward into your esophagus, which wasn't designed to handle the extreme acidity of stomach juices. Taking antacids may protect the esophagus and quiet-down the digestive alarms, but **remember one important thing—these digestive symptoms are just peripheral alarms signalling** *liver trouble!*

When the muscles of the intestine are irritated, they can either spasm—resulting in constipation—or they can try to flush the irritant out, thus creating diarrhea. Of course, if spasming and flushing were to occur at the same time, then cramping would result. Alternating constipation and diarrhea with cramping is commonly called **irritable bowel**, but should really be called *irritable bile*.

In Western medicine, there is no diagnostic test to check for toxic bile. Digestive symptoms are usually overlooked until there is sufficient damage to justify removing the "offending" body part, such as the duodenum or gallbladder. After the gallbladder is removed, the digestive symptoms usually continue or even worsen because the liver will still be spilling toxic peroxides into the bile; this toxic bile will continue to create aggravation somewhere in the digestive system.

The stomach and intestine are only reacting to toxic, peroxide-laden bile, so all these digestive symptoms are completely reversible—including the hiatus hernia—if you stop spilling peroxides into the bile!

LIVER DUMPING INTO THE LYMPH ACTIVATES AN IMMUNE RESPONSE

At the bottom of each of your liver sinusoids is the **space of Disse**, where excess fluid is shunted out of the liver into the lymphatic system. In fact, 50 percent of your lymphatic system originates at these sinusoids. The slightest back-pressure in your liver from the closing of your sinusoid outlet valves, due to peroxide irritation, will open the gaps between the liver cells—enough to allow proteins and lipid peroxides to spill from the space of Disse, directly into your lymphatic system.

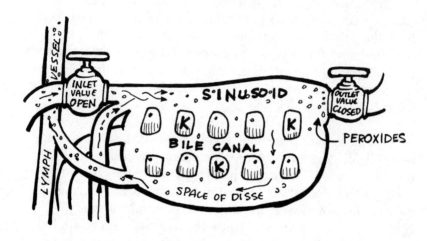

Because some of these proteins will not have been certified as harmless by your liver's immigration department, your immune system will immediately attack these proteins as alien invaders. A wall of fibrin will be put up around them; this obstruction of flow can create swelling throughout your lymphatic system.

Swollen lymph glands are most noticeable in the neck area because of the narrowing at the neck. It is literally the bottleneck to the lymph drainage out of your head. This blockage of your head's lymph drainage can contribute to sinus and nasal allergy symptoms, and can affect the Eustachian tubes that drain your middle ear into your throat. The resulting blockage of your Eustachian tubes can lead to congestion, hearing problems, noises in the ear, infection, or rupture of your eardrum. Your inner ear, which plays an important role in balance and equilibrium, can also be affected; dizziness and vertigo can result.

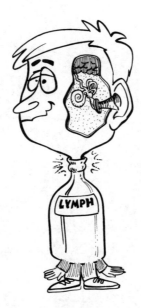

Remember that these head symptoms originated in the liver because excess peroxides caused a spillover into the lymph.

T and B cells will be activated to search out and attack the "invaders." The B cell antibodies used in the lymph are mainly small **two-pronged IgG "harpoons"** that stick this alien debris together into clusters, called **immune complexes**.

Once it has identified an invader, your immune system will attack anything that resembles that invader—your immune system begins to cross-react with a lot of harmless substances. This is the root of allergies. Because not all of these immune reactions are detected by skin-patch allergy tests, they are sometimes called sensitivities or intolerances.

As the antibodies cluster the invaders into immune complexes, their tails become "hot" to activate the **complement system**, which will damage the invaders further. Because your lymph system eventually drains into your circulation system near your left collarbone, any undestroyed immune complexes will drift from your lymph into your bloodstream, and circulate in your body until they are finished off by your liver's Kupffer cells—or until they lodge in an area of poor circulation, such as in a joint, a muscle, or an area of old injury.

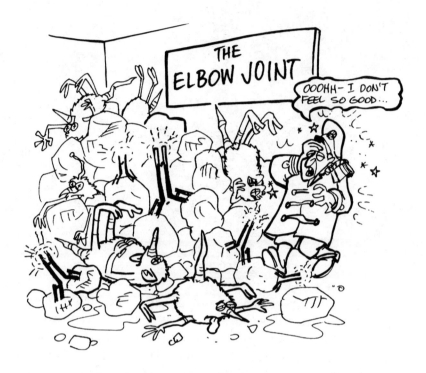

The hot tails of the antibodies themselves can make you feel achy, but if your immune system brings in even more armament to destroy these immune complexes, your joints, muscles, or skin can become severely aggravated.

You have a big **five-pronged antibody** called **IgM**—or Big Momma, as she is more affectionately called by those who know her best. She rumbles around in your larger blood vessels, and if she comes across any IgG immune complexes that trickled out of your lymph system into your circulation system intact, she may set upon them with a vengeance. This is what is known in medicine as **rheumatoid factor**—an indication of one type of **autoimmune disease**.

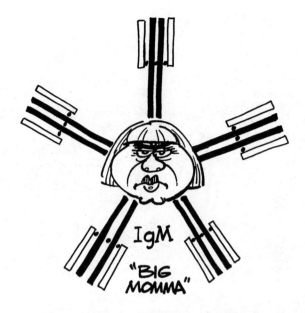

Later on, I'll discuss another type of autoimmune disease, but for now, notice that there is a fairly thin line separating an *allergy* from an *autoimmune disease*. Allergies and autoimmune diseases both involve the immune system's desperate attempts to rid your body of invaders, although it often aggressively attacks things that are quite harmless.

If we step back a minute, we should quickly realize that many things that are called immune system problems really *aren't*. Your immune system's IgM and IgG antibodies—and B and T cells—are just doing their job of trying to clean up "aliens" in your lymph and circulation systems. Your immune system doesn't know that the stuff it is identifying and attacking as "foreign" actually started off "innocent"—until your poorly functioning liver spilled it into your lymph system. Because you don't have an early-stage alarm system in your liver, you might not notice your congested lymph system until your immune system has laid you low with achy joints and muscles, or other autoimmune symptoms.

Treating allergies or the joints or skin with an anti-inflammatory will never cure the problem, but if you could get your liver to stop making lipid peroxides and spilling things into your lymph, your immune system would willingly call a cease-fire—there would soon be nothing left to shoot at.

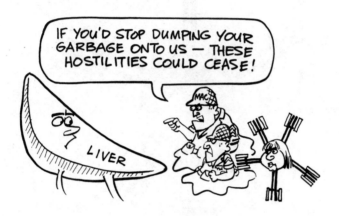

There are other indirect ways you might find out about your liver's trouble with peroxides. The back-pressure that occurs in your liver sinusoids can interfere with some of your liver cells' other jobs. Protein, sugar, or fat levels in your blood can get too high or low if your liver cells' function is hindered. This can manifest as weight loss or gain, hypoglycemia, or sugar cravings.

Your breakdown of steroid hormones can also be interfered with. Because women also have testosterone (6 percent of the amount that men have) and men also have estrogens (20 percent of the amount that women have), poor liver function can wreak havoc with the hormones in both sexes.

The ideal way for your liver to break down female steroid hormones is through what's known as the C-2 pathway, in which the end-products are mild hormones. The alternative breakdown pathway, which is more commonly used when there is a build-up of peroxides in the liver, is known as the C-16α (alpha) pathway. This pathway breaks down female steroid hormones into products such as 16α-hydroxyestrone, which can aggravate the reproductive organs.

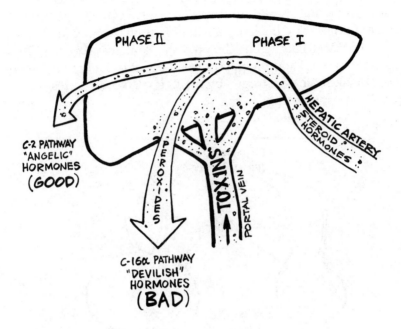

The 16α-hydroxyestrone hormone is considered by many researchers to be the cause of cancers of the female reproductive organs. In practice, I have seen that virtually all female complaints stop—such as menstrual cramping, PMS, and fibrocystic problems—if the liver can regain its proper breakdown of hormones through the C-2 pathway, by improving the way your liver handles peroxides. I've also seen dozens of women with unexplained infertility get pregnant after improving their liver function—and therefore improving their breakdown of female hormones.

In men, dihydrotestosterone (DHT) is the very strong
testosterone that should be quickly broken down by the liver
into a milder form. If a sluggish liver is slow to break down
DHT, the DHT will irritate the prostate gland, causing the
prostate to swell and pinch off urine flow. It is likely that the
poor breakdown of estrogen by the liver also contributes to
prostate problems.

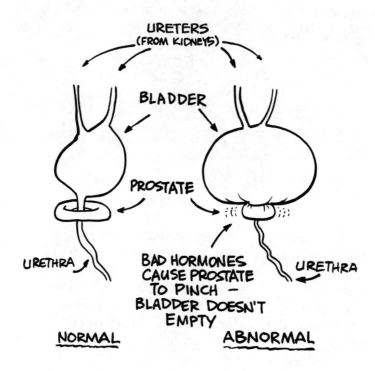

URETERS
(FROM KIDNEYS)

BLADDER

PROSTATE

URETHRA

BAD HORMONES
CAUSE PROSTATE
TO PINCH —
BLADDER DOESN'T
EMPTY

URETHRA

NORMAL   ABNORMAL

When your liver sinusoids are subjected to back-pressure—from closure of the outlet valves, due to peroxides—the millions of swollen sinusoids can create considerable swelling of the liver itself, which can pinch the **inferior vena cava** against your spine. The inferior vena cava is the vein that takes the blood from your lower body back to the heart. When it is pinched by a swollen liver, this can block the drainage from your lower body—including the legs, pelvis, and kidneys—and can lead to varicose veins and pelvic congestion, which can contribute to problems with the reproductive organs.

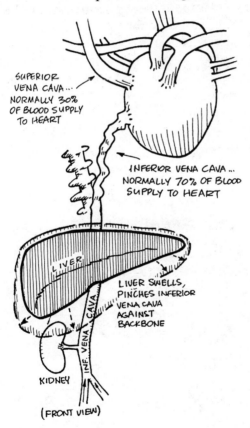

SUPERIOR VENA CAVA...
NORMALLY 30% OF BLOOD SUPPLY TO HEART

INFERIOR VENA CAVA ...
NORMALLY 70% OF BLOOD SUPPLY TO HEART

LIVER

LIVER SWELLS, PINCHES INFERIOR VENA CAVA AGAINST BACKBONE

INF. VENA CAVA

KIDNEY

(FRONT VIEW)

The kidneys can respond to the blockage of their drainage route by making **renin**, which increases blood pressure. This type of blood pressure may fluctuate with the hour-to-hour effects of diet and stress on the liver.

The closing of the inlet valves creates back-pressure on the portal vein itself—called **portal vein hypertension**. This can cause problems anywhere in the digestive system, although the most common symptom is **swelling of the hemorrhoidal veins. Proctitis, colitis, diverticulosis, Crohn's disease, fissures, fistulas, gastritis, and swelling of the esophageal veins** will also have some degree of peroxide-induced portal vein back-pressure associated with them.

When a swollen liver interferes with both the inferior vena cava and the portal vein, up to 70 percent of the venous blood flow—the blood returning through the veins to the heart—can be trapped below the liver, leaving the entire abdomen bloated like a drum. This proverbial "bay window" is not made of fat, even though the person carrying it often thinks it is. Tapping on it will show little of the jiggle for which fat is notorious. Rather, there is a firm tension to it, like an overly inflated beach ball. This abdominal swelling is another of the liver's peripheral alarm systems, notifying you that it's having trouble handling peroxides.

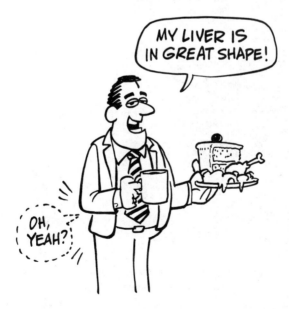

If most of your venous blood flow is trapped below the liver, the only way that blood can reach your heart's **right atrium**, uninhibited, is via your **superior vena cava**. This large vein drains your upper body, but it only carries about 30 percent of the blood returning to the heart. If the other 70 percent—carried by your inferior vena cava—is dammed up below a poorly functioning liver, this reduced blood flow into your heart may be inadequate for proper heart function.

The right atrium has the "electronic switches" that set the beat for the heart. It is the filling of your right atrium with blood that activates the **SA node** to stimulate the simultaneous contraction of the right atrium and **left atrium** at the top of the heart; they quickly pump blood into your **right and left ventricles**. The **AV node** is then activated, which leads to the contraction of the two ventricles together to send blood to your lungs and the rest of your body.

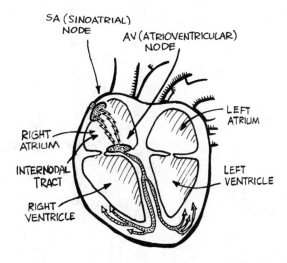

Inadequate filling with blood of the right atrium of your heart can lead to **irregular heartbeats**. So, irregular heartbeat is another peripheral alarm going off—indicating trouble at the liver.

While digestive and allergy symptoms are by far the most common chronic health problems, let's look at what many people consider the most frightening disease—cancer—before we show what can be done at the liver to prevent cancer and perhaps even reverse it.

Virtually every cell in your body has a nucleus that contains your genetic blueprint—the accumulated wisdom of thousands of your ancestors. This blueprint is called **deoxyribonucleic acid (DNA)**. Each DNA molecule has two long "backbone" strands that consist of alternating sugars and bases; these strands are twisted into a helix shape. The backbone strands run parallel to each other and are like the legs of a ladder. They are connected by **base pairs**, which form the "rungs" of the ladder.

Your genetic code consists of a sequence of bases on one strand that are bonded to different bases on the other strand. The four bases are always paired the same way: **Thymine (T)** is always linked to **adenine (A)** with a double bond, while **guanine (G)** is always linked to **cytosine (C)** with a triple bond.

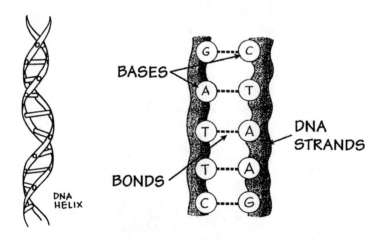

It was this precise combination of DNA bases that your ancestors used to create the enzymes they needed to survive the incredible hardships they confronted over tens of thousands of years on this planet.

Before your cells divide, they **replicate**, or copy, their DNA. The two strands separate, splitting between the base pairs. The sequence of bases on each separated strand then serves as a template for the formation of a new DNA molecule. If one of the bases is damaged, the DNA may be copied with an error— called a *mutation*.

If one of your precious DNA molecules were to have four or more mutations, it could run wild in your body as cancer. While certainly thousands of DNA bases are damaged in each cell every day, don't go getting all nervous and worried—you're not likely to get mutations from this damage. Your ancestors supplied you with **DNA repair crews** that can remove and replace thousands of damaged DNA bases per cell per day.

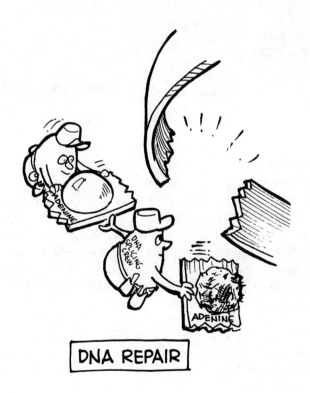

DNA REPAIR

Also, to prevent your DNA from making a faulty copy of itself with unrepaired damage, you have a very efficient and thorough DNA supervisor—called **p53**. It allows no copies, or replication, to be made until all errors are corrected.

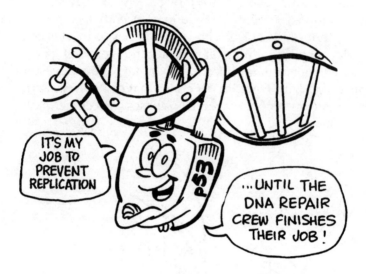

This p53 supervisor, together with your active DNA repair crews, is there to prevent mutations, so that you won't get cancer. So how can cancer possibly occur, and be so common, when the body has so many inherent defences against it? The answer is that **lipid peroxides rip up the membranes of p53**, leaving it dazed and confused and unable to stop its **evil twin—bc12**—which whips your DNA into replicating wildly, even if there are still unrepaired bases in your DNA. Thus are born the mutations that can go on to create a runaway cancer cell.

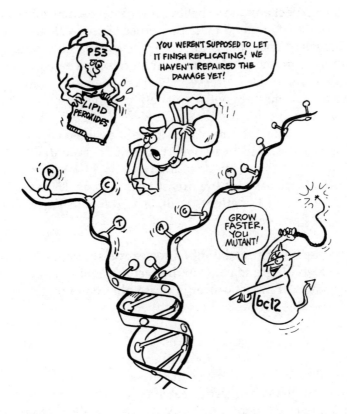

   Some cancer researchers believe that if they could find a way to genetically re-splice p53 back into shape, they might stop a cancer's growth, and perhaps even reverse it. Here's what I say: until genetic re-splicing of p53 is mastered, why not stop the liver from making lipid peroxides?

   In patients who are making dietary changes and taking herbal extract remedies for cancer—as well as supplements that neutralize peroxides before they can spill out of the liver—I've seen **remission** of the following cancers.

- Mouth cancer
- Bile duct cancer that had spread to the lymph
- Prostate cancer that had spread to the bone
- Bone marrow cancer
- Breast cancer

I don't expect anyone to believe anecdotal evidence like this, but I would recommend that you peruse the book, *Spontaneous Remissions*.[124] This interesting book gives many hundreds of examples, from the world's medical literature, where cancer and other "incurable" diseases have been seen to go into remission—sometimes with explanation, and sometimes not. Permit me to provide a short excerpt:

> **"The dramatic but rare regression of a verified case of breast cancer...has been observed and documented by clinicians over the course of many years. In my practice, limited to diseases of the breast over the past 25 years, I have observed 12 patients with...spontaneous regression of breast cancer.**
>
> **"Despite widespread doubt and scepticism, there is ample clinical evidence to confirm the fact that spontaneous regression of breast cancer is a rare phenomenon but is real and does occur."** [125]

So cancer can be a reversible disease. Yet I don't tell my cancer patients to discontinue conventional cancer treatments because they only have one chance to beat it, and most of the billions of dollars of cancer research money have gone into conventional treatment. Currently, conventional treatment has the research advantage and is—for now—the way to go until research on alternative treatments is completed.

Unfortunately, researchers and the medical community don't seem willing to believe cancer—or any other disease—is reversible. They still consider patients to be hapless victims who need some heroic treatment or remedy from the medical profession. One of the main criteria of medical research seems to be that the end-result must be something patentable. Good for business—but is it really good for the patients' long-term health?

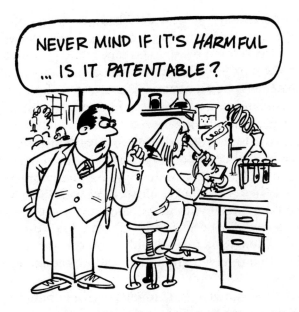

If that treatment happens to destroy the patient's immune system in the process, the attitude seems to be, "oh well, it's the best treatment that research could offer." Even if the treatment does kill the cancer, will the person's defences be better equipped to fight off a return of cancer? Remember, the basic tenet of physiology is homeostasis—that the body wants to and knows how to heal itself, if given the opportunity. But in medicine, pathology overrules physiology.

It is stated in *Spontaneous Remissions* that about 2 percent of cancer patients spontaneously shed their cancer, even in the latest of stages. If 2 percent of cancer patients can reverse cancer spontaneously, surely putting a little thought behind it could raise it to 20 percent, or perhaps much higher.

More important, if the concept that cancer can be reversed in even a small percentage of the population is true, then it must be close to 100 percent *preventable*—given the appropriate insight and motivation. My experience with cancer remission is that it occurs **after** the liver has completely stopped making lipid peroxides.

Earlier in this chapter, we saw that the increase in lipid peroxides in brain and liver disease correlates with low levels of glutathione. Here's some research on cancer and glutathione.

Studies by Milner, in the early 1990s, showed that the p53 gene controls the replication rate of DNA, and that oxidation (such as lipid peroxidation) can lock p53 into a growth-promoting (cancer-inducing) shape, while reduction (the opposite of oxidation) by **glutathione can restore DNA protection**, giving anti-cancer properties.

In a 1980 study of rats, **cancer of the liver** was induced using aflatoxins, but treatment with glutathione resulted in the shrinking of some of the cancers; the untreated rats died.

In 1993, hamsters were treated with chemicals to induce **oral cancer**. Those that received glutathione developed fewer and smaller cancers.

In 1985, Beutler showed that humans with a variety of cancers had decreased levels of glutathione. Donnerstag, in 1996, showed that **glutathione induced cancer cells to die.**

Humans with cancer of the stomach or ovaries, being treated with chemotherapy (cisplatin), were also given glutathione. Those treated with **glutathione showed less nerve and kidney damage from the chemotherapy**—without reducing the effectiveness of the treatment.

A 1992 study showed that **endometrial cancer** patients treated with radiation and glutathione had much less diarrhea from the radiation than those not given glutathione.

A number of studies have linked low levels of glutathione with **cataracts, macular degeneration, asthma, chronic obstructive pulmonary disease, pulmonary fibrosis, pancreatitis, lupus erythematosis, rheumatoid arthritis, ulcerative colitis, Type II diabetes, and myocardial infarction.**

Lenzi found in 1993 that males with deceased sperm motility showed significant improvement from glutathione treatment.

In 1995, Svardal showed that patients with **Common Variable Immunodeficiency** had **increased production of tumour necrosis factor** and **decreased production of interleukin-2** associated with **low glutathione levels.**

Supplementation with **glutathione** increased interleukin-2 and decreased tumour necrosis factor, and apparently **corrected the immune problem.**

In 1994, *Journal of Clinical Epidemiology* showed that **glutathione levels decrease with ageing;** those with the lowest levels were more prone to **arthritis, diabetes, high blood pressure,** or **heart disease**, while those elderly people who maintained their **glutathione levels retained their health.**

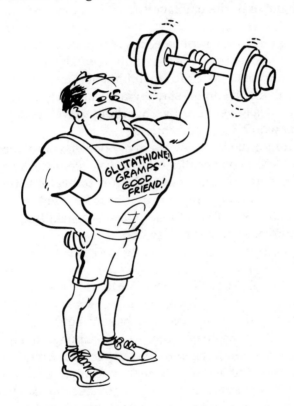

From this brief overview of some of the research, you should see that there is little reason to treat different degenerative diseases as separate entities.

- If you have to stop making lipid peroxides to reverse cancer; and
- if lipid peroxides spilling into the bile are creating stomach and intestine problems; and

- if lipid peroxides spilling into the lymph are activating your immune system to create allergies and autoimmune diseases;
- then **lipid peroxides must be the root of virtually every disease.**

In my practice, it's not unusual for me to treat a patient who's been seen by three or four specialists. Perhaps the gastroenterologist prescribed antacids for reflux indigestion; the rheumatologist prescribed anti-inflammatories for the joint pain; the dermatologist prescribed cortisone cream for the skin inflammation; and of course, the psychiatrist will have prescribed a serotonin recycler for mood imbalances.

I always say that you should stay on medication that you need, but the goal is to get your liver working so well that eventually, you won't need medication.

As I have said for the last 15 years in my books, your liver function is the key to your health. Now the biochemistry is becoming clear as to why that is true: **the key to health is to reduce the production of peroxides by Phase I enzymes, while enhancing the ability of Phase II enzymes—especially glutathione enzymes—to neutralize peroxides.**

BACK TO THE LIVER

When fatty toxins enter your liver, they have to be made water-soluble so they can be neutralized and eliminated. First, the Phase I enzymes add oxygen to the fatty toxins, which makes them water-soluble. The interim oxygenated products made by your Phase I enzymes include peroxides that can be up to 60 times more toxic than the original fatty substance.

LIVER

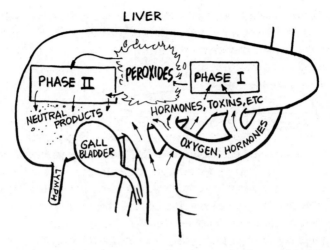

As long as your Phase II enzymes are quickly neutralizing the peroxides being made by the Phase I enzymes, your body will run as smoothly as the proverbial Swiss clock. Homeostasis will prevail; your body will be self-regulating—able to function, heal, and replicate without any problems. In other words, you will be free of disease—healthy as you were designed to be.

Because your Phase I and Phase II enzymes were designed to run at the same speed, **problems in your liver can occur for two reasons:**
1. **when your Phase I enzymes make peroxides too quickly,** or
2. **when your Phase II enzymes neutralize peroxides too slowly.**

Cancer research clearly shows that some commonly ingested substances can affect the speed of these two enzyme systems.

The Phase I enzymes have been shown to be *stimulated*, by both **tobacco** and **alcohol**, to increase peroxide production—which has cancer-inducing properties.

Naringen, a bioflavonoid found in grapefruit, *inhibits* the Phase I enzymes so that they make fewer peroxides. Naringen gives grapefruit its anti-cancer properties. **Wheat grass juice** also has anti-cancer properties because of its abilities to decrease the liver's production of peroxides.

The Phase II enzymes have one of the toughest jobs in the body—neutralizing the myriad toxins thrown at them every minute, night and day, from the gut.

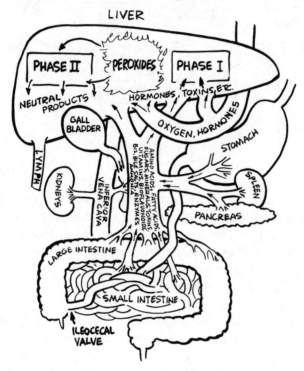

Cancer research has shown that high-carbohydrate, low-protein diets inhibit the function of the Phase II enzymes. The reason that protein is so important for the function of your Phase II enzymes is that it's made up of chains of amino acids, several of which contain sulfur. The two key sulfur-carrying amino acids are **methionine** and **cysteine**, both of which are crucial to your Phase II enzymes' ability to neutralize toxins.

Methionine is converted into **SAMe (S-adenosylmethionine—** pronounced "sammy"). A deficiency of SAMe can cause bile trouble, joint pain, depression, attention deficit disorder, and anxiety. These symptoms are seen in individuals with Gilbert's syndrome—those whose livers don't make SAMe effectively. In some European countries, SAMe is the most widely prescribed supplement for depression, though it is a liver remedy.

If it seems strange to you that a physical problem with the liver can create a symptom normally treated by psychotherapists, consider the word **melancholia**. This is a word that has emotion and mood oozing from it, yet its Greek roots mean **"black bile."** Thousand of years ago, physicians did not separate the body and the mind; they knew that problems with the body's organs can create emotional states, and that emotional states can create organ problems.

The second sulfur-carrying amino acid—cysteine—can bind with the sulfur of another cysteine, forming **cystine**. The binding of two sulfurs—called a **disulfide bridge**—adds stability to the structure of many proteins. While cystine plays a passive, strengthening role, cysteine has a much more active part to play by being incorporated into three key enzymes: **coenzyme A**, **glutathione transferase**, and **glutathione peroxidase**.

Coenzyme A is the most active enzyme in your body. It is the **initiator** of over 100 processes that mainly involve the conversion of fats, carbohydrates, and proteins into energy. Therefore, inadequate amounts of sulfur-containing coenzyme A can cause a lack of energy and an increase in body fat. While coenzyme A isn't one of the Phase II detoxification enzymes, it plays a big role in helping deal with stress, and keeping the immune system strong and alert.

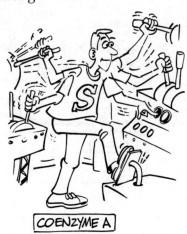

COENZYME A

Glutathione is made of three amino acids—the central one being sulfur-containing cysteine, with glutamate on one side and glycine on the other. It is found in high amounts throughout your body, but is especially important to protect your mitochondria.

Mitochondria are found inside your cells where they function as your cells' power plants. The final stage of digestion takes place inside your mitochondria. They take the food you've provided, add in oxygen, and give you tremendous quantities of ATP—the fuel your body needs to run everything, from your brain to your immune system to your internal heating system.

Mitochondrial DNA is different from the DNA of your cells' nucleus. Your mitochondrial DNA comes only from your mother. It is a more primitive form than your cellular DNA, which comes from both parents.

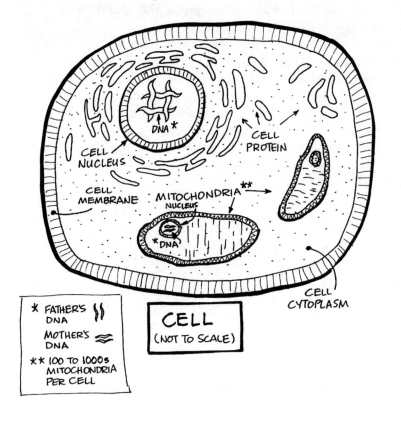

   Mitochondrial DNA has no protective spool—called a
histone—on which to safely wrap itself. Mitochondrial DNA
lacks the diligent DNA repair crew that your more advanced
cells contain, and it's unable to make glutathione, to protect
itself from free radicals.

   In fact, your mitochondria look a lot more like bacterial cells
than human cells. Here's a point to ponder: is it possible that
in some long, forgotten past, a marriage of convenience was
entered into—in which these "energizer bacteria" would come
live inside our cells, to provide us with the most advanced ATP
energy production, while we would provide them with food,
shelter, oxygen, and glutathione?

   The mitochondria inside your cells use over 90 percent of
your oxygen intake to turn your food into energy through the
production of ATP. One of the steps involves **coenzyme Q_{10}**
(**CoQ_{10}**), which passes two electrons down the mitochrondrial
membrane. Sometimes CoQ_{10} is overworked or inadequate, and
it fumbles an electron, generating a free radical and peroxides.

   It's been calculated that up to 5 percent of the electrons
passing through your mitochondrial power plants can end up
as lipid peroxides—capable of causing tremendous damage to
your mitochondrial membranes and DNA, if antioxidants are
not present in adequate amounts.

   Vitamin E is situated in the fatty membranes and vitamin C
is in the watery inner cell, while **lipoic acid** functions in both
areas. All these antioxidants need glutathione to recycle them.

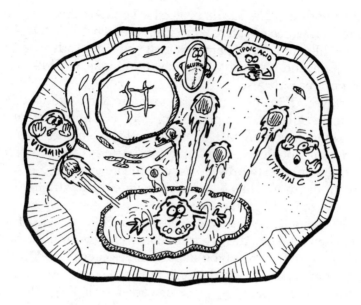

Our failure to provide adequate glutathione protection for our hard-working mitochondrial tenants would increase the lipid peroxidation of the mitochondrial DNA ten-fold, resulting in low energy, degenerative disease, and ageing. **The majority of your body's glutathione is made by your liver cells, but 80 percent is exported—mainly to protect the mitochondria of other cells, such as those of your kidneys.**

While your liver exports most of the glutathione it makes, the 20 percent it keeps is put to good use in your liver's Phase II enzymes. **Glutathione transferase** is the second of your key cysteine-containing enzymes, accounting for 60 percent of the neutralized substances dumped into your bile. Glutathione transferase can grab and neutralize hydroxyl radicals and peroxide radicals from inside the cell, from the cell membrane, or from DNA. It can also pull radicals from vitamins E and C, so they can be recycled back to work.

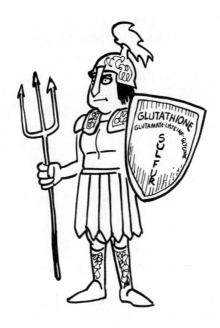

Glutathione peroxidase enzyme contains glutathione plus a sword of selenium, to make the Phase II enzyme most adept at chopping hydrogen peroxide into harmless water, thus preventing the formation of deadly lipid peroxides. This crucial enzyme is found throughout your body, but especially in your key detoxification organ—your liver—and also in your thyroid.

It quickly becomes clear that your two sulfur-carrying glutathione enzymes—glutathione transferase and glutathione peroxidase—are the keys to your Phase II enzymes' ability to neutralize the peroxides made by your Phase I enzymes, thereby maintaining your homeostasis and your health. If health has already been lost, then these two enzymes must be revived in order to reclaim it.

To simplify things, when discussing these two key enzymes in the future, they will collectively be referred to as glutathione peroxidase.

SLOW DOWN PHASE I PEROXIDE PRODUCERS AND SPEED UP PHASE II PEROXIDE BUSTERS

To slow down the Phase I enzymes to their normal speed, you have to stop using stimulants like **tobacco, alcohol, coffee (even decaffeinated), and other chemicals** that increase your liver's production of peroxides. To speed up Phase II enzymes, you have to stop eating the foods that have had their key vitamins or minerals stripped from them—such as **white sugar, white flour, and white salt**—because your Phase II enzymes need every known nutrient to neutralize peroxides.

Of course, many will look at these two lists and compromise, saying, "If I remove the others, I can still keep one bad habit." They may be right; maybe they can get away with a little compromise. More likely, however, they have no leeway at all, as you will see later.

If you have an "irreversible" disease, you must use extraordinary resolve if you want to reverse it. Recently I've seen complete remissions of terminal bile duct cancer, mouth cancer, silicone breast implant syndrome (which caused fibromyalgia, chronic fatigue, and rheumatoid arthritis in one patient), and schizophrenia (as seen in one patient with 40 years' history of the disease). These individuals didn't compromise and they earned their way back to health from diseases that others might have given up on.

There are a few things—like grapefruit and wheat grass juice—that have been shown to slow down the Phase I enzymes. Caution must be used with these if you are taking drugs (pharmaceutical or otherwise), because slowing down the Phase I enzymes will also slow down the breakdown of drugs—increasing their effects on your body. Reduction of some prescription-drug doses may be necessary.

As you slow down the Phase I enzymes' production of peroxides, the next step is to increase the activity of the key Phase II glutathione enzymes, which help neutralize peroxides. Phase II enzymes need nutrients. Of all the nutrients they require, **sulfur** is the most critical. In fact, the need for sulfur is about a million times greater than the need for vitamin E, and

100,000 times more important than vitamin C. This is likely one reason why naturopathic medicine originated in the sulfur hot springs area of central Europe, hundreds of years ago.

As mentioned earlier, glutathione is comprised of cysteine—a sulfur-containing amino acid—sandwiched between two other amino acids, glycine and glutamate. Glutamate has a strong relationship with the membrane of the small intestine, and is readily invited through the membrane. The attached cysteine and glycine slip in, as well, without being digested.

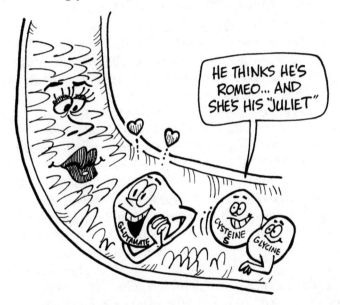

While the small intestine can absorb glutathione intact, the rest of the body must assemble it from its basic components—of which the sulfur-containing amino acid cysteine is the most crucial. Cysteine, however, cannot be taken in its pure form because it is highly toxic on its own.

N-acetylcysteine (NAC) is a form of cysteine that is readily absorbed. One problem with NAC is that it can aggravate some people, so I have stopped recommending it for my patients. For the same reason, I have also stopped recommending cilantro, chlorella, and various homeopathic remedies that are touted as mercury detoxifiers.

One nutritional source of cysteine that I *do* recommend is **whey protein powder**. Whey is the protein left over after milk has been curdled to remove the protein **casein** during cheese-making. It is important that the whey is not overprocessed—especially by overheating—because the proteins can be easily denatured. Whey contains two cysteines joined together in the form of cystine, which makes it both readily absorbed and non-toxic. Your body can split the cystine into two cysteines, as needed. Whey is lower in lactose and casein than milk, so it is less likely to be an allergen than whole milk.

For those who can't take whey, they can use more **MSM** (methyl-sulfonyl-methane). MSM is a sulfur compound made from tree lignin, to which few people are allergic. It helps build up and protect the body's supplies of sulfur. MSM also appears to be a more passive sulfur, unable to "stir up" mercury in the body, which is good when first starting a detoxification program.

While I look at whey as supplying the *liver* with the exact sulfur it needs, MSM works more on the *membranes and joints*, although it also supplies the liver. In practice, I find MSM far more effective than glucosamine sulphate or chondroitin sulphate for strengthening joints, and far less expensive. It is also available in a cream that will often soothe strained soft tissue overnight.

Taurine is a sulfur-containing amino acid that helps protect membranes from lipid peroxidation. Its effects are most pronounced in the eye, heart, and central nervous system. Taurine has been shown to help with epilepsy; eye problems such as cataracts; anxiety; indigestion from low bile flow; heart weakness; and blood sugar and blood pressure problems.

A whole family of vegetables—called the **Cruciferae** family—contain sulfur that can improve the function of both your Phase I and Phase II liver enzymes. The cruciferous vegetables include cabbage, cauliflower, broccoli, bok choy, kale, kohlrabi, brussels sprouts, collards, rutabagas, turnips, and the mustard family, (which includes radish and watercress).

The cruciferous vegetables contain **glucosinolates** that are converted by your digestive system into **isothiocyanates**. Isothiocyanates can aid your Phase I enzymes as they begin the breakdown of your steroid hormones, and also stimulate your Phase II enzymes to finish breaking them down into harmless substances.

The two most active ingredients of the cruciferous vegetables—**indole-3-carbinol** and **sulforaphane**—are found in the highest quantities in broccoli, cabbage, and brussels sprouts. Indole-3-carbinol is most noted for its ability to aid the breakdown of strong hormones into milder hormones through the C-2 pathway—thus protecting against breast, cervical, and prostate cancers. Sulforaphane helps fight a wider range of cancers by directly stimulating the immune system, and enhancing the Phase II enzymes.

Many cancer researchers suspected that **human papilloma virus** was the cause of cervical cancer and genital warts in adults, and respiratory papilloma in children, and that the majority of the North American population is carrying at least one of the 70 strains of this virus. Strains HPV-16 and HPV-18 have the greatest ability to suppress p53, thereby allowing cancer of the cervix to develop.

But don't think you're the helpless victim of a vicious killer-virus; there's new research that shows you can be in charge of the situation.

In the introduction to *The Secrets to Great Health*, I mentioned that two of my patients had recently reversed early-stage breast cancer. One of the things I had recommended to them at the time (about eight years ago) was to take a new supplement containing indole-3-carbinol (I3C). More recently, in the August 2000 *Gynecologic Oncology*, Dr. Maria Bell, of Louisiana State University, gave her findings of a study that involved 27 women with carcinoma of the cervix, 80 percent of whom cultured positive for human papilloma virus.

Eight women received I3C extracted from broccoli at a dose of 200 mg per day, nine received 400 mg of I3C per day, and the ten in the control group received a placebo. **Of the women**

receiving the I3C from broccoli, 47 percent had their cancer of the cervix completely disappear! The improvement was generally greatest in the group receiving the higher dose of I3C; this correlated with the improvement in the liver's ability to break down the estrogen hormones through the C-2 pathway, rather than the 16α pathway. The women in the placebo group showed no improvement in hormone breakdown or in cancer inhibition.[126]

This shows some remarkable things.

- Elements in your daily diet can aid the breakdown of hormones by your liver in a way that can minimize stress on your reproductive hormones.
- The human papilloma virus is not the cause of cervical cancer, but instead is an opportunist that takes advantage of organs damaged by hormones that are produced by faulty liver function.
- Because I3C can reverse cervical cancer in a significant number of women, cervical cancer should be a preventable disease in virtually all women if their livers break down hormones properly.

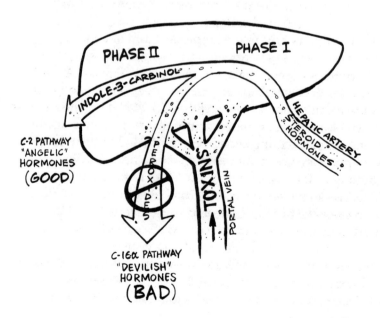

The improved liver function with indole-3-carbinol should not be confined simply to preventing cancer of the cervix, but also diseases of the other female reproductive organs, such as the breasts, the endometrium, and possibly the ovaries. In fact, these cruciferous extracts have shown promise in treating lupus and colon and lung cancers, as well.

Another product of nature that may prove to have similar anti-cancer properties is pollen from rye plants. In numerous Swedish and international studies over the last 50 years, rye pollen has been shown to aid in prostate health.[127]

Unlike most other herbal prostate remedies, rye pollen not only improved urine flow, but also reduced the enlargement of the prostate and reduced **prostate specific antigen (PSA)** readings. Rye pollen has been shown not only to improve the breakdown of DHT—the strong form of testosterone—into milder forms that are less irritating, but also to inhibit the production of DHT. One of the ways rye pollen does this is by increasing the levels of zinc in the prostate, and also by inhibiting the absorption of heavy metals from the small intestine.[128] If you've read Chapter 1 and Chapter 2 of this book, you'll quickly realize how crucial this can be to your health.

Other researchers have been studying rye pollen to find its active ingredients; they have discovered **FV-7, DIBOA,** and **secalosides**. Studies involving these extracts have shown they have the ability to induce apoptosis (suicide) in prostate cancer cells, and also in breast cancer cells.[129]

Rye pollen has also been shown:
- to protect against a wide range of chemicals and drugs;
- to lower cholesterol and triglycerides;
- to raise HDL cholesterol; and
- to reduce artery plaque.[130]

You should know by now that the benefits seen from using rye pollen must be due to increasing the liver's ability to neutralize peroxides. Rye pollen is another one of nature's many gifts to you.

Some compounds called bioflavonoids can help protect and even recycle glutathione. Bioflavonoids are made by plants for protection during photosynthesis, carried out by the plants' chloroplasts. The chloroplasts make carbohydrates using sunlight, water, and carbon dioxide. During this process, oxygen is released into the atmosphere. This tricky job of converting sunlight into carbohydrates also creates free radicals. Bioflavonoids surround the chloroplasts, and capture and neutralize different types of free radicals that might escape from the chloroplasts.

Because different plants use various frequencies of light for their energy source, a wide range of flavonoids has evolved. The 4,000 or more bioflavonoids have acquired various colours to match the different light frequencies in which they work. For example, **lutein** is green; **lycopene** is red; **quercetin** is yellow; and **malvin** is an anthocyanidin that is deep-blue to purple.

All these bioflavonoids have been known to have protective effects for humans. For example, lycopene—found in tomatoes, watermelon, and ruby red grapefruit—has anti-prostate cancer properties. Lutein and zeaxanthin—found in steamed greens (especially kale)—have been shown to help protect the macula of the eye. Quercitin—found in yellow onions—is the most common bioflavonoid; it has a protective effect throughout the body.

The **anthocyanidins**, however, were shown by Kamei in 1995 to have the greatest cancer-suppressing effects of the more common bioflavonoids. A year earlier, Ohlenschager showed that **anthocyanidins have the ability to protect and recycle glutathione** and optimize its ability to detoxify free radicals.

This ability of anthocyanidins to recycle glutathione is surely what gives them their extraordinary anti-cancer properties. The foods highest in anthocyanidins are blueberries, bilberries, blue elderberries, black currants, and beets.

Eating a variety of vegetables—that are all the colours of the rainbow—will give you a wide range of antioxidant activity from all their bioflavonoids.

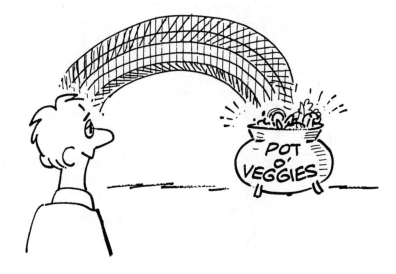

Other plant products known to increase glutathione levels are **proanthocyanidins**. These are stronger than anthocyanidins, but are generally found in much lower quantities in the diet. They can, however, be supplemented. Examples include pycnogenol from pine bark, grape seed extract, turmeric from the ginger root family, the Chinese herb *Hachimijiogan*, and melatonin.

In 1995, a study in *Neurochemical International* showed that melatonin could double the amount of glutathione peroxidase enzyme in the brain within 30 minutes. The drug acetaminophen, however, has been shown in *Drug and Chemical Toxicology* to deplete glutathione levels by over 70 percent, within four hours after ingestion.

The greater the age of the drug-taker, the slower the recovery of glutathione levels after taking acetaminophen. In spite of this evidence, acetaminophen is for sale in any drugstore, yet if a Canadian health food store operator were to sell melatonin, he or she would be quickly arrested.

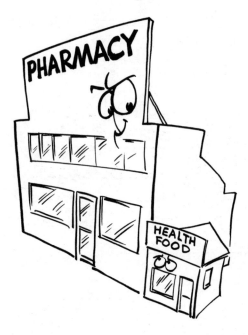

The plant that performs a number of positive functions in the body—and thus may benefit your health in many ways—is **Camellia sinensis**. Its leaf contains 25 percent medicinal bioflavonoids—such as quercetin, myricetin, and rutin—which activate both of your glutathione enzymes, giving a degree of anti-cancer protection. It also contains **catechins**, which can neutralize toxic epoxides before they can bind to your DNA. Camellia sinensis can also knock out lipid peroxides and toxic **nitrosamine compounds** formed from nitrate preservatives.

In Southeast Asia thousands of years ago, it was known that tea made from the leaf of Camellia sinensis had tremendous medicinal properties when used in its fresh green form. When picked, it would quickly oxidize and lose much of its medicinal properties—until a way was found to neutralize the enzyme **polyphenol oxidase** by steaming the leaf shortly after picking. This allowed the tea to retain its green colour and medicinal properties during storage and shipping.

Shipments of Camellia sinensis from Asia to Europe by slow-sailing ship, however, inevitably led to fermentation and oxidation, which turned the green tea leaf black. This degraded product was introduced to a gullible European market as quality Asian black tea; the far-superior green tea has six times the medicinal properties.

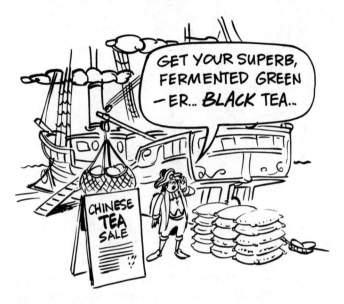

Glutathione peroxidase needs another component, in addition to glutathione, to make it the super peroxide buster that it is. Like many enzymes, glutathione peroxidase works with a metal to make it even more effective—in this case, selenium. It takes four selenium atoms to make glutathione peroxidase so adept at slashing deadly peroxides into harmless water. Without adequate selenium, glutathione peroxidase—and therefore your health—could soon be in big trouble.

In 1996, at the University of Arizona Cancer Center, Clark published his study showing that in patients who had previously had cancer, taking 200 micrograms of selenium per day (*above* what was already available in the diet), correlated with a 50 percent decrease in deaths due to cancer. Lung cancer deaths were reduced 46 percent, prostate cancer deaths dropped by 63 percent, and colon cancer deaths went down 38 percent. Selenium likely plays out its critical anti-cancer role by stimulating glutathione peroxidase enzyme to neutralize peroxides.

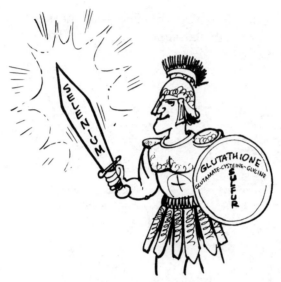

Selenium is normally processed from the soil by plants.
Ingestion of those plants should give you adequate selenium.
Some soils, however, have notoriously high selenium levels;
foods grown in them could be hazardous, since too much
selenium is toxic. Volcanic soils, on the other hand, are known
to be very low in selenium, giving low levels of selenium to the
plants grown in them.

The Pacific Northwest of North America, the Rift valley of
Africa, and Keshan county in China are a few of the areas
renowned for the low selenium levels in their soil. **Keshan
disease** is a heart disease that doesn't involve blockage of the
arteries; studies eventually found the **Coxsackie B virus** to be
involved. Beck did animal studies, and showed that a relatively
harmless form of Coxsackie could become deadly by inducing
selenium deficiency in the animal—another sign that viruses
are more opportunistic than predatory.

Other regions of China with known low-selenium levels have
higher levels of hepatitis B virus and liver cancer. Five-year
studies, in which residents in these areas were supplemented
with selenium, have shown significantly lower incidences of
both hepatitis B and liver cancer, indicating again that
susceptibility to liver diseases can result from inadequate
protection against lipid peroxide damage.

Outbreaks of **Hantaan virus** occur in China periodically, and result in a fever associated with severe hemorraging. One study showed that 38 percent of those with the fever died, while those who were given 2 milligrams of sodium selenite per day, for nine days, had only 7 percent fatality. This disease is very similar to the **Ebola virus Zaire strain**, which also causes hemorraging and has been shown to have a genetic coding that requires selenium, while the **Ebola virus Reston strain**, which is basically harmless, doesn't have genetic coding for selenium.

In 1996, Moss, of the National Institute of Health, showed that the pox virus *Molluscum contagiosum* contains a gene that produces a selenium-containing enzyme similar to glutathione peroxidase. A similar gene has been identified in the **hepatitis C virus**, as well. The hepatitis C **genotype 1b** is the one with the highest risk of progression to cirrhosis and liver cancer, and is the least likely to benefit from interferon treatment—yet it is the one with the genetic ability to make selenium-dependent glutathione peroxidase, which it uses to help defend itself against your immune system. **Therefore, selenium-using viruses drain this crucial nutrient out of your own system, leaving you much more vulnerable to peroxide damage.**

In clinical practice, most cases of viral hepatitis respond dramatically if the production of lipid peroxides by the liver is stopped through supplementation with selenium and herbs to activate glutathione peroxidase enzyme. The virus seems to go dormant in many patients when lipid peroxides aren't weakening the cells' membranes.

Kaposi's Sarcoma has recently been connected to a herpes virus. While seen commonly in carriers of HIV in "civilized" populations, it has long been endemic in subsistence farmers of the African Rift Valley, known for its low levels of selenium.

A number of studies have shown that selenium levels in HIV carriers are steadily depleted, and that the levels of selenium in the blood indicate the outcome of the disease. At the University of Miami, Baum found that low levels of selenium were 15 times more significant than low helper T cells as a risk for mortality in HIV carriers.

A considerable amount of research thus shows that **peroxidation stimulates viruses to replicate and, because selenium plays a key role in assisting glutathione to block peroxidation, selenium has significant antiviral activity.**

This fits the notion that viruses are simply recyclers of abused DNA—that if a DNA molecule is being lipid-peroxidized out of shape, then it has failed in its mission of supplying you with a viable blueprint for survival. So, the virus comes in and changes the genetic structure of the DNA—like a fervent gambler might spin the slot machine handle, trying to find the lucky match-up that might be a winner.

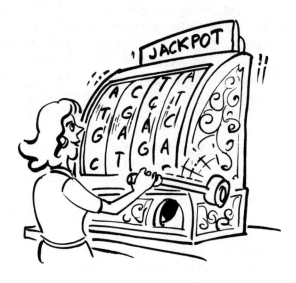

Many vaccinations have either intentionally contained viruses, or have accidentally been contaminated with them, so that millions of people of my age group (50s) have been exposed to a wide range of exotic viruses, including 40 from culturing polio vaccines on monkey kidneys.

These Simian Immunodeficiency Viruses (SIV), numbered 1 to 40, have been implicated in a wide range of diseases, most notably brain cancer and mesothelioma—a cancer of the lungs. The origin of the AIDS virus has also been proposed to have resulted from the accidental transfer of monkey viruses to humans, via vaccinations.

A stronger claim is made by Leonard Horowitz in his book *Emerging Viruses*.[131] He points out that when Nixon declared war on cancer in 1971, it was soon stated that the National Cancer Institute (NCI) would have a vaccine for cancer by 1976, based on the belief that viruses caused cancer. As billions of government dollars became available to researchers, the race was on to identify the cancer-causing viruses so that the appropriate vaccines could be developed.

Researchers began to cross-breed viruses, thereby increasing their deadliness, to save time in this race for fame and fortune. They were successful in creating deadly viruses through genetic manipulation. Horowitz shows how this could have been the origin of the AIDS virus, and how it could have been slipped into vaccines given to African blacks and North American homosexuals.

This plot involved Nixon, Kissinger, the CIA, pharmaceutical companies, the war industry, racism, homophobia, ex-Nazi biological warfare researchers, and the National Cancer Institute—interwoven in a web of intrigue so bizarre it might be true, because who would make up such a wild tale?

Nobel Prize-winning geneticist Joshua Lederberg, of Stanford University, gave fair warning of the possibility of viral warfare.

"In a word, the intentional release of an infectious particle, be it a virus or bacterium, from the confines of a laboratory or of medical practice, must be condemned as an irresponsible threat against the whole human community... ."

"And the potential undoubtedly exists for the design and development of infective agents against which no credible defense is possible, through the genetic and chemical manipulation of these agents."

He also attacked the business of injecting viruses into people via vaccinations.

"Live viruses are themselves genetic messages used for the purpose of programming human cells for the synthesis of immunogenic virus antigens."

"...Many of us carry viruses in our body cells of which we are unaware for years, and which may be harmless—though they may eventually cause the formation of a tumor, or of brain degeneration, or other diseases. At least in the laboratory, we can show that such latent viruses can still cross-breed with other viruses to give rise to new forms... ." [132]

Rutgers University professor, R. Simpson, said: "Immunization programs against flu, measles, mumps, polio, and so forth may actually be seeding humans with RNA to form latent proviruses in cells throughout the body. These latent proviruses could be molecules in search of diseases, including rheumatoid arthritis, multiple sclerosis, systemic lupus erythematosus, Parkinson's disease, and perhaps cancer." [133]

So we don't have to travel to faraway lands to pick up new exotic viruses to develop serious health problems. We've already been seeded with them via our childhood vaccinations. If these viruses are dormant now, the way to keep them dormant is to minimize the production of peroxides in the body, by slowing down the liver's Phase I enzymes and increasing the activity of the Phase II enzymes—especially glutathione peroxidase, armed with sulfur and selenium.

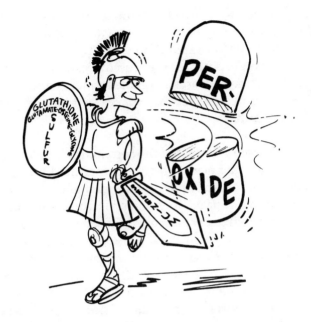

SELENIUM CRITICAL IN THYROID AND SPERM

The thyroid has a selenium-containing enzyme called **iodenase**, which converts the inactive thyroid hormone T_4 into the active T_3 hormone. This process creates peroxides from which the thyroid needs to be protected by glutathione peroxidase enzyme.

The body is set up like a military hierarchy. The liver, being the front line of defence against invaders, gets first pick of recruits. If the liver needs selenium to arm its glutathione peroxidase enzyme against dangerous peroxides, then the thyroid gets what's left over.

If there is no leftover selenium to help the thyroid fight the peroxides, the thyroid can become "barbecued" by its own peroxide production. The tremendous quantities of thyroid hormone that are used in prescription medicines are just another example of how the many peripheral liver alarms are being shut off. The symptoms are being masked, without getting to the root of the problem—trouble at the liver, involving peroxides.

Another product of the body—the male body, that is—that
needs a lot of selenium is sperm. The research showing a 50
percent decline, since your grandfather's day, in the average
male's production of sperm is surely an indicator of trouble
with peroxides. Because Danish organic farmers haven't had
this decline in sperm production, it makes sense to see if the
food chain is at fault.

In 1987, Frost pointed out that modern agricultural practices,
fossil-fuel burning, and acid rain have contributed to the
formation of elemental selenium in the soil that plants have
difficulty absorbing. In 1997, Rayman showed that the selenium
levels in the British diet have declined 50 percent in the last 22
years.

While selenium—one of our important protectors against
chemical toxicity—has been steadily decreasing in the food
chain, the use of chemical fertilizers, herbicides, and pesticides
has been steadily increasing, especially since World War II. A
study by Davis, published in *Journal of the American Medical
Association (JAMA)*, in 1987, showed that men born in the 1940s
had twice the cancer incidence as those born from 1888 to 1897
(after removing the smoking factor), while women born in the
1940s had 50 percent more total cancer.

In 1982, the EPA began to search thousands of tissue samples
taken nationally, for 54 different environmental chemicals. **Five
chemicals were found in every sample** tested. One chemical
was a **dioxin**; the other four were **solvents**. Another nine
chemicals showed in over 90 percent of the samples and
included more solvents, including **toluene** and three more
dioxins, and a breakdown product of **DDT**, called **DDE**.
Eighty-three percent of samples showed **PCBs**.[134]
Many of these chemicals were found to be common in indoor
air, although incidence was much higher during painting, or in
the chemical or plastics industries.

While DDT has been banned in some countries, it is still used
in others. The FDA Total Diet Survey has found chlorinated
pesticides such as DDE in 100 percent of samples of raisins,

spinach, chili con carne, and beef. Of the many other foods tested, 42 had DDE in over 60 percent of the samples.

In people with malignancies, the chemicals found to be present in the highest levels were DDT, DDE, PCBs, and HCH (hexachlorocyclohexane, used to treat lice infections). Also correlated with an increased risk of cancer were termite treatments, pet flea collars, home pesticide bombs, and garden use of pesticides or herbicides.

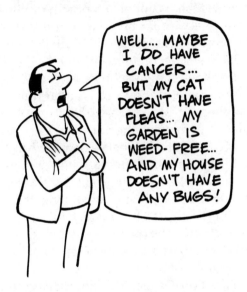

Moving to the country won't necessarily get you away from chemical exposure, because many chemicals are airborne and move world-wide. Hot weather tends to lift chemical and mercury vapours up into the atmosphere.

Winds can carry them great distances. Cool weather tends to drop them back to earth so that they tend to accumulate in the colder regions of the planet. Canadian studies have shown that in the spring, as the Arctic ozone layer gets buffeted by the sun, mercury vapours solidify and fall to the earth like rain.

Native women of the Canadian Arctic have been shown to have very high levels of **organochlorine compounds** and mercury that originated in the south, but that accumulated in the northern food chain. High levels of these estrogen-enhancing chemicals can result in increased **infertility, stillbirths,** and **miscarriages.**

The majority of the chemicals originate from the oil and coal industries, and most of the processing takes place in the country. Farmers—once some of the healthiest people on the planet—are now among the hardest hit by the use of chemicals.

Kansas farmers who use herbicides more than 20 days per year have six times the risk of developing **lymphoma** and **soft tissue sarcomas.** Swedish farmers exposed to **2,4-D or DDT** showed an increased incidence of **multiple myeloma.** Exposure to **pesticides** has been documented in 280 cases of **aplastic anemia. Painters** have shown an increased incidence of **multiple myeloma** and **kidney and bladder tumours.**

Hexachlorophene is added to soap for its antibacterial properties, but it can damage the **nerves to the eye,** as can many of the solvents. **Hearing-nerve damage** can also occur from **solvents.** The **trigeminal nerve** is vulnerable to damage from **trichlorethylene,** which is used in **dry cleaning fluid.**

Formaldehyde is in the glues that hold together the chipboard and particleboard from which our houses and cabinets are built. Synthetic carpet reeks from plastics and glue. Every car that drives past blows a stream of combustion hydrocarbons and fuel additives into our faces.

The movie based on the Erin Brockovich story is only one example of thousands of industrial chemicals that have leaked into the environment—it is only the tip of the iceberg. On March 26, 2001, PBS aired a program titled "Trade Secrets," in which host Bill Moyer exposed the chemical industry and how it manipulates researchers and politicians to hide the hazards of their products, all in the name of profit. Moyer himself was tested for the presence of over 150 industrial chemicals and was positive for 84 of them—many of them known cancer-causers.

It looks as if Sweden will be the country that will set the example and lead us out of the chemical nightmare—the Swedes are increasingly converting back to organic farming and in doing so, have noticed an increase in profits.

We are exposed to a daily onslaught of invisible chemicals—with known and unknown toxicities. They're in the air, the food, the water, and even the medicine you take. (It has recently been calculated that 100,000 Americans lose their lives each year from normal side-effects of medical drugs.) It is the duty of your liver to filter out and neutralize this array of man-made chemistry.

Virtually all of these chemicals are fat-soluble phenols, to which your Phase I enzymes must add oxygen so that your Phase II enzymes can neutralize and eliminate them. This process creates peroxides. If your glutathione peroxidase enzyme handles the peroxides effectively, you maintain your good health. If it doesn't, you lose at least your health—and perhaps your life.

So your whole physical, mental, and emotional well-being hinges on the abilities of two enzymes—both carrying shields of glutathione sulfur and one also carrying a sword of selenium—to chop hydrogen peroxide into water.

The tragedy of mercury exposure is that mercury that enters the body binds strongly to sulfur, disrupting the activity of many enzymes.[132] Binding of mercury to the cysteine-containing amino acid of glutathione cannot only lead to the development of a wide range of diseases,[133] it can further decrease the body's ability to handle heavy metals other than mercury—leading to further toxicity.

The inhibition of glutathione peroxidase enzyme can have a particularly profound effect on kidney function. Mercury also displaces lighter metals, such as selenium, leaving your critical guardian against lipid peroxides—gallant glutathione peroxidase—as powerless as Sampson after a crewcut.

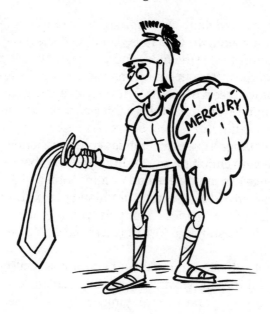

When I wrote *The Secrets to Great Health*, I knew there was still a missing piece in my understanding of the disease process. This quote is taken from the Introduction of that book.

"There are other patients where the results weren't quick, weren't easy, and weren't complete. Or where the results seemed complete, but the symptoms soon returned. They're the patients with the unhappy faces and the frustrated voices. Patients with difficult problems help keep a doctor from becoming complacent; their needs motivate the doctor to constantly search and experiment—adding to and subtracting from both the diagnosis and the treatment—to create improvement in their conditions."

The missing piece to the health puzzle has been found. That piece is heavy metals—and in particular, mercury.

Anyone with a history of mercury exposure—primarily from mercury fillings and vaccines—is in a bit of a dilemma. Having your mercury fillings replaced, if you have the money to do that, can increase your exposure to even more mercury, although that can be minimized with proper removal technique.

The accumulated mercury in the liver can be reduced by chelation, but that can take a few years. Some people are also allergic to the chelation substances.

Clinically, you don't usually hear people yelling, **"Yahoo, do I feel great!"** after they do chelation for a short period of time. What you more typically hear after a year or more of chelation is, "You know, I think I'm feeling better."

There *is* something, however, that *does* make most people with chronic health problems go **"Yahoo!"**—when they have killed off the yeast in their intestine.

Letter from a Patient

In the Fall of 1997, I was diagnosed with primary sclerosing cholangitis (scarring of the bile ducts). The prognosis was not good: five to 15 years until complete liver failure.

The only option I got from conventional medicine was to treat the symptoms. This seemed to improve the numbers, but not enough—nor did it address the disease.

In the spring of 1999, I became aware of Dr. Matsen's book, *The Secrets to Great Health;* during the summer, I acquired the book. I read it through and was intrigued enough by the principles set forth to set up an appointment with the good doctor. It was October 1, 1999, when I made the first trip to North Vancouver. Little did I know the effect this would have. I followed Dr. Matsen's regime to a "t" and improvement began almost immediately.

In the spring of 2000, I began the process of removing the silver amalgam filings and the detoxification of mercury. This continued until the summer of 2001. My blood test in September showed all levels normal for the first time since the summer of 1997! *My gastroenterologist told me he had never seen a response like this before.* My first thought was *a response to what?* I told him I had been doing some work on the side, and that I would tell him about it someday.

Many thanks to Dr. Kinne McCabe for his help with the DMPS injections and hair analysis, and to Dr. Mitch Marder for his excellent work with my filling removal.

I must give my heartfelt thanks, however, to Dr. Jonn Matsen and the entire crew of The Northshore Naturopathic Clinic for their dedication. You have proven to be my *Liver Saviour.*

Walter Gray
Seattle, WA

Liver Function

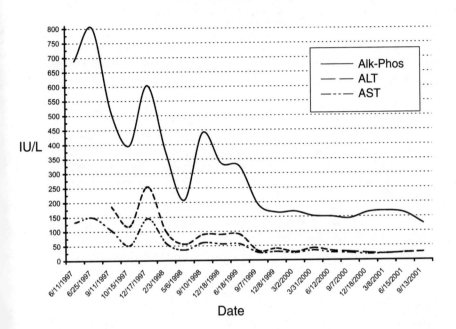

CHAPTER 4

The Yeast are Back

"A disease does not change its state to accommodate itself to the knowledge of the physician, but the physician should understand the causes of the disease. A physician should be a servant of Nature, and not her enemy; he should be able to guide and direct her in her struggle for life, and not throw, by his unreasonable interference, fresh obstacles in the way of recovery."

Paracelsus, 1493–1541

In all my 17 years in practice, after treating over 40,000 patients, the biggest improvement in a patient's recovery—almost universally—is seen after he or she has completed a yeast-killer. Just as universally, the return of the patient's symptoms is accompanied by the return of the yeast. Active yeast make tremendous quantities of phenols, from which the liver makes peroxides during detoxification.

Remember that I started on this investigation into mercury—which led to the writing of this book—because I was trying to understand why a patient with five years of chronic fatigue was able to return to work after taking a yeast-killer, yet relapsed several months later. He denied taking any antibiotics that might have caused the yeast to flare up. Subsequent removal of his mercury fillings led to his return to work again.

Could the mercury fillings have caused the regrowth of the yeast and the return of his chronic fatigue?

473

I know now that mercury vapour leaking from amalgam fillings can be transported by the saliva to the stomach, where it reacts with stomach acid to form **mercuric chloride**. Some of the commercial uses for mercuric chloride are: preserving wood and anatomical specimens, embalming, and disinfectant. Signs and symptoms that could occur due to acute mercuric chloride exposure include: **"salivation, foul breath, inflammation and ulceration of the mucous membranes, abdominal pain, bloody diarrhea."** [135]

Obviously, mercuric chloride is not nutritious, and has potent antibiotic (anti-life) properties that will kill off your good intestinal bacteria. "The Yeast Are Back" sign will go on again, and the liver's production of peroxides will soon shoot up.

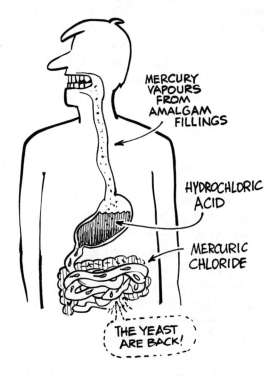

We already know that mercury binds to the sulfur of glutathione, inhibiting the Phase II glutathione enzymes from neutralizing peroxides. Replacement of mercury fillings might stop the addition of more mercury to the glutathione enzymes.

Caution: sloppy removal of amalgam fillings by a dentist who underestimates the toxicity of mercury can dramatically increase the mercury load on the liver.

Because glutathione peroxidase's job is to chop hydrogen peroxide into water, if you were to totally stop making hydrogen peroxide, wouldn't that give the same result—though perhaps much more quickly—as trying to totally regain the function of glutathione peroxidase?

To see if we can find out more about this, let's take a closer look at **the most fatal form of lipid peroxide damage**—killer of over 750,000 North Americans per year, and crippler of just as many—**atherosclerosis**.

Atherosclerosis is the cause of most deaths in the civilized world through heart attacks and strokes. Because it begins quietly without symptoms, and takes place in arteries throughout the body, symptoms can be nonexistent or vague for years, depending on the location and degree of the problem.

If one of the two carotid arteries carrying blood to the brain is narrowed by atherosclerosis, the symptoms might be one-sided—such as loss of vision to one eye, or weakness or numbness to one side of the body—because one side of the brain gets less oxygen from decreased blood flow. Decreased blood flow to the brain can cause decreased mental acuity, light-headedness, or personality changes.

Decreased blood flow to the kidneys can result in unremitting high blood pressure or even kidney failure.

Blockage of blood flow to the pelvic area can decrease sexual function in men. Blockages to the legs can cause **claudication**, which is severe muscle cramping that gets worse with exertion. Extremities can be more sensitive to cold temperatures, and possibly numbness or tingling will be present.

Blockage of blood flow to the heart causes **angina**—a hot, pressing, constrictive pain that can be felt in the left arm, shoulder, or neck, and is generally worse under stress or exertion; angina lessens when the person is calm and at rest.

All of these symptoms can improve, rapidly and dramatically, with increased oxygen.

Atherosclerosis is not a new disease, but only within the last 50 to 100 years has it become a killer of gargantuan proportions. The great writer of medical texts, Sir William Osler, wrote in 1892 that coronary artery disease was relatively rare; in his long and illustrious career, he had only seen a few dozen cases.

By the end of World War I, 12 percent of the population of "advanced" countries was dying of coronary heart disease. That number skyrocketed after World War II, until it reached 30 percent in the 1980s. If you consider that heart attacks and strokes are generally the result of the same thing—blocked arteries, just affecting different parts of the body—then you can say that 50 percent of the people who die annually in industrialized countries, die of these diseases of the circulatory system, while many more individuals are disabled by them.

Atherosclerotic deposits consist largely of cholesterol—a soft cholesterol called **cholesterol ester**, and harder cholesterol called **crystalline cholesterol**. There is often a **fibrous cap** overlying the cholesterol, with an intense immune war going on beneath it, as **macrophages** and **T cells** struggle mightily against a would-be invader.

Occasionally the fibrous cap breaks off or a clot is thrown out; it drifts with the blood flow until the artery gets so small that the clot dams it—blocking the flow of red blood cells and their oxygen cargo from reaching their destination.

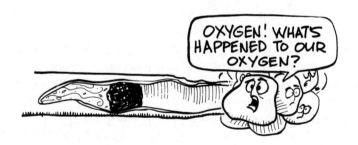

This blocking of oxygen flow kills brain cells or heart cells whose death is called an **infarct**—more commonly known as a stroke or heart attack. The predominance of cholesterol in the atherosclerosis has led to an emphasis on low-cholesterol diets and cholesterol-lowering drugs. However, these changes do not necessarily reduce atherosclerosis.

The deposits that protrude into your arteries are called **plaques**; they can be seen on an x-ray of your arteries, called an angiogram. It turns out that the angiogram is only seeing a very late stage of the development of atherosclerosis.

By the time 25 percent of the artery flow has been blocked by **hard plaque**, 85 percent of the unseen inner artery is filled with soft fatty plaque—called **vulnerable plaque**—which is actually the more dangerous of the two. It doesn't show on an angiogram. The hard plaque may cause discomfort by gradually clogging up your arteries and decreasing oxygen supply, but the soft, hidden plaque underneath is more likely to suddenly release clots that can quickly kill or maim.

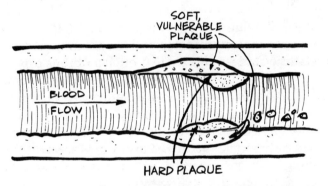

Atherosclerosis doesn't begin when your heart bothers you when you shovel snow at age 65, or when your legs start cramping up after you turn 60. Atherosclerosis can now be found regularly in children, on autopsy. It is, however, is a reversible disease, particularly in the earlier stages.

I had a patient in his late 50s come in with 85 percent blockage to the arteries in his legs; he was losing his ability to walk. He had been told that surgery was out of the question in his case, and that he should buy a wheelchair and get used to it. We changed various parts of his diet, got his digestion working properly, and added a few supplements (vitamins, minerals, herbs, etc.). He had another angiogram four months later, and was down to 35 percent blockage. He experienced no more circulation symptoms.

Since atherosclerosis is a reversible disease, it must also be a preventable disease. This shouldn't come as a surprise if you've read about the Pritikin Diet or the Dean Ornish diet, which have proven that atherosclerosis can be reversed with a very low-fat, high complex-carbohydrate diet. It gets puzzling, however, when Atkins claims to prevent hardening of the arteries with a high-protein, high-fat, low-carbohydrate diet.

CAUSES OF ATHEROSCLEROSIS

Because so many millions of lives are affected by atherosclerosis, let's look at some of the research that's been done world-wide, to see if we can understand the cause and cure of atherosclerosis. If you're not interested in this, you can skip over the following section. Right now, I'll try to put this mish-mash of research into an explanation of how atherosclerosis occurs.

- In the mid-1850s, Virchow pointed out that fat deposits in the arteries were secondary to an original inflammation. More recent studies have shown that the inflammatory response in the arteries mainly involves macrophages and T cells.
- While cholesterol-lowering drugs do reduce the incidence of death, they don't stop the immune response in the artery. In other words, the cholesterol problem seems to be secondary.
- The **cow's milk** protein, **casein**, has been shown, since 1908, to **cause atherosclerosis** more than vegetable proteins, such as soy.
- Willis published studies of Canadian war vets in the 1950s in the *Canadian Medical Association Journal.* He showed on x-ray that **500 mg of vitamin C, three times per day, reduced thigh-artery plaque** in six of ten individuals, after two to six months.
- Willis also showed that feeding guinea pigs a diet that was low in vitamin C resulted in atherosclerosis. Like

the human body, the guinea pig's body is unable to make vitamin C and must get it from the diet.

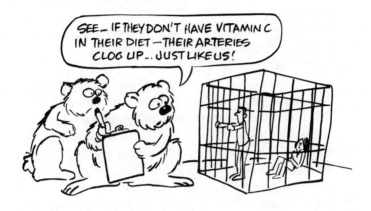

- Nobel Prize winner Linus Pauling repeated Willis's guinea pig studies, and found that as levels of vitamin C *decreased*, levels of **lipoprotein(a)** *increased*, which correlated strongly with the increased incidence of atherosclerosis. This research won Pauling his second Nobel Prize.
- In 1953, Enos found that Korean War **autopsies on Americans** (average age 22.1 years) showed that **77 percent had coronary artery disease**, which wasn't found in the Asians that were studied.
- The Japanese have a higher-stress lifestyle than North Americans, but have far fewer problems with coronary artery disease—unless they adopt the Western diet.

- In 1973, Ross found the enzyme **xanthine oxidase, from homogenized cow's milk, in artery plaque.**
- In 1979, Taylor pointed out that tests begun in 1912— showing that cholesterol caused atherosclerosis in rabbits—had used *rancid* (oxidized) cholesterol, and that newer studies with *pure* cholesterol didn't show the same results.

- In 1980, Velican found hardening of the arteries in adolescents as young as age ten, in Europe and North America, particularly if they smoked. This was not found in Japan.
- In 1984, Murata induced **coronary artery disease** in mice by repeatedly injecting an extract of the **fungus** *Candida albicans* into them.
- In 1985, Toth fed mice **phydrazinobenzoic acid** from the edible **mushroom** *Agaricus bisporus*. After 20 weeks, they developed **severe atherosclerosis**-like problems.
- In 1988, Masycheva showed that **baker's yeast** *(Saccharomyces cerevisiae)* fed to mice, **dramatically reduced their livers' ability to detoxify.** In 1990, Zhikhar fed baker's yeast to rats, and reported **major increases in atherosclerosis.**
- In 1988, Jaskiewicz showed that the toxin **citreoviridin**, from the **fungus** *Penicillium citreoviride*, creates the same **ECG readings as seen in human atherosclerosis.** He also showed that the toxin **cyclopiazonoc acid** from the **fungus** *Aspergillus* caused significant **damage to primate arteries.**
- In 1989, Besson showed that **cholesterol is capable of protecting a red blood cell's membrane from damage by the bacterial toxin mycosublitin.**
- In 1990, Harris showed that **triglycerides, chylomicrons,** and both **LDL** and **HDL cholesterol** help protect the body against toxins.
- In 1992, Weinstock showed that people with very **high levels of LDL cholesterol were able to inactivate more bacterial toxin than those with normal cholesterol levels.**
- In 1992, Fincham and Haschek fed primates and pigs a low-fat diet and the toxin **fumonisin** from the **fungus** *Fusarium*, found in corn products. He saw the development of **high levels of blood fats and atherosclerosis.**
- In 1995, Navah showed that **atherosclerosis begins when the antioxidant properties of high density**

lipoprotein (HDL) cholesterol become overwhelmed by lipid peroxides.

- In 1996, Stevens showed that **vitamin E** supplementation **reduced the death rate from heart attack due to hardening of the arteries.**
- In 1997, a study in *Circulation* showed that lower levels of vitamin D increased the chance that calcium would build up in athersclerotic plaque, while **higher levels of vitamin D would decrease the chances of atherosclerosis.**

- *Cyclosporine* is a **fungus**-derived drug used in transplant patients; it has been shown to cause a **37 percent rise in cholesterol levels** in 82 percent of users.
- *Ergot*, a **fungus** found on mouldy rye bread, has been known to cause **severe circulation disorders, including coronary artery disease.**
- The **fungus** *Aspergillus ochraceus* produces a toxin called **ochratoxin,** which can **create atherosclerosis.**
- New Zealand sheep, exposed to the **fungal** toxin *sporidesmin*, developed **artery damage** similar to atherosclerosis.
- **Aflatoxins** are made by *Aspergillus* **fungus** on nuts and grains not dried properly after harvesting; aflatoxins are known to be **carcinogenic and damaging to the arteries.**
- A World Health Organization study has shown that **excessive lowering of lipoproteins through medication may exacerbate atherosclerosis.**
- Various studies have shown **sugar, unfermented milk,** and **saturated fats** are involved with **atherosclerosis,** while **vitamin E and vitamin A** have been shown to be **preventative.**
- **Animal fats** have been shown to be the greatest **risk for men,** while **sugars** are the greatest **risk for women.**
- **Hydrogenated fats** from food processing have the same **negative effect on the arteries** as saturated fats.

- The 1993 Harvard study of over 85,000 nurses, over five years, showed that those who developed coronary artery disease were the biggest consumers of **cookies, biscuits, cake,** and **white bread.**

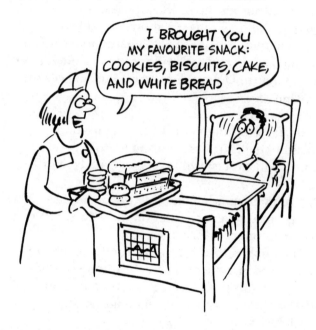

Using the results of the preceding research studies—combined with results I've seen in patients who follow my dietary recommendations—I'm ready to piece together this information into an explanation of hardening of the arteries.

Atherosclerosis must start with irritation to the membrane. An obvious irritant is our old acquaintance lipid peroxide—lipid peroxides are known to damage membranes on contact. They are made when your liver's Phase I enzymes make hydrogen peroxide faster than your liver's Phase II enzymes can chop it into water, causing the hydrogen peroxide to bind to cholesterol or fatty acids (lipids) in your liver, to form lipid peroxides.

If we take a closer look at how lipid peroxides create damage, we'll see how they can be the root of atherosclerosis. Whenever a lipid peroxide comes in contact with a membrane, it can release an OH group—a deadly hydroxyl radical—into the membrane. A hydroxyl radical set adrift in the sea of delicately linked membrane fats can have the effect of a bowling ball hitting pins—knocking fats askew as it rips down the membrane.

The more metals to which a hydroxyl radical is exposed, the more dramatically amplified the membrane damage. Eventually, vitamin E in the membrane will nab the hydroxyl radical, ending its wild, destructive journey—but since vitamin E is only stationed at about every 1,000 fats in a membrane, a sizeable tear can occur in the membrane before the hydroxyl radical is eliminated.

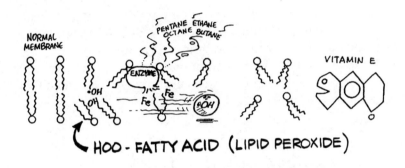

To repair the damage, the blood will immediately deliver a convoy of fats—such as **lipoprotein(a)**, **LDL cholesterol**, and **HDL cholesterol**—to the membrane.

Lipoprotein(a) is like the hospital ship of the blood, carrying **apoprotein**, a sticky substance used to hold the damaged area together, much as you would use a sticky bandage to hold the sides of a wound together.

LDL cholesterol is the freighter that carries the cholesterol needed to repair the damaged membrane. To protect its cholesterol cargo from oxidation (rancidity), LDL cholesterol is only lightly armed with weak antioxidants.

HDL cholesterol is a more heavily armed destroyer, sent to protect both the freighter (LDL) and the damaged membrane from further lipid peroxide damage. HDL is armed with the enzymes **paraoxenase** and **platelet-activating factor**, which can destroy lipid peroxides on contact.

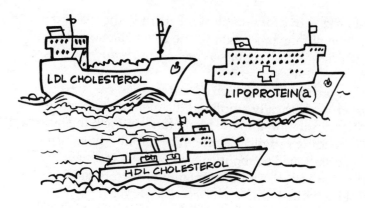

A well-equipped membrane repair crew consisting of these three important fats is more than capable of patching up lipid peroxide damage to your membranes. If lipid peroxides continue to bombard your membranes over and over again, your weakly protected LDL cholesterol can get torpedoed by the peroxides.

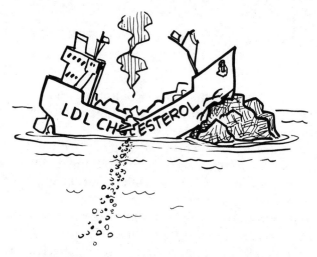

With ongoing lipid peroxide damage to your membranes, your liver will have to increase its production of fats into the blood to meet the demand. The increased levels of LDL cholesterol—if not given adequate antioxidant protection in the face of a barrage of lipid peroxides—will quickly get peroxidized and run aground in your arteries, giving it the unjust nickname "bad" cholesterol. While high levels of LDL have long been considered a sign of pending heart attack or stroke, high levels of lipoprotein(a) are ten times more dangerous because its stickiness can cause clots.

An Oxford University study found that people with high levels of lipoprotein(a) were 70 percent more likely to have a stroke or heart attack because, due to lipoprotein(a)'s stickiness, high levels begin to deposit plaque in the arteries.

In fact, Linus Pauling, who won the 1985 Nobel Prize in Medicine for his research on lipoprotein(a), theorized that vitamin C deficiency weakens the connective tissue—particularly collagen—of the arteries. This deficiency leaves the arteries more prone to damage, and to patch them up requires more lipoprotein(a). Pauling maintained that to keep lipoprotein(a) levels low, 3,000 mg or more of vitamin C daily is necessary, with doses to be taken at four hour intervals.

Because LDL cholesterol and lipoprotein(a) are being produced to help repair the membrane damage caused by *lipid peroxides*, it's obvious that when it comes to creating artery damage, lipid peroxides are at least as responsible as low levels of vitamin C.

The problem in the arteries can become much worse when your immune system gets involved. For one thing, your macrophages go in to rescue the damaged LDL that has been torpedoed by peroxidation. The macrophages eat the damaged LDL, but the rancidity can be so severe that the macrophages themselves can bloat up and die, becoming **foam cells.**

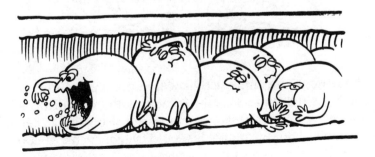

The immune crisis escalates when the immune system attacks the membranes of the endothelial cells lining the arteries. Why would your immune system attack your arteries' endothelial cells? The obvious answer is that they were asked to, by the endothelial cells themselves.

Cells communicate among themselves by several means, including hormones. Short-range hormones called **eicosanoids** can be secreted from the membranes of your endothelial cells, to alert your immune cells that they are being attacked by invaders and that they need immediate help—much as a sinking ship might send out an SOS. The "invader" doesn't have to be a live micro-organism to trigger this response; for example, a phenol can activate this immune reaction.

The endothelial cell membrane can make three types of eicosanoids: **prostaglandins**, **leukotrienes**, and **thromboxanes**. These eicosanoids are made by two membrane enzymes called cyclooxygenase (**COX**) and lipoxygenase (**LOX**) enzymes.

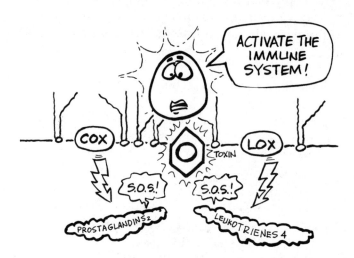

The appropriate immune cells will respond promptly to this distress call, and attack the invader with free radicals— although your own artery membranes are also going to be hit by this volley. But what invader could trigger such a zealous reaction that would result in damage to your arteries' protective endothelial cells?

The research listed earlier shows that the fungus family can cause serious injury to the arteries of mammals. If we also note that macrophages and T cells are the predominant immune cells involved in atherosclerosis, then it becomes more apparent that the immune reaction involved in atherosclerosis is likely that of **delayed-type hypersensitivity**—the same reaction the Swedes found when testing for metal allergies.

This immune response has evolved over thousands of years. Our ancestors' immune systems learned to fight off **mycobacteria**, such as *Mycobacterium tuberculosis* (TB) or *Mycobacterium leprae* (leprosy).

When a macrophage swallows a mycobacterium, the next step is to digest it. But these skillful mycobacteria have found a way to block the macrophages' digestive function, leaving the mycobacteria able to live quite comfortably—and even reproduce—inside the macrophages.

The struggling macrophages then secrete **tumour necrosis factor** and **fibroblast growth factor**, a cry for help in their struggle against mycobacteria. The immune system answers back with interleukin-6, which in turn stimulates the liver to make C-reactive protein. Interleukin-6 and C-reactive protein are substances that act as messages between different parts of the body to enhance immune reaction.

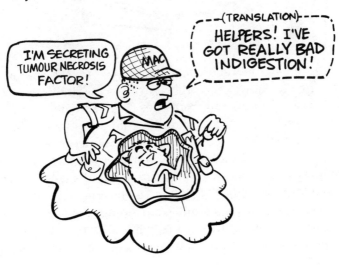

Tumour necrosis factor and fibroblast growth factor are
known to cause fibrotic lung damage and **granulomas**—
attempts to surround and imprison the bacteria with a wall
of fibrous tissue—seen in tuberculosis and leprosy.

Autoimmune damage from tumour necrosis factor is also
suspected in scleroderma, rheumatoid arthritis, lupus, asthma,
Crohn's disease, and Alzheimer Disease, and—because tumour
necrosis factor is renowned for being destructive to the
endothelial cells that line the walls of the arteries—
atherosclerosis.

The last-ditch response of a delayed-type hypersensitivity
immune reaction is to entomb the invader in a calcium coffin,
from which, hopefully, it will never escape. This is why TB
patients often develop calcified nodules in their lungs.

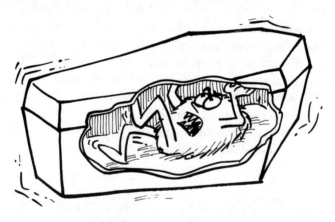

Does this mean that tuberculosis or leprosy mycobacteria
are attacking the endothelial cells of everyone with
atherosclerosis—and the macrophages are desperately trying
to root them out, damaging the endothelial cells in the process?
No, there's no leprosy or TB involved in most people's
atherosclerosis, but let's take a look at that word *myco*bacteria.

Myco is from the Greek word for fungus, so it's long been
recognized that tuberculosis and leprosy bacteria have a close
resemblance to fungus. Certainly, your immune system
responds to mycobacteria and fungus in the same way, with
the delayed-type hypersensitivity reactions. Does this mean

that the arteries have been invaded by hordes of deadly fungi? Not necessarily.

There are more than 70,000 species of fungus, including **moulds, mildews, yeasts, mushrooms,** and **puffballs.** Indoor air usually contains about 155 species; approximately 17 of these are potentially disease-causing, but dryness normally limits their ability to grow. Wet conditions indoors, and a food source such as cellulose, can bring a dramatic increase in such species as *Stachybotrys atra,* which makes plentiful and deadly fungal toxins called **mycotoxins.**

While your endothelial cells and immune cells react to and attack mycobacteria with the delayed-type hypersensitivity reaction, **they react more to the *toxins* made by fungus than to the fungus itself.**

The ironic thing about this is that the fungal toxins entering your body, through food or air, can therefore cause you more harm than if the fungus were actually in your body. In other words, fungus doesn't have to actually be in your arteries to activate the endothelial cell/macrophage/T cell delayed-type response—only their toxins have to be present.

Let's look at toxins made by *Aspergillus flavus*, because they've been so well researched. Toxins made by *Aspergillus flavus* are called **aflatoxins**; they are commonly found in peanuts, grains, and beans that weren't dried thoroughly before storage. When you open a peanut shell, aflatoxins are the mouldy-looking stuff on the inside of the shell.

Aflatoxins are a big problem in warm, humid climates that favour the growth of this fungus—especially in undeveloped countries where they don't have the ability to dry food properly. It's believed that many of the liver cancers and childhood liver cirrhoses in Africa, south of the Sahara, are directly related to aflatoxins in the food. In addition, many studies show that aflatoxins can cause atherosclerosis.

The aflatoxins are relatively harmless as they enter the liver's Phase I enzymes, but like benzopyrene, after they've been bound with oxygen and leave the Phase I enzymes, they've

formed deadly carcinogenic epoxides and peroxides. If the
liver's Phase II enzymes don't promptly and completely
neutralize the peroxides, they can tear apart liver cells, their
DNA, or the membranes of the arteries, as is shown clearly in
the research.

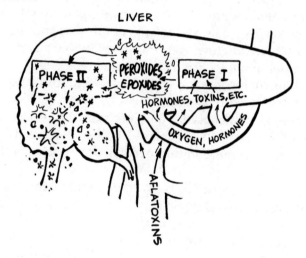

Of course, the endothelial cells will scream for help with their
eicosanoid SOS, and the immune system will rush to the rescue.
Spotting aflatoxins in the area will set the macrophages to
gobbling them up. If unable to completely digest them, the
macrophages will secrete tumour necrosis factor—which
inadvertently causes further damage to the artery membranes.
The liver makes more LDL cholesterol and HDL cholesterol to
repair the damaged membranes, but if the LDL becomes
peroxidized, the macrophages go into the membrane to dig it
out, thus increasing the problem.

Eventually the fibrosis and calcification stages of delayed-
type hypersensitivity reactions create the hardened outer layers
of atherosclerosis. Underlying the hard outer plaque is the
softer plaque, where the macrophages and T cells are
continually attacking fungal invaders, and trying to dig out
damaged LDL.

This plaquing process may continue until the arteries are so
narrowed that red blood cells are blocked, and are unable to

deliver their precious oxygen cargo, creating angina or brain dysfunction. Or the softer, underlying **"vulnerable plaque"** breaks off and blocks a small artery, creating a stroke or heart attack.

As you can see, aflatoxins, while being processed by your liver, create peroxides that can cause atherosclerosis. However, aflatoxins aren't likely associated with the epidemic of heart and stroke disease in the industrialized countries of the world, because aflatoxin levels are monitored in these countries. What, then, is contributing to atherosclerosis in the developed world?

The apparent success that I've seen with a certain supplement does give an important clue as to the culprit. There are a number of "herbal heart remedies" on the market, some of which are claimed by their respective manufacturers to cure heart disease. Of course, it's impossible to confirm such strong claims without seeing any studies that have been done on these remedies.

However, I've prescribed one brand in particular for a number of my patients; I've seen some cases of stubborn cholesterol lowered to normal, heart patients walking uphill after a few months, and a diabetic chasing his wife around after years of erectile dysfunction.

So definitely, it does reverse atherosclerosis in some people. I also know of several people who've had strokes after taking this remedy for several months, but their symptoms were mild. And it's impossible to tell if the remedy contributed to the strokes' occurrence, or if it actually reduced the severity of what could have been much more serious strokes.

Of the six ingredients in the herbal heart remedy, the main one is garlic oil. Garlic oil is a mild killer of a fungus called Candida, indicating that Candida toxins are the main trigger for these immune reactions. Since Candida—also called yeast—are normal denizens of the intestinal tract, how can they become such a deadly killer of thousands of people every year?

When you were born, your intestine was sterile. It soon began collecting a wide array of intestinal colonizers from your mother, your food, your fingers, and the air. By adulthood, your intestine had collected over 400 species of bacteria and several species of Candida yeast. Of the billions of bacteria in your large intestine, **Bacteroides** and **Escherichia coli** (**E. coli**) are the most numerous species. Lactobacillus species such as acidophilus, though less numerous, distinguish themselves by fermenting carbohydrates into lactic acid, which maintains an acid pH in your colon.

Candida yeast are strongly inhibited by acidity, and they are content to hide away in the nooks and crannies of your large intestine—wherever the pH is acceptably alkaline. Because Candida, like other fungi, are unable to produce their own food, they bide their time waiting for you and your acidophilus allies to die, so they can compost you.

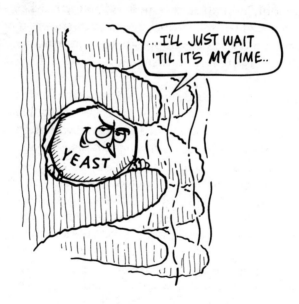

Anything that interferes with the health of your friendly intestinal bacteria can let the Bad Guys, namely yeast, begin their sordid party prematurely. If you've ever taken antibiotics for an extended period of time, it's bye-bye to your good bacteria, because antibiotics can kill your good bacteria along with the bacteria for which they were prescribed. This makes your colon more alkaline—and thereby more inviting—for the yeast.

They crawl out of their dark holes, squint a couple of times, and say, "Well, this one ain't dead yet, but we can speed that up." Since yeast are sucrose specialists—able to ferment sucrose into toxins faster than any other organism—they shout out, "Hey, buddy, we need booze down here so we can party. All right, all right, if you can't get booze, send sugar, white flour, or our favourite snack—chocolate—and we'll make our own damn booze. After all, we're fermenters."

Unfortunately, **yeast are the "Party Animals" of the gut: the nicer the party you throw for them, the more phenol toxins they are going to make—which are going to beat up on your liver!**

The food-refining industry has gone out of its way to increase the sucrose content in our diet—and white sugar, white flour, and white rice have created the perfect food for a yeast party.

Also, the refined-food industry has successfully penetrated the entire social and festive calendar, from birth to death, while the medical community has pretty much ignored a patient's dietary habits in favour of a quick pharmaceutical-fix. Ever since the introduction of antibiotics some 50 years ago, all the ingredients have been in place for the yeast to have a rocking and rolling party in your gut.

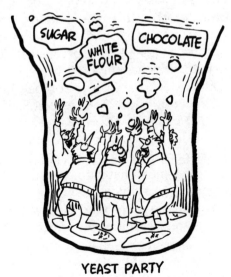

YEAST PARTY

The book, *The Missing Diagnosis*,[136] published in 1983 by Dr. Truss, was one of the first in a long line of books warning the public about the physical, mental, and emotional symptoms that can be a result of "chronic Candidiasis"—which is still generally ignored by the mainstream medical community.

While the medical community has generally downplayed the increase of Candida yeast that has occurred since the advent of the antibiotic and refined-food era, members of the general public have not. They have so often gone to their MDs and found no answers to their myriad complaints.

Yeast, especially when well-fed, make copious quantities of phenols—such as **cinnamic acid**, **gallic acid**, and **acetaldehyde**—which will be charged with oxygen by your liver's Phase I detoxification enzymes, creating a flood of deadly peroxides that must be neutralized quickly by your liver's Phase II enzymes.

If not promptly neutralized, the peroxides can go on to create the bounty of degenerative diseases so common in "civilized" society, such as coronary heart disease, stroke, cancer, diabetes, MS, asthma, fibromyalgia, chronic fatigue, arthritis, allergies, etc.

If you eat a lot of refined carbohydrates and other processed foods, your health could be in big trouble. Your Phase II enzymes need every known nutrient—vitamins, minerals, etc.— to neutralize the peroxides made by Phase I enzymes. Refined carbohydrates have had these precious nutrients stripped from them during the refining process, so that manufacturers could extend the shelf-life of their products.

Asthma deaths in young adults and children have increased 118 percent from 1980 to 1993.[137] Many would say that the increase in asthma is due to exposure of the lungs to more air pollutants. Researcher Scott Weiss at Harvard, however, reports that preliminary studies show that women who ate green, leafy vegetables and fatty fish had children who were less prone to developing asthma. He also said, **"One thing we do know: as the Western diet spreads around the world, so does asthma."** [138]

Fish and green vegetables are not what yeast prefer. Obviously it's the sugars found in refined foods and drinks that they want you to eat. A former professor at Harvard, who was once a spokesperson for American nutrition, was known to recommend a well-known soft drink as the ideal between-meals beverage.

This is perfect propaganda for the soft drink companies as they steadily infiltrate markets world-wide; a recent example is the bribing of school boards to grant exclusivity to specific soft drink companies' installation of machines in schools.

Recent studies by D. Grace Wyshak—ironically, also a Harvard professor—found that teenage girls who drank soft drinks were three times more likely to break bones than those who didn't. For athletes, this likelihood increased five times. The sugars in soft drinks deplete calcium in the body. This is hardly the type of nutrition that schools should be encouraging! (And don't think that it's safe to switch to sugar-free varieties, because other ingredients in the soft drink also deplete calcium.)

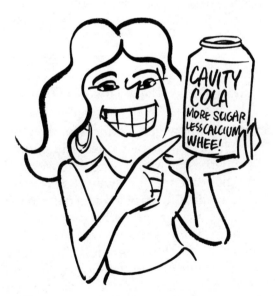

The same sugars that weaken bones and form cavities also feed the yeast so they can make the phenols that your liver turns into peroxides. And, as mentioned earlier, these peroxides can damage your artery membranes and raise your cholesterol, and then kill or damage your heart or brain by blocking the flow of blood.

Let's look at the herbal heart remedies again, and see if we can better understand why such a simple formula can work minor miracles in lowering cholesterol and cleaning out arteries. The brand I prescribed for my patients contains garlic, which inhibits or kills the activity of yeast in the intestine— reducing their production of phenols, thereby reducing the liver's need to make peroxides.

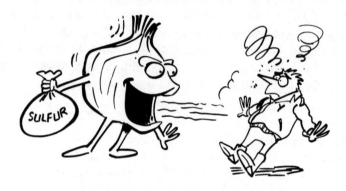

GARLIC..... KILLS OFF YEAST

Garlic also carries sulfur, which is critical for the glutathione peroxidase enzyme to neutralize peroxides. The sulfur has metal-chelation properties, as well.

The remedy also has cayenne in it, which opens up the blood flow, increasing the availability of blood and oxygen to the organs. In addition, it contains four herbs; two of them are bilberry and hawthorn. These herbs are known for their bioflavonoids, which have antioxidant properties stronger than vitamin C. They are capable of stimulating collagen production in the artery membranes, so they become thicker and stronger and less easily damaged by peroxides that have strayed out from the liver.

SUMMARY OF PREVENTING ATHEROSCLEROSIS

Atherosclerosis can begin with yeast toxins from the gut stimulating the liver's Phase I enzymes into producing peroxides which, when not quickly neutralized, spill out of the liver—creating membrane damage and immune reactions in the arteries. Here are suggestions to help prevent atherosclerosis.

- Keep the yeast in your gut under control with garlic, acidophilus, and yeast-killer. Don't feed them the refined sugars on which they thrive.

- Keep your liver's production of peroxides down by slowing Phase I enzymes, while increasing the activity of the Phase II enzymes, especially glutathione peroxidase. To do this, avoid refined carbohydrates, tobacco, alcohol, and coffee, and use antioxidants such as green tea, onions, apples, berries (especially blue and purple berries), ginger, and turmeric. Remember that the more metals there are in the liver, the harder it is for the Phase II enzymes to neutralize peroxides, so a healthy diet is even more important!

- Strengthen your arteries' connective tissue with vitamin C and plant bioflavonoids that assist vitamin C. Take doses four hours apart. This will also help to recycle vitamin E.

- Use healthy oils such as fish oil, Udo's Choice Ultimate Oil Blend®, and olive oil, which reduce inflammation in the artery membranes. Avoid hydrogenated oils and saturated fats. Minimize frying oils. A study showed that in a group of healthy men who were supplemented with 50 grams of olive oil per day for two weeks, there was a 73 percent reduction in risk of LDL to peroxidation.[139]

- A fermented rice product called **red yeast rice** has been shown to lower cholesterol without any liver or kidney side-effects.[140]

PLANTS OFFER PROTECTION

Herman Adlercreutz was a practitioner whose exceptional curiosity led him into nutritional research. He was brought up in the countryside of Finland. While attending medical school in Helsinki, Adlercreutz was aghast to learn there was a disease like cancer. Growing up, he'd never seen or heard of it. He found that when country people moved into the city, they didn't want to be looked upon as "country bumpkins." One of the first things they gave up was the dark rye bread of the peasant countryside—in exchange for the French croissants and Danish pastries of the sophisticated urban coffee houses.

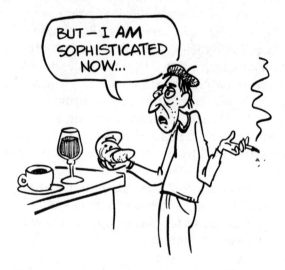

Little did they know, they were giving up one of their key defences against cancer. The outer fibrous coating of a seed, grain, berry, or nut is its physical line-of-defence against micro-organisms. Just underneath, but bound to it, is the **aleuron layer**, the chemical line-of-defence.

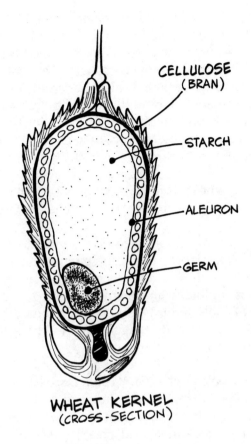

CELLULOSE
(BRAN)

STARCH

ALEURON

GERM

WHEAT KERNEL
(CROSS-SECTION)

Adlercreutz's curiosity led him to discover that, bound tightly to the aleuron layer of the rye bran, is a group of **phytoalexins** called **lignans**.[141] When lignans are eaten by your intestinal bacteria, they are converted into **phytoestrogens**, which act like very mild estrogens—they balance out your hormones and protect against cancer.

Milling of the grain into white flour removes the protective benefits of phytoalexins. In addition, vitamins—especially vitamin E—and minerals are found in the germ of the grain. After milling, these vitamins will be exposed to oxygen from the air, which can soon make them rancid, so the vitamins are removed during processing to increase the shelf-life of the food product.

So people take vitamin E supplements to make up for what's missing in the foods. The problem with vitamin E *supplements* is that they only contain alpha tocopherol, while *foods* contain alpha, beta, delta, *and* gamma tocopherol. Only gamma tocopherol can intercept the deadly chemical toxin peroxynitrite, which can be at the root of cancer and heart disease in smokers. Too much supplementation with alpha tocopherol can reduce the amount of gamma tocopherol in your membranes. Foods that are high in both alpha and gamma tocopherol are fish, soy, leafy greens, wheat germ, avocados, and mangoes. Wheat germ oil is not only high in tocopherols, but also octacosenol, which may help prevent infertility and miscarriage.

There's also another neglected side of vitamin E: the four tocotrienols—alpha, beta, delta, and gamma tocotrienol. They're similar to the four tocopherols, but they can lower cholesterol by inhibiting an enzyme that's involved in the production of cholesterol. Tocotrienols also block the eicosanoid that's responsible for platelet aggregation. Whole grains, especially rice, contain tocotrienols.

Let's take a look at what Dr. Weston Price had to say about the role of refined carbohydrates in the diet 70 years ago. In the 1930s, he took much time out from his busy LA dental practice to see what the rest of the world's teeth looked like. In studying 14 "primitive" tribes, from the Arctic to the Equator, this is what he found:

"In many groups, the primitive stocks showed as few as one tooth per thousand teeth attacked by dental caries before the contact was made with modern civilization, and an increase for the highly modernized groups to 400 and even 600 per thousand.

"Similarly, the health of the supporting tissues, as expressed in loosening of the teeth…often changed from a very high immunity to an exceedingly low immunity in a short time after a group made contact with modern civilization."

Dr. Price also noted:
"It is particularly tragic that whereas many of the primitive races studied have had practically no delinquency problems prior to their contact with the white race, serious problems have arisen with the processes of modernization.

"A chemical analysis of the primitive foods provided in the various native dietaries when compared with the foods of commerce has disclosed a much higher level of minerals and vitamins in the native foods, as selected in accordance with the accumulated wisdom of those tribes, than in the foods of commerce." [142]

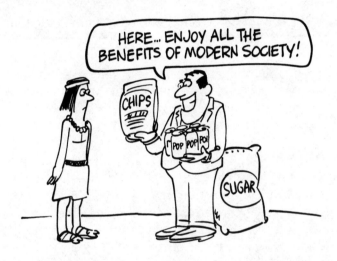

The following photos are taken from Dr. Weston Price's classic book, *Nutrition and Physical Degeneration*.[143] They are just a few of the many photos in his book that demonstrate the effect of the Western diet on dental health. *Nutrition and Physical Degeneration* is available from:
Price-Pottenger Nutrition Foundation
7890 Broadway
Lemon Grove, California 91946
(619) 462-7600
www.ppnf.org

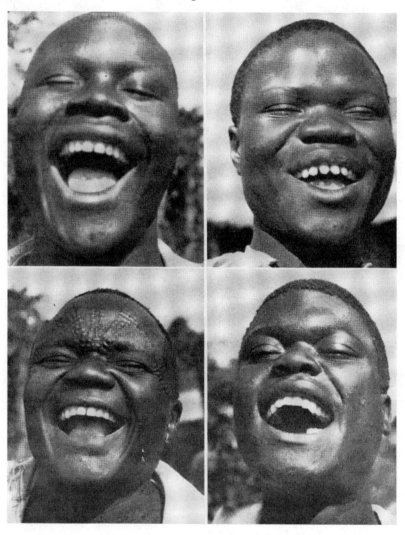

The reward of obeying nature's laws of nutrition is illustrated in this West Nile tribe in Belgian Congo. Note the breadth of the dental arches and the finely proportioned features. Their bodies are as well built as their heads. Exceedingly few teeth have been attacked by dental caries while on their native foods.

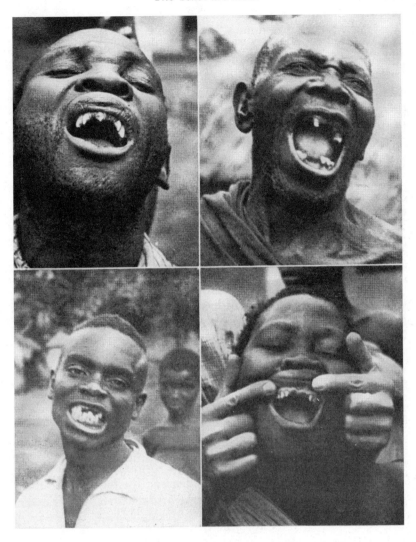

Wherever the Africans have adopted the foods of modern commerce, dental caries was active, thus destroying large numbers of the teeth and causing great suffering. The cases shown here are typical of workers on plantations which largely use imported foods.

It seems that whenever a culture embraces the "Western" diet, the Western diseases and Western medicine soon follow.

A study done by Marks, published in 1975 in the *Journal of Pediatrics*, found that **of children with cancer, 74 percent carried Candida yeast in the mouth. Of children entering hospital, 30 percent carried Candida on admission, but after three days, 64 percent carried Candida.**

This study shows that children with cancer have a weakened immune system, making them more prone to Candida overgrowth, or vice versa. Because a three-day stay in a children's hospital more than doubles the activity of Candida yeast, doesn't that also infer that these children's immune systems have been dramatically weakened by this short hospital stay? Of course, it has to be asked if it was the *hospital food* or the *hospital medicine* that doubled the yeast activity in these sick kids in only three days.

Other research found that children who were given one or two courses of antibiotics in the first year of life had a 225 percent greater chance of developing asthma than those who had no antibiotics. Three or more courses of antibiotics in the first year of life gave a 400 percent increase of the risk of asthma. If one or two courses of antibiotics were given *after* the first year, the chances of asthma were 65 percent greater than those who had no antibiotics.[144] Therefore, as the presence of yeast increases with the increased use of antibiotics, the incidence of asthma also increases.

Let's go back to dentist Weston Price, and see what else he might have learned from a study of New Zealand Maori children in the 1930s.

"The skulls of the native New Zealanders before the coming of the white race...showed that only one tooth per thousand teeth had been attacked by dental caries. My studies of the modernized Maori revealed that from 30 to 60 per cent of the teeth had been attacked by dental caries, or from 400 to 600 teeth per thousand teeth. The present Maori dietary is very similar to that of the whites of New Zealand. In contrast with the original high immunity of the natives

to caries, the modern whites of New Zealand are credited by their own dentist with having the poorest teeth of all groups in the world."

The students at the Hukerara Girls' School in Napier switched back to their native diet, which **"included a liberal increase of sea foods and seeds as used by the original Maori."**
The result was a 75 percent reduction in the occurrence of new dental caries. A nearby boys' school—which remained on a processed-food diet—was used as a control, and those children showed no decrease in cavities. Results were seen beyond dental improvement, however, as:
"a flu epidemic in which not one of the girls in this group under the nutritional program contracted the flu, whereas in the Maori boys' school in the same vicinity, approximately half of the boys developed influenza. Similarly diphtheria, which was epidemic, failed to attack any of the girls on this special dietary program."

"The failure to establish complete immunity was limited to those persons who did not cooperate properly."

What was it in the girls' diets that improved their immune system defences against flu and diphtheria? The increase in sea foods and seeds would increase their intake of omega 3 fatty acids—these help release anti-inflammatory hormones (eicosanoids) from the cell membranes. In addition, they were probably getting more vitamins and other nutrients from these whole foods, compared to their previous diet.
In 1937, M. Ormerod and associates published two articles in the *Canadian Medical Association Journal* showing that vitamin C administered orally to 29 pertussis patients markedly decreased the intensity and duration of the symptoms.[145] In the 1940s and 1950s, F. Klenner, an MD in North Carolina, used vitamin C extensively as an IV treatment, claiming results with a wide range of viral diseases, including measles, polio, encephalitis, and diphtheria.[146]

Also, vitamin A deficiency has been implicated in susceptibility to measles, respiratory infection, diarrhea, and blindness in young children. Beyond the obvious benefits of increased vitamins A and C in whole foods, there is the whole range of B vitamins and a long list of minerals, all of which are critical for the proper functioning of the body's enzymes—especially the liver's Phase II enzymes whose job is to neutralize peroxides.

As you can see, research done in the 1930s found that following a native ancestral diet (eating foods that are unprocessed) showed promising results in preventing dental cavities and childhood infections. So then why did the dental profession choose to use amalgam fillings and fluoride—and the medical profession choose to use vaccinations and antibiotics—when good nutrition may have avoided the need for much of this?

It doesn't take much digging to find that after World War II, nutrition classes were virtually tossed into the scrap-heap at medical schools, and replaced with more classes in pharmaceuticals. A cynic might think that physicians aren't much more than sales agents for the drug companies and their researchers. Robert Mendelsohn, MD, certainly thought so in his book, *Confessions of a Medical Heretic*:
"I once believed in Modern Medicine.
But I no longer believe in Modern Medicine.
I believe that despite all the super technology and elite bedside manner that's supposed to make you feel about as well-cared-for as an astronaut on the way to the moon, the greatest danger to your health is the doctor who practices Modern Medicine. I believe that Modern Medicine's treatments for disease are seldom effective and that they're often more dangerous than the disease they're designed to treat. So when you go to the doctor, you're seen not as a person who needs help with his or her health, but as a potential market for the medical factories' products." [147]

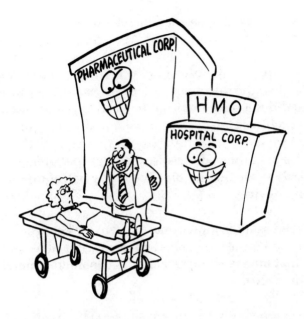

Or, as Mahatma Gandhi once said, "I believe that a multiplicity of hospitals is not a test of civilization. It is rather a symptom of decay." [148]

Even the *New England Journal of Medicine* seemed to go through a crisis of conscience on May 18, 2000, when the editor, Marcia Angell, MD, made some enlightening statements— as shown in these excerpts from her editorial, entitled "Is Academic Medicine for Sale?" (Bold print is my addition.)

"In 1984, the *Journal* became the first of the major medical journals to require authors of original research articles to disclose any financial ties with companies that make products discussed in papers submitted to us. We were aware that such ties were becoming fairly common, and we thought it reasonable to disclose them to readers. Although we came to this issue early, no one could have foreseen at the time just **how ubiquitous and manifold such financial associations would become.** The article by Keller *et al.* in this issue of the *Journal* provides a striking example. The authors' ties with companies that make antidepressant drugs were so extensive that it would have used too much space to disclose them fully in the *Journal*. We decided merely to summarize them, and to provide the details on our Web site.

"But as we spoke with research psychiatrists about writing an editorial on the treatment of depression, **we found very few who did not have financial ties to drug companies that make antidepressants….** . The problem is by no means unique to psychiatry. We routinely encounter similar difficulties in finding editorialists in other specialties, **particularly those that involve the heavy use of expensive drugs and devices.**

"It is argued that the more contacts there are between academia and industry, the better it is for clinical medicine; **the fact that money changes hands is considered merely the way of the world.**

"What is wrong with the current situation? Why shouldn't clinical researchers have close ties to industry? One obvious concern is that these ties will bias research, both the kind of work that is done and the way it is reported. Researchers might undertake studies on the basis of whether they can get industry funding, not whether the studies are scientifically important. **That would mean more research on drugs and devices and less [research] designed to gain insights into the causes and mechanisms of disease.**" [149]

I think Marcia Angell just summarized the last 50 years of medical practice and research. I think she gave out way too much "secret" information, and I bet she's about to leave her job! Oh, look, she did! Well, at least she went out honestly.

An accompanying article by Thomas Bodenheimer, entitled **"Uneasy Alliance–Clinical Investigators and the Pharmaceutical Industry,"** went into more detail on the many tricks the pharmaceutical industry uses to **"provide the spin on the data that favors them"** by manipulating research and researchers.

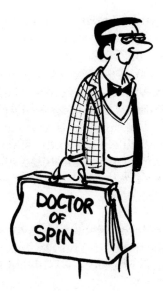

Why would a researcher want to find out that people could stay healthy inexpensively—with proper nutrition and exercise—when he or she could get paid big bucks to find something patentable—like a drug—to treat their diseases so that everyone can cash in? So, perhaps the researchers may be less interested in your health than in the financial health of their career and the drug company that is sponsoring their research.

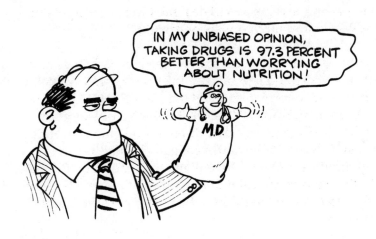

In the US, over **160 men and women per hour have heart attacks, for a total of over 1,500,00 per year. About half survive their first heart attack, but still 750,000 die.** Over half of those who die never even knew they had heart disease—and of the women who die from heart disease, 28 percent are under 55 years of age. Cost in treatment and lost productivity is $40,000,000,000.

Cancer kills 500,000 American men, women, and children each year. Cancer is the leading cause of death in children between the ages of three and 14. Cost of cancer treatment in the US is $100,000,000,000 per year.

Fortunately, government bodies like the FDA are keeping a close eye on the drug companies, to make sure they're not trying to pull a fast one that could jeopardize the health of innocent American citizens, **right?**

ABC News reported, on Sept 25, 2000:
"More than half of the experts hired to advise the US government on the safety and effectiveness of medicines have financial ties that will be affected by their decisions, *USA Today* reported today."

"These conflicts include helping a pharmaceutical company develop a medicine, then serving on an FDA advisory committee that judges the drug; holding stock in the company; consulting fees or research grants."

"Federal law generally prohibits the FDA from using experts with financial conflicts of interest, but the paper said the agency had waived the restriction over 800 times since 1998.

"The pharmaceutical experts, about 300 on 18 advisory committees, make decisions that affect the health of millions of Americans and billions of dollars in drugs sales. With few exceptions, the FDA follows the committees' advice. "

"At 55 percent of meetings, half or more of the FDA advisers had conflicts of interest, the paper said." [150]

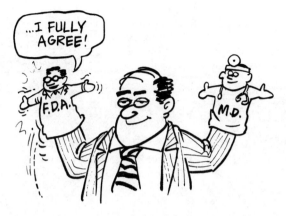

Of course, a little creative manipulation of a few bureaucrats by the drug companies couldn't seriously affect your health, **right?**

On April 15, 1998, the *Journal of the American Medical Association* had this to say: "We estimated that in 1994 overall, **2,216,000 hospitalized patients had serious ADRs (adverse drug reactions)** and **106,000 had fatal ADRs**, making these reactions between the fourth and sixth leading cause of death." [151]

Deaths per year from heart disease	**750,000**
Deaths per year from cancer	**500,000**
Grand total dead from US hospital care in one year	**225,000**
Total dead from normal drug side-effects[152]	106,000
Add in dead from hospital infections[153]	80,000
Add in hospital error[154]	20,000
Add in dead from medication error[155]	7,000
Add in dead from unnecessary surgery[156]	12,000

Deaths from car accidents in 1998	43,400
Deaths by gunfire in 1998	14,088
Deaths from food contamination	9,100
Deaths from boating accidents	2,064
Deaths from household cleaners	74
Deaths from acute pesticide poisoning	12
Deaths from vitamins, herbs, minerals, and amino acids	0

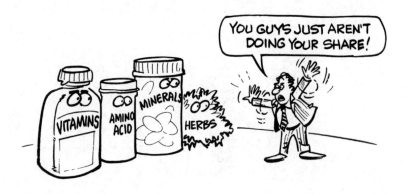

Hospitals are the third-largest source of mortality after heart/stroke attacks and cancer. Because these statistics are readily available—and no one seems to bat an eye—it seems there has been some sort of political immunity purchased, which makes it all the easier to understand how similar immunity has been accorded to purveyors of mercury-amalgam fillings and vaccinations.

Here's another statistic: a 1996 *JAMA* study showed that of the Americans who weren't in hospitals or other institutions, 45 percent suffered from chronic health conditions.[157] By now it must be clear that the medical model of "health" care is not only dangerous, but extremely ineffective—no matter how many billions of dollars are thrown at it.

While the average MD may still be naïve enough to think that he or she got the best medical education money can buy, it doesn't take much digging to find that the medical education process was hijacked by the pharmaceutical industry, long before the students entered medical school. Medical school provides the best education for treating injuries such as those sustained in car accidents, and for treating acute stroke patients and the like. It does not, however, provide the best education for maintaining good health. As the pharmaceutical industry barged into the front doors of the medical schools—especially after World War II—nutrition was tossed out the back door.

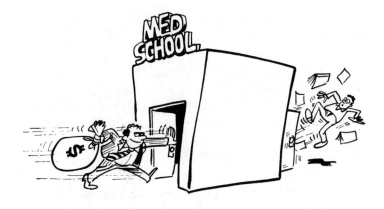

Any medical doctor who wrote that diet and/or vitamins were beneficial to health would soon discover that his or her receptive audience was the general public—not those who were reading the medical journals. The Shute brothers promoted vitamin E; Linus Pauling promoted vitamin C; Abram Hoffer promoted the role of vitamin B_3 in mental disease; etc. Other unpatentable things, like herbs, were also looked upon with derision.

Let's take a brief look at what happened to Harry Hoxsey and his herbal formula. His grandfather, John Hoxsey, was a horse breeder in Illinois in the mid-1800s, whose prized stallion developed a cancerous growth. The horse was put into a small fenced field and, to Hoxsey's amazement, the tumour gradually disappeared.

Thinking it could only have been the plants in the field that brought about this cure, he began to try the different herbs in various combinations, until he was able to repeat the results with other horses. His reputation spread, and other horse breeders soon requested his formula. This is a classic story of American insight and ingenuity.

His son, also named John, became a veterinary surgeon; he continued the use of the Hoxsey formula. In 1901, under the supervision of two MDs in Gerard, Illinois, human cancer patients began using the herbal formula, as well. Harry Hoxsey, John's son, grew up assisting his father with his veterinary practice, but also helping him with more and more human patients who requested the various herbal formulas that had by now been developed.

After his father's death in 1919, Harry Hoxsey took training as a naturopathic doctor, and opened his first clinic in Taylorville, Illinois, in the 1920s. This was the beginning of a long and brutal battle with the American Medical Association (AMA) and the FDA.

His main critic was Morris Fishbein, former long-time editor of the *Journal of the American Medical Association (JAMA)*, and writer for the Hearst newspaper chain under the moniker, "Voice of American Medicine." Through *JAMA* and the mass media, Fishbein called Hoxsey a "cancer charlatan" and stated, "Of all the ghouls who feed on the bodies of the dead and the dying, the cancer quacks are most vicious and most heartless." [158]

A court in Texas upheld Hoxsey's claim that he had successful treatment for skin cancer. Hoxsey won a libel suit against Fishbein, *JAMA*, and Hearst, but the court only awarded him a $1.00 settlement. During a court case in the 1950s, Harry Hoxsey revealed the ingredients of his formula as varying proportions of potassium iodide, cascara sagrada, poke root, burdock root, barberry, buckthorn, stillingia root, and prickly ash bark.

The Bureau of Investigation of the AMA immediately dismissed the formula as worthless—as any intelligent physician could testify that all of these substances were useless in the internal treatment of cancer.

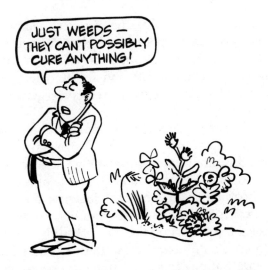

Other plants summarily dismissed as worthless in that hostile era were mistletoe, periwinkle, cinchona, and chaulmoogra—now used in treatments of cancer, malaria, and leprosy. Many of the herbs used by Harry Hoxsey are now undergoing study, especially in Japan, and are showing promise as anti-cancer agents.

In 1956, the FDA posted a "PUBLIC WARNING AGAINST HOXSEY CANCER TREATMENT" in 46,000 US Post Offices. Hoxsey closed his last clinic in Dallas soon afterward, worn out by decades of political battle. He gave his formulas to one of his nurses, Mildred Nelson, whose mother had been cured of cancer by Hoxsey. Mildred opened the Bio-Medical Center in Tijuana, Mexico, which is still an economically priced cancer clinic today, even though Mildred Nelson has passed away.

Hoxsey was only one of many doctors who used herbs and nutrition in the 1950s, and subsequently experienced the wrath of medical politics. In fact, the right to practise naturopathic, homeopathic, and herbal medicine was outlawed in many states, until only a few small enclaves remained in the northwest and the northeast.

Today in North America, the primary treatments for most types of cancer are surgery, chemotherapy, and radiation—all available at great expense and none of which will actually improve your overall health and ability to fight off future cancer or any other disease. Prevention of cancer…well, that requires more research, **right?**

So, corporate medicine has taken over the education of medical students, as nutrition and herbs have been quietly eliminated from the curriculum. Of course, you can't totally remove nutrition; people do have to eat something, even if they are in a hospital, **right?** You can't just give them drugs all the time. Of course, because disease is still a mystery, researchers have to keep working on the mystery, **right?**

So you need a research journal. And you're going to need some money to pay those researchers, so you find companies with big bucks to give generous support. Here's an example: In *The American Journal of Clinical Nutrition*—the official publication of *The American Society for Clinical Nutrition, Inc*—the Society lists its sustaining members, and acknowledges their generous support. This list includes, among others, the Coca Cola company, the Nutrasweet company, Kraft General Foods, the Carnation company, and Nabisco Brands Inc.

Since researchers can't be swayed by monetary considerations in their determined search for the true causes of disease—and these big companies won't mind if it's proven that their products are bad for your health—then there won't be any conflict of interest, **right? Disease is still a mystery, right?**

If you would like to see how nutritional research can be manipulated through money and connections, check out www.truthinlabeling.org. Research psychologist Dr. Adrienne Samuels gives an account as to how the monosodium glutamate (MSG) industry has manipulated and influenced research, the media, the FDA, the USDA, the National Institute of Health (NIH), and the EPA into downplaying the health hazards of MSG. She says, "few will notice…in that wasteland of ponderous detail and scientific terminology…a program of deception has been executed." [159]

While Dr. Weston Price proved in the 1930s that refined carbohydrates dramatically increased the incidence of dental cavities, the incidence of cavities in recent years has been greatly reduced by the additions of **fluoride** to drinking water.

As fast as governments add fluoride to North American drinking water, however, the populace rises up and insists on its removal; they, like the Europeans, read a wider array of literature than that presented by the pro-fluoride lobby. One of the key problems with fluoridated water is that, while it may improve the resistance of children's teeth to cavities, it decreases the tensile strength of bones in the elderly, making them more susceptible to fracture.

Studies by the New Jersey Department of Health showed that fluoridation also increased the likelihood of male children under the age of 20 of getting **osteosarcoma**—cancer of the bone—from two to seven times. This matched earlier laboratory studies with rats.

Russian studies in the 1970s indicated that workers exposed to fluoride exhibited signs of impaired mental function, but this was ignored in the West, because fluoride was considered a stable molecule that couldn't affect biological systems. In 1981, however, in *The Journal of The American Chemical Society*, Dr. John Elmsley wrote that "we have found an explanation of how this reputedly inert ion could disrupt key sites in biological systems," by forming strong hydrogen bonds with molecules such as proteins.[160]

Dr. Phyllis Mullinex, head of the department of toxicology at the Forsyth Dental Institute in Boston, conducted research on the effects of fluoride on rats. The studies showed that fluoride accumulated in the rats' brains at relatively low levels of exposure, and disrupted their behaviour.

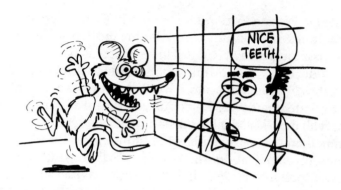

Publication of this research in *Neurotoxicology and Teratology* resulted in Dr. Mullinex's dismissal from her job at the dental institute.[161] The old saying, "there's no scientific proof of harm," is still used as the reason why fluoridation should continue.

We took this little detour to show you that there are political and economic reasons why so many of the treatments that are claimed to improve your health actually *decrease* it.

While a hospital stay may save your life if you've just been run over by a bus, your likelihood of Candida yeast overgrowth—due to the antibiotics or steroids you are given—is greatly increased. There is, however, an even more serious threat from antibiotics that has been well-documented, but about which little action has been taken. That threat is the creation of killer bacteria that are resistant to antibiotics.

Remember that bacteria have been one of the most primal adversaries we have ever faced in our relatively short span on this planet. Even today, over 20 million people die each year from infections.

Medicine has long searched for weapons to fight and kill these bacteria and, with the advent of antibiotics in the 1940s and 1950s, it was thought the war had been won—only to find that the bacteria quickly presented resistance to the antibiotics.

- **Sulpha drugs** were introduced in 1943; major resistance was reported by 1963.
- **Sulphonamide** was marketed in 1948; major resistance was reported in 1959.

- **Penicillin** also was marketed in 1948; gonorrhea became resistant to it in 1966. *Staphylococcus aureus* became resistant in 1989.
- **Tetracycline** was marketed in 1953; resistance was reported within ten years.
- **Ampicillin** came out in 1963; several bacteria had developed resistance by the early 1970s.
- **Vancomycin** was introduced in 1957, and has been considered the "last resort" antibiotic. Enterococci developed resistance to it in 1988. *Staphylococcus aureus* showed resistance in 1997.

Combinations of antibiotics were then used, yet the ability of bacteria to develop resistance has been greater than our persistence at finding things to kill them.
- INH began to be used against tuberculosis in 1951; major resistance occurred by 1953.
- INH was combined with Rifampin; resistance to this combination was present by 1988.

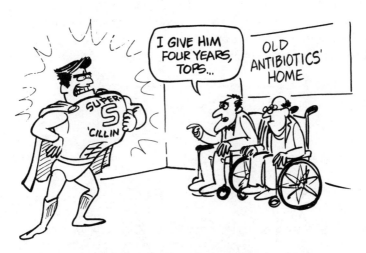

There are more antibiotics on the market now than ever before, but deaths from infectious disease are up more than 50 percent in the last 20 years. *Enterococcus*, a relatively rare bacteria, has developed resistance to a wide range of antibiotics; this bacteria killed thousands of hospital patients in the 1990s.

The hallowed halls of hospitals—intended as a sanctuary for the sick and maimed—have again become a source of disease and pestilence, much as they were before Semmelweis and Lister introduced antiseptics.

The very common **staphylococci bacteria** have become resistant to some of the basic antibiotics. Penicillin is now useless against staphylococci bacteria, and it takes a thousand times more penicillin to fight *Streptococcus pneumoniae*.

What if *Enterococcus* were to pass on its resistance to *Streptococcus pneumoniae*? This has already been done in a laboratory, and it's probably only a matter of time before it occurs in nature.

The reality is that bacteria don't develop resistance—they already have it. When we use antibiotics to kill bacteria, we are only killing the bacteria that *don't* have the genes to create the particular biochemicals needed to block the effect of the antibiotics.

The ones that *do* have the right biochemistry will survive. These survivors can not only multiply to take the place of those killed off, they also have the ability to pass these bits of genes to other bacteria. This is the bacterial version of sex—their way of exchanging genetic material—and it doesn't have to be with bacteria of the same species.

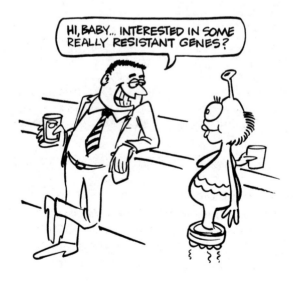

For example, hundreds of tons of antibiotics are used annually in animal feedlots on healthy animals, to increase their growth rate. This blatant misuse has strongly affected the intestinal flora of the animals. *E. coli*, normally a docile intestinal bacteria that quietly ferments cellulose into sugars, has been so disrupted by this bombardment of antibiotics that it has "mated" with the *Shigella* (dysentery) bacteria, to "inherit" its antibiotic-resistant gene.

Along with the antibiotic resistance, however, it also got some of *Shigella*'s "mean streak." This new *E. coli* strain— known as 0157.H7—when spilled onto meat during sloppy slaughtering of cattle, gave birth to "hamburger disease," which has infected hundreds of people, killed some of them, and has probably driven thousands more toward vegetarianism.

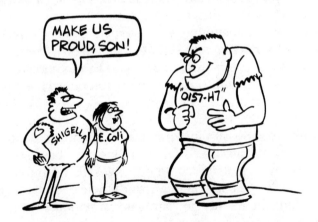

About 5 percent of people infected with this bacteria, usually children under the age of five, develop **hemolytic uremic syndrome (HUS)**. HUS destroys red blood cells—in turn, this damages the kidneys, causing a wide range of symptoms. Ironically, giving antibiotics to kill this bacteria seems to increase the incidence of HUS.

The incidence of tuberculosis, mankind's biggest killer, decreased dramatically with the advent of antibiotics in the 1950s. Using combinations of antibiotics against TB was even more effective—for a while.

In the last ten years, tuberculosis has been steadily increasing, particularly in Europe. Weakened immune systems due to drug and alcohol use have been partly to blame, but bacteria that have increased their resistance to numerous antibiotics is an all-too-common observation.

While research is going on to find newer and ever-stronger antibiotics, it's becoming clear that the whole philosophy of this approach was wrong to begin with. The bacteria were here billions of years before we were, and they outnumber us by the trillions. One bucket of garden soil contains more bacteria than the total of all people who have ever lived on earth.

Bacteria are biochemical wizards; they can live *off* things, *in* things, *in spite of* things, and *they can create things* that would stagger our comprehension. There is probably not a biochemical pathway they haven't discovered.

While there are seemingly endless species of bacteria, they share a "group intelligence"—that is, they will exchange genetic biochemical blueprints from one species to another. We, however, are biochemical rookies who don't have the ability to match biochemical wits with them.

Because we were *born* into this sea of potentially deadly micro-organisms, we are not helpless. We have been supplied with allies to adequately defend ourselves. For example, your skin contains more bacteria than your whole body has cells; these bacteria are mainly on *your* team. **Staphylococcus epidermis**, the most common skin bacteria, helps defend your skin from harmful bacteria and fungi. Killing off the staph with topical antibiotics weakens your skin's defences.

Many of the skin bacteria live under the skin, at the openings to the hair follicles. One of the bacteria found deepest under your skin is **Propionibacterium acnes**, which inhibits bacterial growth with the production of **propionic acid**. Acne only forms when internal fat/hormonal imbalances—which, of course, means liver trouble—cause this bacteria to become a glutton. The use of tetracycline antibiotic to kill this skin bacteria is one of the main causes of Candida overgrowth in the gut.

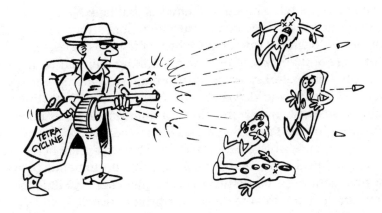

Fungus is also normally found on your skin in small amounts. Disruption of the skin's normal bacterial defenders—or weakening of the body's internal immune defences—allows the fungus to penetrate the skin or along the nails. The fungus is often seen as white skin patches that don't tan, or as a yellowy-orange-to-black discolouration around the nails.

Your most obvious bacterial allies are your very own intestinal flora. Your large intestine is filled with billions of bacteria whose vested interest is to keep you alive and healthy, so you can carry them around to buffet lunches.

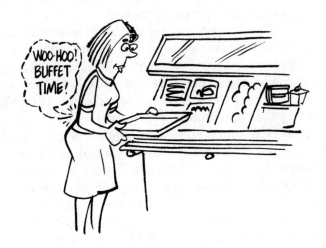

They make a wide range of chemicals that help keep "order" downstairs. When we keep our intestinal flora strong, we are part of the "bacterial universe," which enables us to take advantage of their prodigious talents. Killing them off with antibiotics only weakens your gut and makes it susceptible to overgrowths of Candida yeast and *Clostridium difficile* (the main cause of diarrhea from taking antibiotics), to invasion by viruses, or to infestation by parasites.

In my clinical experience, almost universally, the main improvement in stubborn health problems is seen **AFTER** elimination of any internal yeast overgrowth problem. In theory, it should be simple: kill the yeast in the large intestine, replace them with the good acid-forming bacteria, and things will quickly resolve. Sometimes it works that simply, but more often than not, it doesn't.

First, yeast make a lot of toxins when they're alive in your gut—but they can be even more toxic when they die. The membranes of dead yeast are fat-soluble. If not quickly flushed out of the bowel when they die, they will be another fatty burden that your liver has to make water-soluble—which means that more peroxides are going to be formed. Also, 78 percent of the cell wall of fungus is **mannan** which, if dumped by your overloaded liver into your lymph system, could result in **hives** as your immune system attacks it.

Taking yeast-killers over long periods of time is often not successful; the main reason is because the yeast problem is not in the large intestine. When I wrote *EATING ALIVE* 15 years ago, I mentioned that people who were reading the most health books seemed to have the worst health problems—and they all were showing trouble with the **ileocecal valve (ICV)**.

"The symptoms can be identical to those associated with yeast problems. I find many patients are taking large quantities of yeast-killers with little improvement, as the malfunctioning ileocecal valve is the source of their toxicity. "

"Often the person with ileocecal valve problems looks quite healthy, so this barrage of symptoms seems very out

of place. It is seldom that anything shows on conventional blood tests, CAT scans, ultrasound, or even on physical exam, though a closer look will usually show tenderness deep in the lower right abdomen."

The ileocecal valve is located between the small and the large intestine. This valve is usually kept closed so that the food that you've eaten stays in the small intestine long enough to be digested and absorbed fully. It also prevents the good micro-organisms in the large intestine from getting into the small intestine, where their waste products could easily be absorbed.

As digestion and absorption are completed in the small intestine, the ileocecal valve opens, and the smooth, rhythmic waves of contraction move the food into the large intestine or colon.

In people who have ileocecal valve problems, this valve has become weakened. The normally "good" bacteria of the large intestine get through the ileocecal valve, up into the small intestine—where they're not supposed to be—and now they are "Bad Guys." Once your good bacteria become bad, yeast soon join the party.

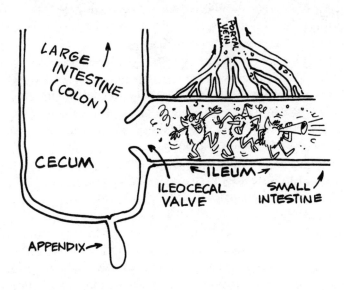

These Bad Guys then begin plundering and pillaging. They:
- eat the sugars, from which they make alcohol;
- eat your fats and your minerals;
- steal your vitamin B_{12} as well as tryptophan and other amino acids;
- deconjugate the bile salts in your upper small intestine, which further disrupts your amino acid absorption;
- destroy the enzymes of your digestive tract so you can't digest lactose or maltose or gluten any more; and most important,
- can overwhelm the glutathione enzymes in your liver.

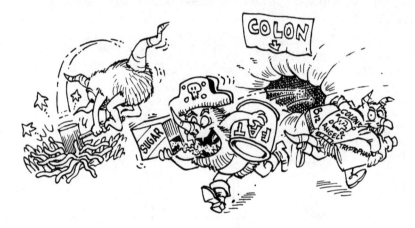

Your digestive system consists of an alternating alkaline/acid medium. For example:
- your mouth makes alkaline digestive enzymes;
- your stomach makes strong acid;
- your small intestine is alkaline; and
- your large intestine is made acidic by your acidophilus bacteria.

This alternating of pH levels between acidity and alkalinity improves the extraction of nutrients from various types of food—but it also puts great stress on any would-be invader trying to ride into your body in your food. Yeast can't stand acid, so both the stomach acid and the colon acid strongly inhibit them.

If, however, the flora in your large intestine move into the alkaline environment of the small intestine, the yeast can grow as if by magic. Taking antacids that lower your stomach acid production can quickly increase the range in which the alkaline-loving yeast can continue their partying.

Mercury from amalgam fillings can react with the hydrochloric acid of the stomach to create mercuric chloride, which also can devastate your normal intestinal flora, allowing the yeast and other Bad Guys to party.

Yeast are not innocent bystanders. They have ways of letting you know that they need alcohol to keep their party going. But hey, if you can't get alcohol, then sugar will surely do; they can ferment it into alcohol themselves. One of the chemicals that yeast secrete is **salsolinol**, which has the ability to turn your brain into their bartender, commanding you to fetch them their treats. High levels of salsolinol can lead to extreme cravings for, and even addiction to, alcohol or sweets.

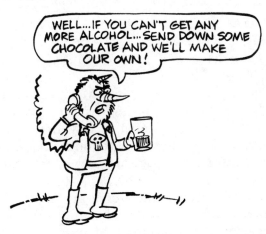

Sweetened chocolate is gourmet dining to yeast. It's quite common to see a person diagnosed with a fatty liver or a cirrhosed liver who has never touched a drop of alcohol in his or her life—but who did have a sweet tooth and a belly full of yeast. The phenols that the yeast make will be turned into peroxides by your liver. If not quickly neutralized, these peroxides will destroy any membranes they contact—including those of your liver—also leaving it more vulnerable to viral infections, such as hepatitis viruses.

Once the small intestine party really gets going, the bacteria and yeast will steal a lot more than just the refined carbohydrates present in your small intestine. They will soon start making off with your amino acids.

Your rarest amino acid is **tryptophan**, so it is usually the first one to show signs of deficiency. Normally, about 10 percent of tryptophan is converted into the neurotransmitter **serotonin**. This conversion takes place mainly in your small intestine; however, 1 percent of the serotonin in your body is made in the brain.

Since serotonin is made in your brain under the stimulation of sunrise, it is, in a sense, your "on" switch in the morning. Because serotonin also overlaps from the physical into the mental and emotional realms, deficiencies of brain serotonin can create appetite and mood disorders, emotional instability, depression, anxiety, memory loss, learning disorders, physical weakness, a sense of inadequacy, suicidal tendencies, and obsessive-compulsive disorders. Earlier in this book, we saw that mercury inhibits serotonin production.

At sunset, the brain begins the conversion of serotonin into **melatonin**, which is your "off" switch. Melatonin penetrates the blood-brain barrier into the brain and central nervous system, and begins shutting down your nerves and adrenal hormones, to prepare you for sleep. Melatonin's strong antioxidant properties scavenge any free radicals that might be threatening your delicate nerves.

When you're asleep, melatonin brings on the repair crews to fix the wear-and-tear that your body has endured during the day. Growth hormone repairs damaged proteins throughout your body, and thymus hormones activate your immune system to kill any invaders and repair any damage—so that when dawn approaches, you are rested, repaired, and recharged, ready for another busy day on planet Earth. This is why it's so important that you get adequate sleep every night.

If bacteria and yeast are stealing your tryptophan, you may not be able to make adequate amounts of serotonin and melatonin, which could result in emotional instability and inadequate nightly regeneration. Since 90 percent of tryptophan is made into other important substances, a lack of it may cause you to develop other problems.

Nicotinic acid—otherwise known as niacin or vitamin B_3—is the main product of tryptophan. From nicotinic acid, your body makes **NAD** (nicotinamide adenine dinucleotide) and **NADP** (nicotinamide adenine dinucleotide phosphate).

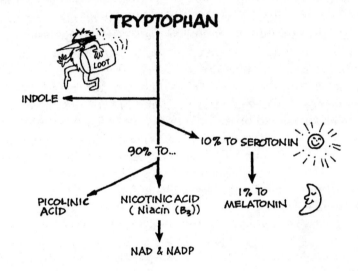

Famed psychiatrist Abram Hoffer treated Canadian soldiers who had suffered through years of malnutrition in Japanese Prisoner of War camps. He found that some schizophrenics can benefit from supplementation of niacin (vitamin B_3). From this insight developed a field of medical practice called Orthomolecular Psychiatry, which uses large doses of vitamins to treat mental illness.

Niacin has also been shown in a number of studies to lower cholesterol. Here's what Dr. Hoffer says, in the year 2000:

"In high tech societies, starvation is relatively rare, except in chronic drug and alcoholic addicts and other street

people. It has been replaced by affluent malnutrition, by a diet too rich in calories from the sugars and their offspring: alcohol, free fats, and white flour. An obese person eating a doughnut provides a perfect example of the modern affluent diet consisting of white flour soaked in oil which is cooked (heat treated), and reinforced with sugar. I think this diet will also produce a niacin dependency, although it will come on more insidiously." [162]

Deficiencies of NADP have been found in a wide range of chronic diseases. The main benefit of NADP in the body is the alleviation of fatigue. NADP helps your mitochondria produce energy. NAD and NADP have inherited a special gift from tryptophan that makes them crucial to hundreds of enzymes involved in important energy reactions.

Tryptophan is the amino acid that absorbs the most ultraviolet (UV) wave energy; NAD and NADP use this special energy-absorbing ability to hold onto—or give up—energy for the enzymes while they perform their chemical wizardry. Thus NAD and NADP have official **coenzyme** status. NADP is a coenzyme for enzymes that *build things up*, while NAD is a coenzyme for enzymes that *break things down*.

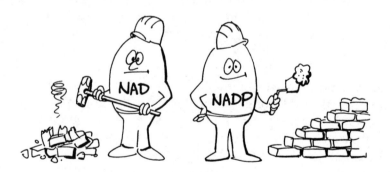

Tryptophan is also used in the production of **picolinic acid,** which is crucial for zinc absorption. So you can see that if bacteria and yeast get into your small intestine and start partying—and steal your tryptophan—you could find yourself with some fairly serious deficiencies.

If that isn't bad enough, these Bad Guys can turn your tryptophan into a number of **toxic indoles**—fat-soluble toxins that your Phase I enzymes must make water-soluble, creating peroxides in the process. Indoles can contribute to constipation, sinus congestion, allergies, asthma, fatigue, and depression.

The very last nutrient to be absorbed from your small intestine—and therefore the one that is very vulnerable to bacterial and yeast overgrowth in the small intestine—is vitamin B_{12}. Vitamin B_{12} can also be made into a coenzyme for energy transformations. In some people, the conversion of B_{12} into the active coenzyme methylcobalamin seems to be blocked by heavy metals, particularly mercury.

Coenzyme B_{12} isn't content to hold onto energy, the way NAD or NADP do; B_{12} juggles free radicals around like a circus performer handling flaming torches. Its extreme talent is crucial in strengthening and protecting your nervous system.

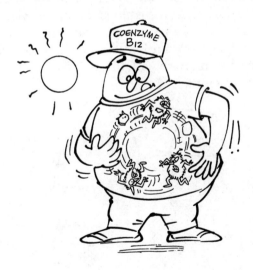

The earliest signs of vitamin B_{12} deficiency might be a sore tongue, or numbness, tingling, or burning in the extremities. This may or may not be accompanied by apathy, mood changes, memory weakness, and paranoia—which can occur before the vitamin B_{12} deficiency shows on a blood test.

You can see that allowing bacteria and yeast into your small intestine is not a good thing. Not only do you lose nutrients of tremendous value, you also get a terrible burden of toxins delivered to your liver via the portal vein. This does explain, however, why some people experience dramatic improvement from taking antibiotics for perhaps a cold or flu or acne; the antibiotics will kill some of the bacteria that are inappropriately in the small intestine.

So what causes the ileocecal valve to weaken, thereby allowing billions of bacteria from the large intestine to stampede into the small intestine, where they quickly become Bad Guys? The most common cause is low calcium levels in the body. Calcium is what keeps the ileocecal valve strong. It only takes about five days of low calcium levels to weaken this valve.

Calcium is a large molecule that can't get through the intestinal membrane on its own, so it must be transported through the membrane, into the blood. Stomach acid can chelate calcium—that is, bind it to a carrier. The carrier can then transport calcium across your intestinal membrane. Of course, taking antacids can interfere with this process by blocking the chelation of the calcium.

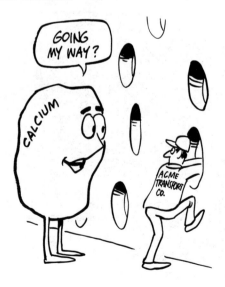

Most of your calcium absorption depends on vitamin D. Vitamin D stimulates your intestinal cells to make a calcium-binding protein that dramatically increases your absorption of calcium. Vitamin D is made in your skin when exposed to the ultraviolet rays of the sun, and then it is stored in an inactive form in your liver.

When vitamin D is released from liver storage, your liver converts it into **calcidiol**. Calcidiol, a weak form of vitamin D, activates calcium absorption to a small degree. This might be sufficient activation if you were out in the sun regularly, when your skin can make a lot of vitamin D.

The really strong (active) form of vitamin D is created when your kidneys—in the presence of **parathyroid hormone**—convert calcidiol into **calcitriol**. Calcitriol can improve calcium absorption up to 1,000 times more than calcidiol. This strong activation of vitamin D is especially crucial for wintertime when there is little sun around to make vitamin D directly through the skin.

Your kidneys are in charge of regulating calcium levels by altering the activation of vitamin D with the changes in the seasons. But how do your kidneys know what the seasons are? They can't see outside—they're stuck in the dark basement of your abdomen.

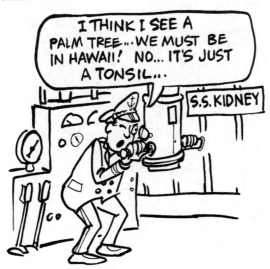

Besides calcium, your kidneys monitor and adjust the levels of other ions in your body. The kidneys have become masters at judging the outside weather by the ratio of sodium and potassium ions they detect in your incoming foods.

The kidneys need to maintain an equal balance between sodium and potassium, and as the seasons change, so do the levels of sodium and potassium in the foods that we eat. When spring sunshine arrives, plants grow. As a plant grows from the stimulation of the sun, it accumulates potassium. The more sun it gets, the more potassium it acquires. For example, a banana requires a tremendous amount of sun to grow, and therefore has a very high level of potassium.

Eating high-potassium foods tells your kidneys that there is plenty of sun available from which your skin must be making vitamin D, so your kidneys will decrease the activation of vitamin D.

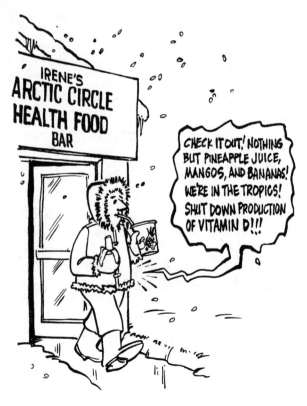

Because the body needs an equal amount of sodium and potassium, a vegetarian animal that eats a high-potassium diet will have a tremendous drive to obtain sodium in the form of salt. Eating appropriate amounts of salt creates the same 3 percent salt ratio in the blood that ocean water contains, thus giving animal meat a salty flavour.

In the winter, an Inuit will eat a high-sodium diet of meat and fish, which will inform the kidneys that the growing season is over, and that there isn't much sun. The kidneys will then activate vitamin D very strongly.

Your kidneys don't really know where you are in the world, and therefore, they don't know how much sunlight you're being exposed to. If you're eating foods high in potassium, like bananas, your kidneys simply assume that you must be out in the hot tropical sun, so they activate the vitamin D *less*. And if you're eating more sodium, then they assume that you're *not* out in the sun—and that your skin is not making vitamin D—so they *increase* your activation of vitamin D.

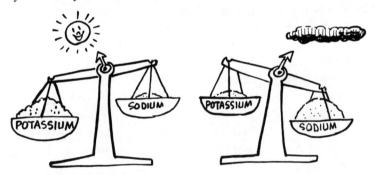

Our ancestors were aware of the importance of sodium in the diet, so they salted their vegetable products accordingly. Only in recent times could people in northern climates get tropical produce in the winter and, at the same time, read books (that were written by people living in the south) telling them that raw fruits and vegetables are good for them—and that salt is bad. This is the beginning of the ileocecal valve problem, or what I also refer to as **EATING TOO WELL!**

In 1987, in *EATING ALIVE*, I stated that about 50 percent of the people I see for the first time have an ileocecal valve problem. Today that number is over 90 percent. In the medical journals, this problem is referred to as "small intestine bacterial overgrowth"; it is considered common in the tropics in all age groups—and considered normal in the temperate zone in people over 60.

The reason that researchers consider small intestine bacterial overgrowth to be somewhat "normal" in the tropics, even in kids, is that the inhabitants eat so much fruit and sugar that it disrupts their calcium absorption. Low calcium levels lead to the weakening of the ileocecal valve, allowing the good bacteria from the large intestine to get up into the small intestine where they become Bad Guys.

In the temperate zone, only older people commonly had this problem because, with age, the kidneys were less able to hold onto their calcium. Now, with the dramatic increase of fruit and juice consumption in the temperate zone, this tropical condition of calcium deficiency and resultant small intestine bacterial overgrowth is common in the temperate zone in people of all ages.

Obviously, you want to get rid of any Bad Guys that have made their way into your small intestine. Trying to kill bacteria and/or yeast in the small intestine is an endless task, however, if the ileocecal valve remains open—because as fast as you kill them, they will be replaced by others moving in from the large intestine.

Before even trying to kill the yeast, it's important to first strengthen the gate—the ileocecal valve. This will block any further Bad-Guy reinforcements from entering the small intestine from the large intestine. The gate can be strengthened by improving your calcium absorption. Calcium absorption can be improved by increasing your activation of vitamin D. Increasing your kidneys' activation of vitamin D can be achieved by balancing your sodium and potassium intake to match the weather to which you're exposed.

Killing the yeast gives the most noticeable improvement in stubborn health problems, yet over and over again, I've seen that if you *don't do* this first step—closing the ileocecal valve by improving calcium absorption—the net improvement may be minimal or short-lived.

I live in Vancouver, British Columbia. Our weather comes off the North Pacific Ocean. We have a mild climate, but it can be prone to long spells of cloudy weather, particularly in the winter. Vancouver is a fairly affluent area, and people tend to travel in the winter, especially to the south. They primarily go to Hawaii, Mexico, California, and Arizona.

While there, they eat a lot of fruit and salad, and feel really good doing so. When they return to our cloudy weather, they continue to eat those foods that made them feel *good* in the south and, within a week, they usually end up feeling *bad*— their ileocecal valve usually weakens after about five days of low calcium levels.

Over and over again, I patch them up by telling them to eat fewer fruits and salads, and by encouraging them to eat more "warming," salty foods, like soups and fish. Also, as the calcium levels plummet from *EATING TOO WELL*, the ileocecal valve becomes very sensitive to coarse, rough fibre, as is found in bran, popcorn, granola, coarse-grain breads, etc.—so it's best to avoid these foods when you have ileocecal valve problems.

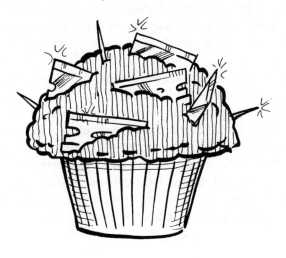

Over the years, patients who live in Hawaii, California, Arizona, Texas, and Florida have come to see me at my clinic. What I found was that every one of them had an ileocecal valve problem—even though he or she lived in a hot, sunny climate year-round. The insight from this is that you can *EAT TOO WELL*, even in these climates.

This is not to say that our ancestors didn't eat fruit in the winter. In northern climates, berries are the native fruit. Fresh berries in season are as natural as can be. Berries ripen during the longest days of late spring and summer. If you're outside in the heat, going a little brown—the skin goes brown to try to block the production of vitamin D—what could be more natural than to cool down with some local fresh fruit?

Local fruits are also dried, canned, or frozen for winter use. Even the Inuit dried cranberries for winter. Dried, canned, or frozen fruits can be added to cooked cereals in winter to aid the bowels. And because you add salt to the cereal when you cook it, salt will indirectly be added to the fruit, to help balance the amount of sodium and potassium that you're consuming.

Our ancestors had no hesitation about using salt. They were often farmers who were well aware that their vegetarian animals needed salt, so they supplied these animals with salt licks. They also kept table salt handy for their own use when eating high-potassium vegetable products.

Salt was so important in ancient farming societies that it was worth its weight in gold. It's the root of the word "salary," which most people slave away to earn, even today. One of the reasons salt got a bad name is that it has been worked over by the food processors, in the same way that white sugar and white flour have been.

To make them **pure white**, these foods have had their essential minerals, vitamins, and medicinal bioflavonoids stripped away. The same has happened to salt. Even sea salt has had its 60 to 80 protective trace minerals stripped and sold to someone else—while you are left with industrial-grade sodium chloride.

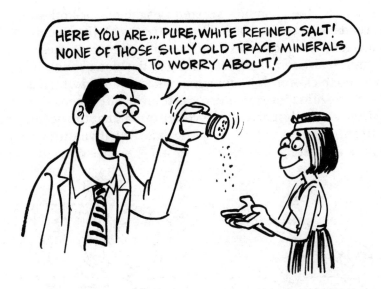

Pure sodium chloride will have some irritating properties that could have been negated by leaving the trace minerals intact. Fortunately, there are still some whole salts left. The one I recommend is called Celtic Sea Salt®; it has been produced in Brittany in France for many hundreds of years. Celtic Sea Salt® contains beneficial trace minerals—chloride, sodium, sulfur, zinc, magnesium, calcium, iron, potassium, manganese, copper, and silicon—as well as numerous micro-elements.

So you can see how important it is that you eat according to the climate to which you're exposed. Once you have your sodium/potassium levels balanced with the amount of vitamin D your skin is making from the sun, your body will be absorbing calcium better. Your calcium levels should be up enough, in a week or so, to toughen up your ileocecal valve.

Another important step in calcium absorption is to get your calcium *from your blood* into your bones, to protect against the development of osteoporosis; this is the job of vitamin K. Vitamin K activates **osteocalcin**, which guides calcium to where it's needed most in the body, reducing the risk of osteoporosis six-fold.

Ironically, the vitamin K also reduces the risk of stroke and heart attack just as dramatically: it activates **MGP** protein, which helps keep calcium from depositing in the arteries. Vitamin K also regulates the clotting of the blood by thinning it, if it's too thick—or thickening it, if it's too thin. So where does this magic lifesaving vitamin come from? Leafy greens! Eat your greens daily. Eat salads if you're out in the sun, but switch to steamed greens with a little sea salt added, if you're not out in the sun daily.

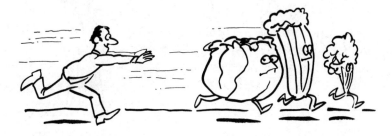

So once you have your calcium levels up and your ileocecal valve is strengthened, you can proceed to kill off the dreaded yeast, **right?**

Not necessarily. There are a few other things to do before you start taking a yeast-killer. Since the yeast are sometimes tough to kill—and toxic when they die—you want to weaken them first. You also need to maximize your bowel movements so the yeast will be flushed out quickly once they are killed. And it's important to get your liver working at its best so it will be better able to handle the yeast die-off.

You can weaken the yeast by *not feeding them* what they like most—refined carbohydrates such as white sugar and white flour. Candida yeast are sucrose (sugar) specialists; they can digest it quicker than any other known organism.

One sweetener that yeast apparently don't digest is **stevia**. Stevia is a plant that grows naturally in South America. Extracts of its leaves have been used for centuries in Brazil and Paraguay as a safe, natural sweetener. Stevia is 200 to 300 times sweeter than sugar and has a slight licorice-like taste. It doesn't feed yeast and other "Bad Guys," doesn't cause an increase in blood sugar levels, and doesn't promote tooth decay.[163]

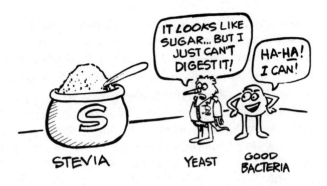

At my clinic, I often recommend a mineral supplement called Minbal™, by Nutri-West, which helps to decrease sugar cravings. If Minbal™ is not available in your area, you could use chromium, but it is slower-acting. Taking acidophilus bacteria also helps to inhibit the yeast by direct competition, and by creating an acid pH, which yeast don't like.

Soft fibres like psyllium or ground flax seeds will often help to maximize bowel movements. Since toxic bile is at the root of most chronic constipation, a daily dose of beets, or purple or blue anthocyanidin-containing fruits, such as blueberries, will often help. Beets work by activating the enzyme that makes SAMe, which is crucial in detoxification.

Regular exercise—especially abdominal exercises—can also help increase bowel frequency. If none of this works, try public speaking—fear or excitement usually gets the bowels going. Toastmasters should be promoted as a cure for stubborn constipation, as well as shyness.

To get your liver working better, stop the sugar, coffee, alcohol, and tobacco—at least as much as you can surrender without experiencing a major withdrawal attack. Also, use nutritional supplements to help support your liver during the detoxification process.

I recommend liver remedies that contain a wide range of ingredients that aid the Phase I and Phase II liver enzymes. In a pinch, you can make your own liver remedy, using milk thistle and selenium, plus whey powder or MSM for sulfur. I also suggest vitamin C with bioflavonoids, as well as a multivitamin/mineral containing B vitamins.

It takes about three days of supplementing with milk thistle for it to activate glutathione peroxidase, so you shouldn't start a yeast-killer before then. I usually have the individual wait one to two weeks before starting a yeast-killer. This reduces some of the liver aggravation that is typical of yeast die-off.

I must emphasize again that almost universally, the biggest improvement in a patient's well-being is seen after the yeast have been successfully eliminated. A return toward health usually follows shortly after their demise. Stubborn problems may not improve until metals are removed.

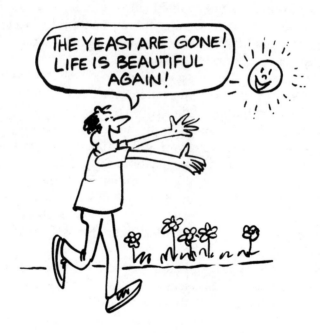

Letter from a Patient

In 1990, I suffered a serious attack of angina. An angiogram revealed I had six partially plugged arteries around my heart. The blockage in one artery was 90 percent, two were blocked 50 percent, and three were 25 percent blocked.

An angioplasty was performed on the most severely blocked artery. The procedure would have to be repeated in two to five years, or alternate by-pass surgery would have to be performed. Treatment for the remaining five arteries consisted of diet, exercise, and two drugs: Cardizam and Entrophen. I was also told that if the arteries' conditions worsened, I would have to be treated with angioplasty procedures or surgery.

After six months passed, I became thoroughly discouraged with the treatment program. The drugs left me feeling groggy and despondent all the time. I decided to look around for alternative treatment. In the course of my search, I came across Dr. Matsen's book *Eating Alive.* The success of his treatment for so many illnesses impressed me. I decided to make an appointment to see him.

Dr. Matsen examined me, and did blood, Candida, and sensitivity testing. He prescribed a program that consisted of a diet (food-combining) and supplements, along with homeopathy remedies. After three months, I felt much better and decided to do away with the drugs.

After six months, I decided to put the success of the treatment to the test. I started at the foot of the banks of the Capilano River and climbed to the top (a distance of some 500 feet almost straight up), without stopping—a feat I had tried and failed many times before. What was even more impressive was that my heart rate quickly subsided after I reached the top. Not bad for a 58-year-old man.

In 1993, I was examined by the cardiologist who first treated me. He put me on a treadmill and through a nuclear testing machine. The results were amazing. The only remaining aspects of the disease were two small scars on my heart, believed to be caused by the original attack of angina.

In the 11 years that have passed, I have not had any further recurrence of angina or any other cardiovascular problem. The natural healing methods used by Dr. Matsen in this case were the answer.

Thank you.

Regards,
Fred Walchli
North Vancouver, BC

CHAPTER 5

Oxygen: Nature's Best Cure

"...I have gratified that curiosity by breathing it [pure oxygen], drawing it through a glass siphon, and, by this means, I reduced a large jar of it to the standard of common air. The feeling of it to my lungs was not sensibly different from that of common air; but I fancied that my breast felt peculiarly light and easy for some time afterwards. Who can tell but that, in time, this pure air may become a fashionable article in luxury. Hitherto only two mice and myself have had the privilege of breathing it."

Joseph Priestley
London, 1774

In the first four chapters, I've primarily told you of things—heavy metals, chemicals, refined foods, tobacco, alcohol, coffee—that limit the ability of your liver to detoxify, and therefore limit your ability to maintain good health. In this chapter, I'll tell you of the one thing *above all* that can increase your likelihood of achieving great health: *oxygen*.

There are two ways to increase the oxygen in your body. One is by increasing breathing through regular exercise, which has

been consistently shown to reduce the incidence of every
known degenerative disease.

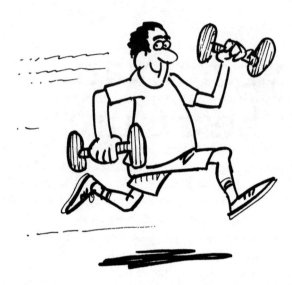

For example, in 1986, Paffensbarger and his associates
showed that Harvard graduates who **exercised regularly had
decreased mortality rates,** compared to sedentary men.

In 1958, Pomeroy and White showed that ex-football players
who continued to **exercise** the most, **were less likely to
develop coronary artery disease**.

Numerous studies like these show that active people are
healthier than sedentary people. For those who are unable to do
active exercise, there are less strenuous ways to increase oxygen
intake, such as Tai Chi, Qi Gong, or yoga.

Since deep breathing is the key to efficient oxygen intake—as
well as functioning as the primary pump for liver function—the
hearty belly laugh that comes with a sense of humour can also
help to maintain health.

For those who have been debilitated by a major disease, there
is a second way to increase your intake of oxygen: **hyperbaric
oxygen therapy (HBOT)**.

A patient with diverticulitis came to my clinic many years ago because his doctor recommended surgical removal of his colon; the man wanted to try an alternative approach. By following my treatment program, he regained normal function of his digestive system.

His name is Gino Gemma. He was one of the earliest SCUBA divers in the province of British Columbia, and later became involved in the development of underwater technology—including modern hard diving suits and mini-subs—which has become a major industry in North Vancouver.

Gino told me a lot about the development of pressure chambers for the reversal of the diving sickness called "the bends," and how he had become interested in developing an improved chamber to treat a variety of health problems. I read widely on the topic of oxygen and oxygen therapy, and Gino and I went to San Antonio, Texas, to take an in-depth course on hyperbaric oxygen therapy.

OXYGEN: THE MOST IMPORTANT NUTRIENT

You can survive for many weeks without food because your body has stores of sugar, fat, and protein that can be used as fuel in time of need. You can also survive for many days without water because 57 percent of your total body weight is water—about 40 litres (10 gallons) in a person weighing 70 kilograms (154 lbs). This can act as a reservoir for a few days, if fresh water is not available.

Without oxygen, however, you will lose consciousness and be dead within five minutes, because you have no reservoir of stored oxygen. This makes oxygen the most important nutrient.

Half or more of the life on this planet exists deep under the ground or under the sea. Those life forms have never seen the light of the sun, and would be repulsed by "a breath of fresh air." Called **Archaea**, these microscopic organisms are the hardy pioneers of this planet.

Archaea have no need for oxygen or the delicate temperatures that surface creatures require. They live in boiling-hot water found in cracks and fissures deep below the earth's surface, at the bottom of the deepest oceans, under the icy glacial mountains of Antarctica, and in hotsprings. They feast on sulfur and hydrogen, and give off large amounts of methane gas which—along with ammonia—formed parts of the earth's primitive atmosphere.

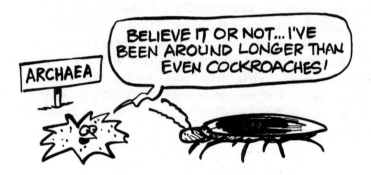

Bacteria—almost as physically tough as Archaea, and perhaps even more adept biochemically—contributed to turning our atmosphere toward carbon dioxide and nitrogen, several billion years before we came along.

Plants came later. Powered by a small electron current generated from sunlight, plants stripped the carbon from the carbon dioxide in the atmosphere to produce carbohydrates and release oxygen (O_2) into the air. Only after our planet had long been blessed with plants could oxygen-breathing animals appear.

Many life forms preceded us, for we are latecomers to this planet—the last born on the sixth day, according to *The Bible*. We were born into a bounteous atmosphere, many kilometres high; its very pressure (760 mm of mercury at sea level) pushes air into our lungs with little effort on our part—beyond breathing in, ever so slightly.

The atmosphere isn't pure oxygen, but 21 percent oxygen is still very rich—50 times more available oxygen than fish get by pumping water through their gills. Inert nitrogen makes up 78 percent of the atmosphere; the other 1 percent is carbon dioxide and other gases.

Every cell of our bodies requires a steady supply of oxygen delivered to it, each minute of our lives. Fortunately, unlike food and water, oxygen was dispersed democratically over the surface of the planet, available equally to all—at least those who live at the lower elevations.

Even on the highest mountains (over 29,000 feet or 8,840 metres), there's sufficient oxygen for life, though it's at the extreme margins for our bodies. Since most of us live at lower elevations, scarcity of oxygen was never a consideration in our body's design, so no "reservoir" of oxygen exists.

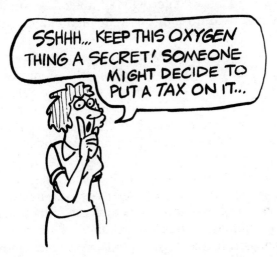

When at rest, we take in about a half-litre of air per breath, averaging 12 breaths per minute, which is 360 litres (about 95 gallons) per hour. During strenuous exertion, that intake can rise to 4.6 litres (1.0 gallon) per breath, 50 times per minute, which would be over 13,000 litres (3,435 gallons) per hour, if we could maintain it for that long.

Air that is breathed in through your nose gets warmed and moistened; **nitric oxide**—which is made in your sinuses—is mixed in with it. The nitric oxide helps control the dilation of the blood vessels of your lungs and heart.

The air passes down the bronchi of your lungs, which then fork 23 times into smaller branches before entering one of approximately 300 million small bubble-like cells called **alveoli**.

The large upper-respiratory tubes are covered with cells that secrete mucous. These cells also contain hair-like **cilia**, which whip the mucous upward and away from your lungs at about 900 beats per minute. This helps move any dust, bacteria, and viruses that might be coming in with each breath, out of your respiratory tract. When the mucous and debris are moved up to your throat, you unconsciously swallow it.

Surrounding your 300 million alveoli are many more millions of tiny blood vessels, called **capillaries**. The oxygen (O_2) molecules of the air entering your alveoli are under enough pressure to readily diffuse through the membranes into your capillaries.

Once in the capillaries, only about 3 percent of the O_2 is able to dissolve directly into your blood plasma. Along come your red blood cells to the rescue, squeezing their way along the narrow capillaries. Your red blood cells are the most abundant of your cells, numbering about 5 million per cubic millimetre of blood or 30,000 billion in total. They are your "packhorses" for oxygen.

Stem cells are your universal mother cells; they have the ability to produce clones of themselves or become **progenitor cells** that can go on to become virtually any other cell. Stem cells are most abundant in areas that have a high turnover-rate of cells, such as your skin, gut, and blood system. Stem cells in your bone marrow generate red blood cells as they are needed.

The stem cells in your bone marrow are relatively rare— one stem cell per every 100,000 marrow cells. When stimulated by various growth factors, stem cells can make numerous progenitor cells that can go through one of three pathways to become either a red blood cell, a white blood cell, or a platelet. Once a progenitor cell has started out on one of these cell pathways, it can't go back; its "career" choice has been made.

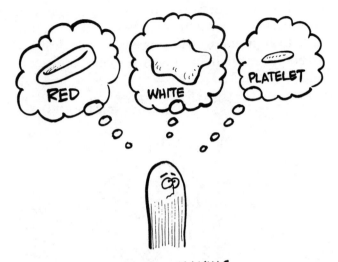

STEM CELL MAKING
A CAREER CHOICE...

A red blood cell is red because it carries iron in its
hemoglobin. While a red blood cell may be your packhorse
for oxygen, the hemoglobin—which covers three-quarters of
the red cell—is the pack. The hemoglobin pack is a four-seater,
capable of loading up four oxygen molecules at a time from the
capillaries of your lungs' alveoli.

This ability of hemoglobin to carry oxygen increases your
blood's oxygen-carrying capacity 70-fold. The now-loaded red
blood cell—its redness brightened by its load of oxygen—
scurries out of the lung capillary, and off to your heart.

The oxygenated red blood cell arrives in the **left atrium** of
your heart, which is the waiting room for the **left ventricle**
below it. The left ventricle is by far the strongest muscle of your
heart. As the red blood cells enter, the door to the waiting room
is quickly closed.

Your massive left ventricle contracts strongly, swooshing
your blood out through your **aorta** to the far-reaches of your
body, where all your busy cells await its prompt arrival. Your
hard-working heart has its **coronary arteries** tapped into the
beginning of the aorta so that it gets first pick of this fresh batch
of precious oxygen.

The second and third branches from your aorta are your two **carotid arteries**, which carry the oxygenated blood up the sides of your neck to your brain—which needs oxygen desperately. Your heart and your brain are your two biggest users of oxygen.

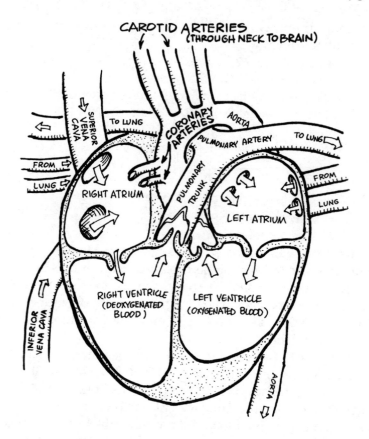

The many other branches from your aorta carry blood to every nook and cranny of your body, where small capillaries squeeze the red blood cells, causing the oxygen to dismount from the hemoglobin and pass through the membranes to your needy cells.

Hemoglobin then picks up carbon dioxide (CO_2) wastes from the cells. Your red blood cells scamper off to the right side of the heart and then to your lungs, to dump their load of CO_2 and repeat the cycle.

The basic tenet of human physiology (the study of human body function) is homeostasis—that your body is a self-correcting mechanism, able to provide and maintain a constant state of ideal conditions for your cells to function at their optimum level. Here is how homeostasis works.

- Your digestive system provides nutrients and eliminates waste.
- Your lungs and circulation system provide oxygen and remove carbon dioxide waste.
- Your kidneys control ion levels and remove waste.
- Your liver cells neutralize toxins entering the body through the digestive system.
- Your immune system destroys invaders and repairs damage, etc.

The proof of this inherent ability of our bodies to heal themselves is obvious by the fact that we are alive, and will probably be alive for a lot longer.

There must also, however, be some basic flaws in homeostasis or there wouldn't be any gastroenterologists, respirologists, nephrologists, or immunologists—not to mention pathologists; proctologists; dermatologists; urologists; gynecologists; rheumatologists; pediatricians; podiatrists; obstetricians; opthamologists; optometrists; orthopedists; osteopaths; psychiatrists; psychologists; registered nurses; practical nurses; psychic healers; physiotherapists; music therapists; art therapists; speech therapists; massage therapists; dentists; dental surgeons; denturists; nutritionists; dieticians; naturopaths; nutripaths; naprapaths; homeopaths; reflexologists; acupuncturists; shamans; touch healers; laser surgeons; plastic surgeons; cosmetic surgeons; psychic surgeons; herbalists; allergists; or all the lay people that sell the latest multi-level marketing health products to their relatives and friends.

For systems designed to be self-healing through homeostasis, our bodies seem to have become very high-maintenance items, often still failing to regain equilibrium, even with the most professional care.

Our advanced design was conceived in an atmosphere so rich in oxygen that survival is totally dependent on using 90 percent of our oxygen intake to convert food into energy.

Let's first take a look at what happens to some of the other 10 percent of the oxygen that you take in.

INJURY OR INFECTION = INFLAMMATION

The two foremost enemies of your homeostasis are injury and infection. The skeletons of Neanderthals, tens of thousands of years old, indicate that it was common for them to have broken and healed bones, many times in their lives. Since they took on large animals—with short, stubby spears, in virtual hand-to-hoof combat—it would be expected that they would receive some injuries.

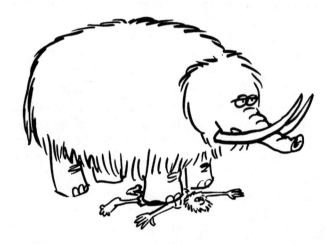

While we weren't as tough as the Neanderthals, we outlasted them because we were smart enough to stand back a bit and *throw* our spears at the animals.

A skeleton found recently along the Columbia River, and carbon-dated to be 9,300 years old, had a spear-tip embedded in the pelvic bone, yet this was an old injury that had healed long before death. Tuberculosis damage has been found in a skeleton 7,000 years old, as well as in some of the Egyptian Pharaohs.

Your immune system treats all injury—whether from bacteria, trauma, burns, or cold—as an invasion attempt. Your immune system's reaction is the same to both injury and infection; it will immediately "wall off" the damaged or infected area by surrounding it with inflammation. Your blood vessels around the site dilate, allowing more fluid to flow into the area.

At the same time, the small capillaries around the site become more permeable, allowing **fibrinogen** and **platelets** to pour out of your blood into your tissue fluid, where fibrinogen reacts with **thrombin** to form sticky **fibrin** threads. These fibrin threads stick to your blood vessels, and then run in all directions, like a spider's web, trapping blood cells, platelets, and plasma in their ever-strengthening mesh. This forms a **clot**, which stops blood from pouring out of your broken blood vessels, and blocks bacteria from entering the body through any wounds.

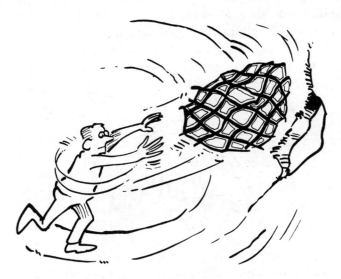

"THE CLOTMASTER"

The swelling that occurs around this wall contributes to its effectiveness, but it also causes much of the pain associated with inflammation or swelling.

As the fibrin wall goes up around the war zone, your immune system's front-line troops, the **macrophages**, slip through the wall into the threatened zone, in search of invaders. Your macrophages are the Sergeants of your white blood cell army. Big, tough, and experienced, they're the first on the scene of an injury or invasion, and quickly take charge.

As it gobbles down a potential invader, a macrophage will show a fragment of it to naïve young **B** and **T lymphocytes**, who will soon join the battle with weapons designed to specifically attack this invader.

If the macrophage needs immediate help, it sends out the messengers, especially **tumour necrosis factor** (**TNF**)—to bring more macrophages rushing to the rescue. Within hours, millions of **neutrophils** can be on the site.

Neutrophils are mini-versions of macrophages—not as big or as tough, but far more numerous. They are able to take oxygen from the surrounding fluids, and convert it into deadly **superoxide radicals** to blast apart the membranes of invaders. These determined white blood cells are protected from the destructive effects of their own deadly bursts of oxygen-powered weaponry by a shield of sulfur, called **glutathione**, which you know well by now.

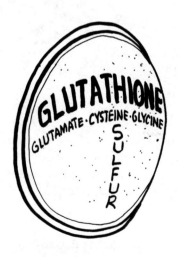

GLUTATHIONE SHIELD

As the invaders are ripped asunder by oxygen free radicals, both macrophages and neutrophils gobble down the remnants.

The B and T lymphocyte immune cells have fully matured and are ready for war. The B cells, now called plasma cells, are making millions of "harpoons" called **antibodies**, with their heads designed to lock onto the specific invader shown to them by the macrophage.

As the antibodies stick into the enemies, they become bound together into clumps called **immune complexes**. The protruding tails of the antibodies become "hot," activating a group of 20 proteins in the blood called the **complement system**. These activated complement proteins:
- help the inflammation response;
- rupture bacterial membranes;
- deactivate viruses; and
- attract more macrophages and neutrophils.

Helper T cells—T_H1 and T_H2—secrete **interferons** and **interleukins** that stimulate and coordinate all the other white blood cell troops. T_H1 cells administer the *coupe de grâce* to the invaders, with their secretion of **gamma interferon**.

Gamma interferon finishes the job in two ways.
1. It activates your **cytotoxic killer T** cells to deliver their lethal one-two punch: they secrete **perforin**, which punches gaping holes in the invaders' membranes, through which the cytotoxic T cell then pours **granzymes** that react inside the invader, to blow it to smithereens.
2. It activates your macrophages to secrete strong enzymes to digest the invaders they've swallowed. **Lysozyme** digests the invaders' fatty membranes, and **proteolytic enzymes** shatter the invaders' proteins. If that doesn't finish the job, the macrophage will produce **superoxides, nitric oxide, hydrogen peroxide**, and even **hypochlorite** to digest the invaders.

So you can see that T_H1 cells' secretion of gamma interferon is crucial to resolving immune conflicts.

If there is damage done to your bone, **osteoclast cells** gobble up the faulty bone tissue so **osteoblasts** can replace it with new bone. Your macrophages secrete **fibroblast growth factor**, which stimulates your **fibroblast cells** along the edge of the injury, to add oxygen to the amino acids proline and lysine, to create **collagen**. Collagen lays the connective scaffolding for new capillaries to be built, which then bring more red blood cells, and that means more oxygen.

Increased oxygen supplies your white blood cells with more ammunition to slay invaders.

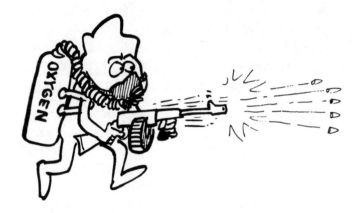

Increased oxygen further stimulates your fibroblasts, osteoclasts, and osteoblasts to work harder at repair; it also causes your dilated blood vessels to constrict, thus reducing the swelling and pain, as inflammation gives way to healing. This is a perfect example of how homeostasis works in correcting injury or infection.

It should be very, very clear that **the amount of oxygen in your tissue plays a key role in its healing ability**. Some tissues—such as ligaments, tendons, cartilage, and intervertebral discs—normally have low oxygen flow, and therefore a reduced healing ability. It doesn't mean they can't heal; it just means they heal more slowly than tissue with higher oxygen flow.

One of the great obstacles to the healing of injury or infection is when the inflammatory wall is erected so intensely that your red blood cells are unable to penetrate it with their life-giving load of oxygen.

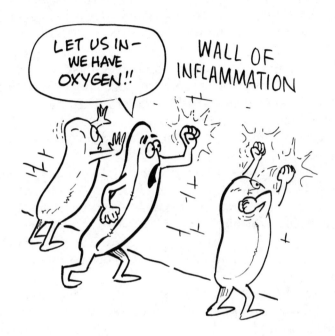

Without oxygen ammunition, your immune cells are unable to attack bacteria successfully. The blood vessels stay dilated, which allows the swelling and pain associated with it to go on, unabated.

Without oxygen, your fibroblasts are unable to produce collagen, and your osteoclasts and osteoblasts are unable to produce new bone.

The inflammatory process—designed as a short-term first step to healing—becomes stuck, and eventually becomes a chronic, lingering disease. Your immune system's response gets snuffed out by its own exuberance.

MILLIONAIRES HAVE FOUND THEIR ANSWER

Let's use a fictional story to illustrate the importance of oxygen in the healing process.

Bart Barnum owns a professional sports team, the Springfield Springs, which plays in the NPL (National Pogo League). He has just brought in the star player from Pogoland, where the sport obviously originated. In fact, Pogo is not only the national sport of Pogoland, it is the *only* sport played there.

Peter Pongo, whose father once led Pogoland to three consecutive World Championships, is considered by many to be the top Pogo player in the world; he has landed himself a guaranteed $5 million contract for the five-month season in Springfield.

At his very first preseason practice, he falls off his pogo stick in a freak accident, lacerating his lower leg, severely spraining his right ankle, and fracturing his tibia. The team doctor says that Peter will be unable to practise Pogo for at least three months, *if* the healing goes well—and even then, there will be a further period of conditioning before he will be able to play full-time.

If the fracture doesn't heal well, he'll be out for at least the season. If the ever-present **staphylococci** bacteria were to get through the wound into the bone, they could create a serious infection called **osteomyelitis**, which antibiotics don't always reverse. That could be a career-ending situation.

It looks like Bart Barnum is going to be out most, if not all, of his $5 million annual investment in his would-be star. Then he has a long talk with his brother-in-law, the renowned LA plastic surgeon, Dr. Morty Lipshitz, Facelifter of the Stars. Morty knows his celebrities don't want to be seen around town in between faces so, immediately after surgery, he puts them into a hyperbaric oxygen chamber to speed their healing.

By using **hyperbaric oxygen therapy** after his nips and tucks, Morty has seen a rapid decrease in swelling and bruising, a healing time shortened by 65 percent, and a dramatic decrease in scarring. Even his skin grafts are "taking" much better. When he uses hyperbaric oxygen treatments before grafting, the failure rate drops from 10 percent to 4.5 percent.

Most important, he's seen virtually no infections. The curse of the surgeon has always been that cutting through the skin has allowed **staphylococci** and **streptococci** bacteria to penetrate the body, where they could spread. Staphylococci (or staph, for short) are rude and crude, secreting extremely toxic compounds that give fair warning to the body to erect an especially strong wall of inflammation around them.

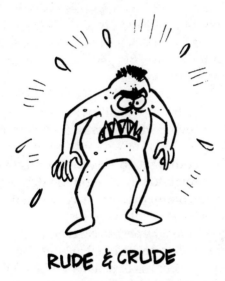

RUDE & CRUDE

Staph's development of antibiotic resistance—and the body's strong walling-off reaction to it—has made staph bacteria tough to treat when they get firmly established inside the body.

Like staphylococci, streptococci (or strep, for short) are common, but their toxins aren't as strong as staph's, and therefore don't stimulate such a rapid walling-off by your immune system. This actually works to their advantage, giving strep more opportunity to spread widely before the inflammation wall is fully established.

Streptococci bacteria used to be less of a concern, because they hadn't yet developed major antibiotic resistance. Recently, however, one form of strep picked up some new genes from a virus. This enabled them to eat through flesh at the rate of

2.5 cm (one inch) an hour. Because the antibiotics usually take 48 hours to start working, this could be tragic to the patient, as well as the career of the cosmetic surgeon.

Dr. Lipshitz tells Bart Barnum that after the hyperbaric oxygen treatments, it seems like the skin has been disinfected. Staph and strep infections have virtually disappeared. While hyperbaric oxygen therapy has even been used with antibiotics to help cure flesh-eating disease and osteomyelitis, Morty finds that using the oxygen treatments routinely before and/or after surgery prevents the development of these diseases in his patients. "An ounce of prevention is worth a pound of cure," he says, chuckling as he quotes his hero, Benjamin Franklin.

And the cost of hyperbaric oxygen therapy is insignificant compared to what these people are willing to pay for their surgery.

Even the skin of his burn patients, whether injured from fire or radiation, heals much faster and with far fewer infections.

Bart Barnum has nothing to lose by trying this treatment on his fallen star. He's going to be out a million dollars each month that his star is out of commission anyway, so what's a few thousand dollars to try and cut his losses!

Peter Pongo goes into a hyperbaric oxygen chamber that is then sealed; air is slowly pumped in. He holds his nose and blows occasionally to clear his Eustachian tubes, so that his inner ears stay balanced with the increased air pressure in the chamber.

This is the same procedure you can use on takeoff in an airplane, but for the opposite reasons. The upper atmosphere has less pressure, so you need to regulate the inner ear to the decrease in pressure. Increasing the pressure in the oxygen chamber is like going underwater, where the weight of the water is added to the weight of the atmosphere—the inner ear must adjust to it.

At 100 metres (33 feet) beneath the ocean surface, the pressure of the water is equivalent to the weight of the entire atmosphere, so you would be exposed to a pressure of 2 atmospheres—1 atmosphere of pressure from the water pushing down on you, plus 1 atmosphere from the air pushing down upon the water.

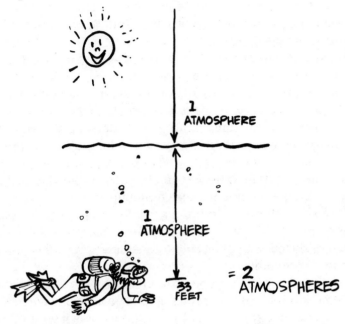

For an hour, Peter breathes 100 percent oxygen through a special oxygen hood. After an hour, the oxygen breathing is discontinued and the chamber pressure is lowered back to the normal pressure of 1 atmosphere; then he leaves the chamber. This procedure is repeated for a number of days in a row.

Within a few treatments, Peter has a reduction in swelling—and therefore less pain—followed by an improvement in healing of both the sprain and the fracture. There are no signs of infection at any time.

Peter is able to resume training a month ahead of schedule, and makes it back in time to lead the Springfield Springs to their first-ever NPL Championship.

Bart Barnum saves a million dollars or more by getting his star back early, and stands to make even *more* millions by having his team win. Bart Barnum thinks hyperbaric oxygen therapy is a good investment, as does Dr. Lipshitz. Their wealthy clients would surely agree.

While the preceding story is fictional, the benefits of hyperbaric oxygen therapy are not. Of the hundreds of hyperbaric chambers in operation in North America, most are operated by research institutions or hospitals; they are not available for private use.

The hyperbaric chambers in US hospitals are used only for the treatment of the 14 conditions covered by Medicare insurance. Most treatments are for severe life-threatening events, such as carbon monoxide poisoning, where hyperbaric oxygen therapy is the only treatment available. Or, treatment in hyperbaric oxygen chambers is used as a last-resort therapy, after the failure of other hospital treatments.

For example, hyperbaric oxygen therapy is only covered by insurance in the treatment of osteomyelitis if it is **refractory**, which means after the condition has failed to respond to a long series of antibiotics. Prevention of disease or treatment of disease in the early stages is not a consideration by the insurance companies.

The privately owned hyperbaric chambers are used primarily by cosmetic surgeons and professional sports teams, where cost is not considered an important factor. So what is it about this treatment that has the wealthy sport and entertainment stars using it?

We already know that oxygen is the key to successful healing—so why not just breathe oxygen through a mask, without the cost and hassle of an expensive hyperbaric chamber? The reason is that the hemoglobin of your red blood cells is usually already carrying its maximum amount of oxygen, so breathing in extra oxygen isn't going to deliver very much more oxygen to your cells. Also, if the wall of inflammation is preventing your red blood cells from getting to the site of injury, the oxygen isn't likely to get where it's needed anyway.

With divers going deep under the water, it was found that as they breathed air under pressure, even the normally inert nitrogen gas would dissolve into their blood. And at great depths—over 30 metres (100 feet)—this would have an effect on their brains that is similar to the effect of alcohol. This is called **"nitrogen narcosis."**

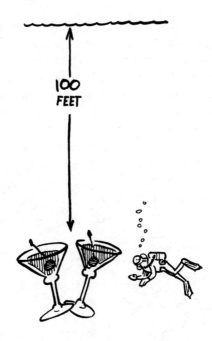

If a diver comes up from the depths too rapidly, the dissolved nitrogen in his or her tissues will expand with the reduced pressure of shallower water, creating gas bubbles that could jam up in the nervous system, lungs, or joints—causing the diver to experience **"hits," "chokes,"** or **"the bends."**

Hyperbaric chambers were first developed to put these divers back under pressure. This shrinks the size of the nitrogen bubbles, enabling them to successfully pass by the joints, thus relieving the symptoms of "the bends." The pressure is then slowly decreased, at a speed that allows the lungs to eliminate the nitrogen gas.

It was later discovered that breathing oxygen while in the pressurized chamber further helped the elimination of nitrogen-bubble symptoms. The reason was that **the oxygen breathed under pressure also dissolved into the blood more readily—and even though the hemoglobin of the red blood cells was already saturated with oxygen, the blood plasma itself**

became a carrier of oxygen, which helped to displace the nitrogen.

In the case of injury or infection, the extra oxygen supplied by hyperbaric oxygen therapy eliminated the difficulty in delivering precious oxygen through the wall of inflammation. **The blood plasma carried the dissolved oxygen to the wall, where it literally "seeped" through into the war zone.**

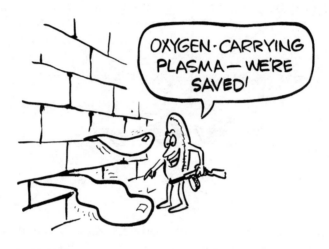

- This fresh supply of oxygen ammunition allowed macrophages and neutrophils to step up their assault on bacterial invaders.
- Then oxygen-powered cells like the osteoclasts could break down old bone faster—while the osteoblasts made new bone more quickly.
- The fibroblasts could make more collagen, faster, which allowed the formation of new capillaries to bring in more oxygen-carrying red blood cells.
- The increase of oxygen constricted the blood vessels so that swelling and pain quickly faded away. In fact, it was found that migraine-headache sufferers experienced almost immediate disappearance of their stubborn headache problems when breathing oxygen under pressure.

You can see that oxygen is crucial to your ability to heal injuries and fight off bacterial infections. Hyperbaric oxygen therapy can dramatically aid in all of this.

OXYGEN AND THE HEART

Let's take a look at an organ to which oxygen is crucial—your heart. Your heart is a strong, tough, hard-working muscle that can run for more years than you could imagine, as long as it gets one important nutrient—you guessed it—oxygen.

Oxygen is supplied to your heart through the small coronary arteries that branch off the aorta. Temporary blockage of these small arteries is usually due to narrowing of the arteries by **atherosclerotic plaque**. Combined with acute stress, this blockage can create a reduced flow of blood—and therefore a reduced supply of oxygen—into the heart, causing a squeezing pain in the left chest, difficulty breathing, and an inability to exert oneself. Commonly called **angina**, this may pass with relaxation.

If a clot were to be released from the artery plaque and clog the coronary arteries, the lack of oxygen into the heart would seriously endanger the heart, possibly destroying vital heart cells. This type of damage to the heart is called an **infarct** or heart attack. In fact, in industrialized countries, about half the deaths that occur each year are due to cardiovascular disease.

If a person survives a heart attack, the medical treatment would be a clot-dissolver called **tissue plasminogen activator** (**TPA**). A study done by Ellestad at the Memorial Heart Institute in Long Beach, California, found the following.
- In 22 heart attack patients treated with TPA, relief of chest pain was felt after 671 minutes, on average; it took 374 minutes for their **electrocardiogram** (**ECG**) to normalize.
- Another 24 patients who received TPA, *plus two hours of hyperbaric oxygen therapy,* experienced relief of chest pain after 271 minutes; their ECGs stabilized after 188 minutes.

So the recovery time after an acute heart attack was shortened by over 50 percent, with the addition of hyperbaric oxygen therapy. The hyperbaric treatment also lowered the blood levels of the enzyme creatine phosphokinase, indicating that the damage to the heart was greatly decreased.

While North Americans may be unfamiliar with these results, hundreds of studies have been done in Russia on hyperbaric oxygen therapy over many years. Here are some of their findings.

- Cardiac pain and difficulty with breathing disappeared with hyperbaric oxygen therapy (HBOT).
- Dmitrieva showed that HBOT had a strong defibrillating effect on the heart.
- Rugenyus showed that the entire heart-conduction system benefitted from HBOT.
- Kolomeitseva and Kulkybaev showed that heart patients treated with HBOT could take on more physical work.

These studies show conclusively that the heart—which normally has such a huge requirement for oxygen—can benefit from additional oxygen, when in distress.

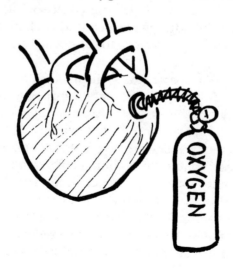

Oxygen is often administered to heart attack patients via an oxygen mask, but a much greater absorption of oxygen actually takes place when oxygen is administered in a hyperbaric chamber.

OXYGEN AND THE BRAIN

Some cells have an even greater need for oxygen than your heart does. Those cells are nerve cells.

Approximately 90 percent of the oxygen entering your body is used to produce energy in the form of **adenosine triphosphate (ATP)**—a type of "super high octane" phosphorus fuel. Without using oxygen, an anaerobic bacteria, yeast, or cancer cell can ferment 1 glucose sugar molecule into 2 ATP, which is 3 percent of the potential energy available.

Our cells can use our new, fandangled, modern, hi-tech, latest-model "turbo-charged" oxygen system to generate 38 ATP from 1 glucose molecule, which is 66 percent of the energy available. This means that we are 22 times more efficient at creating ATP than are bacteria, yeast, or cancer cells.

Still, compared to many of the other species on this planet, we are rather bland and inconspicuous. We weren't born with the colourful beauty of the butterfly or the ability to change our skin colour like the chameleon, so we invented fashion. We couldn't make music like the cricket or the birds, so we invented whistles, flutes, and other instruments, then improved them and combined them to form the symphony orchestra.

We weren't born with the power and weaponry of the lion, so we invented knives, spears, and swords, and eventually atomic bombs that could destroy all life on the planet—at least on its surface. We couldn't run as fast as the cheetah, so we invented bicycles and cars and eventually trains that can travel over the surface of the earth at hundreds of kilometres per hour.

We couldn't fly like the birds, so we invented kites and balloons, then airplanes, and eventually rockets that could travel to the moon and back. We couldn't hover like a bee, so we built helicopters. We saw beavers building dams, so we built Grand Coulee.

We couldn't dive under water like the whale, so we created the nuclear submarine, which can circle the globe without surfacing. We couldn't see in the dark like the bat, so we devised radar. We couldn't see long distances like the eagle, so we invented the telescope, and improved it until now we can see planets spinning around other suns, and galaxies unfolding at distances that stagger our comprehension.

To make up for the fact that we don't have the abilities with which other species are blessed, we use our abilities of observation, analysis, and creativity—all of which take place in our brains. Your brain is only 2 percent of your body weight, yet it draws 15 percent of the blood pumped into your aorta by the left ventricle of your heart.

The carotid arteries in your neck deliver 1 litre (about 4 cups) of blood per minute to your brain, carrying 25 percent of your body's oxygen intake to your 12 billion brain cells, called neurons (nerve cells). So your brain—small as it may be physically—uses a giant's share of the oxygen you breathe in, because of its tremendous activity. **I think, therefore I need oxygen!!!**

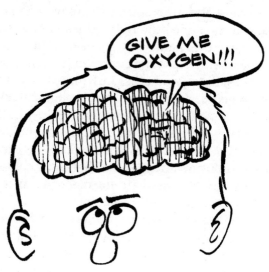

This tremendous activity of our brains gives us the ability to excel in so many areas where we are not inherently gifted. But if the brain's oxygen supply is interrupted, we can become fragile and vulnerable.

If your muscles were to run out of oxygen, they can switch back to the old-fashioned anaerobic metabolism to burn glucose to provide ATP energy—not an efficient system, but it could keep your muscles functioning for a short time. **Your nerve cells don't have the ability to make ATP without oxygen, AND nerve cells use over seven times more oxygen than your muscles do.**

Because your brain is totally dependent on oxygen, if your oxygen levels fall, that can create immediate symptoms. Even a slight reduction in oxygen—from 21 percent found in normal air, down to 18 percent—can cause disorientation and impaired judgment. If oxygen is reduced to 14 percent, that can cause mental failure and fainting.

Complete blockage of oxygen to the brain will result in nerve cell disruption within six seconds, cause brain activity to cease in two minutes, and result in the death of brain cells within five minutes.

There are exceptions. A person who "drowns" in very cold water and is revived ten minutes later, or even longer, may make a complete recovery. One reason for this is that **cold fluid retains more dissolved oxygen than warm fluid.** Someone who drowns in very cold water could retain oxygen in his or her brain long enough to prevent cell death far beyond five minutes. Even if all signs of life are gone, if re-warming of the body brings back the spark of life, the person could very well revive with little or no brain damage.

Another thing that causes fluid to retain more dissolved oxygen is pressure, which is why hyperbaric oxygen therapy has shown some dramatic positive results in people with brain or spinal cord damage.

Loss of oxygen supply to the brain can happen in many ways—including choking, carbon monoxide poisoning, cyanide poisoning, drowning, lightning strike, or cardiac arrest, to name

a few. The birth process can also result in reduced oxygen
supply to the brain of a baby.

During pregnancy, the mother delivers oxygen directly to
the fetus from her placenta, via the umbilical cord. Birth itself
involves the sudden shift away from the mother's oxygen
supply to the newborn's lungs and heart, delivering the oxygen
to the brain.

Early detachment of the placenta, wrapping of the cord
around the baby's neck, strong uterine contractions, or delayed
functioning of the newborn's lungs or heart can all lead to
deficient oxygen delivery to the baby's brain. These
interruptions in oxygen supply, as well as infection and
premature birthing, can contribute to the brain damage
called **cerebral palsy**.

In the middle of the hemispheres of the brain, neurons send
fibres down through the **internal capsules** to the spinal cord,
where they inhibit the spinal cord nerves that activate the
muscles of the arms and legs. The internal capsules normally
have poor blood supply; any further decrease in oxygen causes
them to leak fluid, which pinches-off the oxygen supply to the
myelin sheath.

The myelin sheath coats the nerves like insulation coats an
electrical wire. It begins development before birth, and finishes
by two years of age. Blocking the flow of oxygen to the myelin
sheath before, during, and after birth—by the swelling of the
internal capsules, due to low brain-oxygen levels—results in
atrophy of the myelin, and eventually leaves the nerves
exposed and nonfunctional.

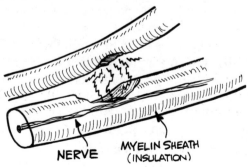

NERVE   MYELIN SHEATH
         (INSULATION)

If the brain's nerves are unable to inhibit the spinal nerves to the arms and legs, symptoms of uncontrolled contraction called spasticity occur in those affected limbs. This is seen in cerebral palsy and other brain injuries, including juvenile multiple sclerosis.

It may take several months to two years after birth for the myelin to disappear, so spastic paralysis, writhing movements, and problems with balance and coordination may not appear immediately. Because the nerves to the legs are closest to the area of poorest blood supply, the legs are most likely to be affected by the swelling of the internal capsules. These physical symptoms may be accompanied by symptoms of mental handicap.

While the condition doesn't worsen with age, there has been nothing to improve the symptoms of cerebral palsy—until the use of hyperbaric oxygen therapy. Hyperbaric oxygen therapy has been shown to increase oxygen supply by constricting blood vessels and thereby reducing swelling. This, in turn, reduces spasticity.

In the late 1980s in Sao Paulo, Brazil, Machaldo treated 230 cerebral palsy patients with 20 one-hour hyperbaric oxygen therapy treatments. In 218 patients, there was clear reduction of spasticity. The 12 patients who had no improvement were the ones with the most severe cerebral symptoms from the beginning.

Six months after completion of HBOT treatments, a follow-up was done on 82 of the patients; 75 percent reported continued improvement of intelligence, fewer convulsions, and less bronchitis.

From 1992 to1999, the Baromedical Research Institute of New Orleans treated 18 children who had cerebral palsy with 40 hyperbaric oxygen treatments. Only two showed *no improvement*, while the other 16 showed improvements in one or more of seven functions: awareness, tone, fine and gross motor skills, communication, balance/gait, overall cognition, and swallowing.

Barrett, at the University of Texas in Galveston, did a study with four children with cerebral palsy, using HBOT at 1.5 atmospheres, one hour per day, five days per week. He saw improvements in motor skills, modest decreases in spasticity, and improvement in the vision of one child who had been diagnosed with cortical blindness.

A pilot study was done at McGill University, Montreal, on 25 children with cerebral palsy, with a mean age of 5.6 years. The study showed that two weeks after 20 HBOTs at 1.75 atmospheres, for one hour, there was significant improvement in card-turning, lifting and stacking objects, and walking and sitting. There were also reduced tendon reflexes and reduced spasticity.

Other brain syndromes that have shown improvement with HBOT are **Rett Syndrome** and **childhood epilepsy**. At the 11th International Congress on Hyperbaric Medicine, a study was presented in which HBOTs were done for 100 children with childhood epilepsy, in Zhujiang, China. Their ages were mainly from one month to nine years; the treatments were 80 minutes at 1.7 to 2 atmospheres, for up to 30 treatments.

- No improvement was seen in 14 of the 100 children, while the rest showed some improvement, and 68 had major improvements in intelligence, personality, and mental function.
- Of the 92 that had abnormal electroencephalograms (EEGs), 45 achieved normal EEGs after treatment.

OXYGEN AND STROKE

Let's take a look at the improvement seen in using hyperbaric oxygen therapy for stroke victims, which may give some insight into how HBOT works in these cases. A stroke is a stoppage of blood flow—usually because of a clot that has been released from atherosclerotic plaque—to a part of the brain that then suffers damage due to the lack of oxygen.

About one-third of stroke victims die from this damage. Of the two-thirds who do survive, about half are confined to nursing homes. Those who survive the stroke are left with damage to their brain cells, called—as in heart damage—an **infarct**. In a sense, a stroke is a brain attack, identical to a heart attack, except that nerve cells are affected, rather than heart cells.

While a heart attack may be preceded by angina, a stroke may be preceded by **transient ischemal attacks (TIAs)** in one-third of people who go on to have a full-blown stroke.

Like angina, TIAs are short-lived blockages of blood flow that usually pass within a few minutes to hours. If no damage is done, symptoms—such as lapses in concentration, memory, and awareness—quickly pass. If damage occurs to the brain, then it is called a stroke.

The wall of inflammation goes up immediately around the area of infarct, to stop fluid leakage from the dying area and prevent bacterial penetration. The swelling that ensues around the injured brain cells can have a profound impact here because the skull will confine the expansion, putting more pressure on the brain's blood vessels—further reducing blood flow and therefore reducing oxygen to the area within the wall of inflammation.

When the brain cells surrounding the damaged area have their blood supply decreased by 85 percent, they stop generating electrical currents in an attempt to conserve energy. These nonfunctioning or "idling" brain cells surrounding the damaged area are called the **penumbra zone.**

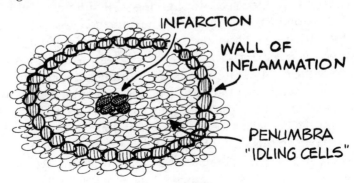

INFARCTION

WALL OF INFLAMMATION

PENUMBRA "IDLING CELLS"

The time when medical intervention can give the greatest help to reduce further damage is during the first three hours of a stroke. About half of stroke victims show some improvement in six hours. Improvement within 48 hours is a good sign for long-term outcome, although 95 percent of stroke victims retain some degree of long-term complication. Symptoms of neurological damage show on the opposite side of the body to the brain damage, due to nerve crossover.

What has been seen with hyperbaric oxygen therapy in rehabilitation of stroke victims is that **all** showed a response with daily treatments at 1.5 atmospheres of pressure.

After six weeks of treatment, most retained the gains they had made. The most noticeable improvement was that of lessened spasticity, allowing physiotherapy to be much more effective. In fact, **those individuals treated within three months of their stroke never developed spasticity**.

Some patients, whose strokes had occurred ten or more years before hyperbaric oxygen treatment, still showed significant improvement. The use of hyperbaric oxygen therapy in stroke rehabilitation has allowed virtually all patients using it to return home.

The proposed mechanism for the improvement in stroke recovery is similar to that of other injuries—with one important addition. As we learned earlier, breathing oxygen under pressure allows your blood to carry far more oxygen, by allowing it to dissolve directly into your blood plasma. This extra oxygen can then seep through the wall of inflammation that your body has erected around the damaged area.

In the situation of brain and spinal cord injuries, there is an added benefit to hyperbaric oxygen therapy. Almost ten percent of the cavity that contains your brain and spinal cord is occupied by **cerebrospinal fluid**. The cerebrospinal fluid flows around and into your brain, draining away wastes, the way your lymphatic system does in the rest of your body. Your brain literally floats in this cushion of protective fluid.

Hyperbaric oxygen therapy not only allows extra oxygen to dissolve into your bloodstream, *it allows even your cerebrospinal fluid to become an oxygen carrier.* In brain or spinal cord injuries, this can be crucial to recovery.

As the dissolved oxygen from the blood and cerebrospinal fluid seeps through the wall of inflammation into the damaged zone, your macrophages and fibroblasts can go to work repairing the damage. The oxygen constricts the dilated blood vessels, thus reducing the swelling, which then allows red blood cells to bring in even more oxygen. With the return of normal oxygen supplies, the area of penumbra around the infarct may regain its function.

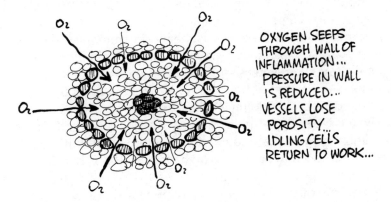

OXYGEN SEEPS THROUGH WALL OF INFLAMMATION... PRESSURE IN WALL IS REDUCED... VESSELS LOSE POROSITY... IDLING CELLS RETURN TO WORK...

The return of the penumbra cells to active generation of nerve impulses is believed to be behind most of the improvement seen with hyperbaric oxygen therapy in stroke rehabilitation. If the improvement is strong enough, and the area of infarct small enough, the **newly rejuvenated penumbra cells may even be able to do some of the jobs of the destroyed cells.** Physiotherapy is believed to enhance this ability.

One part of your body needs even more oxygen than your brain, and that is your eye. The **retina** in the back of your eye works like a television screen, taking signals from the lens of your eye and displaying them as upside-down pictures in miniature, on a bed of **photoreceptors.**

The retina then sends these two-dimensional signals to the cortical area of your brain, where they are converted to three-dimensional upright images. Vision is hard work for your photoreceptors—making them the greatest user of oxygen in your body.

It is believed that low oxygen levels contribute to **retinitis pigmentosa** and **macular degeneration**. An HBOT study done in Yugoslavia, using 2 atmospheres pressure, 90 minutes daily for 30 sessions, showed visual improvement in three out of four cases.

Another study done with patients with visual disturbances from **glaucoma** showed improvement in vision after 20 treatments, without any lowering of the eye pressure. It's likely that the extra oxygen from HBOT was working on the part of the brain that is damaged in glaucoma.

Myopia (short-sightedness) is the most common side-effect of hyperbaric oxygen therapy, seen particularly in older patients. Myopia reverses spontaneously, however, several months after the end of treatment; it's recommended that treatments be limited to fewer than 75.

The increased exposure to oxygen can also contribute to the formation of cataracts by depletion of antioxidants, although this is rarely seen in patients who have had fewer than 200 treatments.

The whole topic of oxygen toxicity in HBOT has been thoroughly evaluated. Oxygen toxicity can be avoided by limiting the length of exposure and the amount of pressure used, by avoiding coffee, alcohol, and narcotics, and by taking antioxidant supplements.

Breathing oxygen under pressure has been shown to increase the absorption of oxygen 14-fold, which can help dramatically in a number of chronic infections and degenerative diseases. For example, Kjeldsen showed, in 1969, that **decreasing oxygen increased atherosclerosis** in rabbits—while **increasing oxygen with hyperbaric oxygen therapy (HBOT) reversed atherosclerosis**. Okamoto repeated these results in 1983.

Russian studies have shown the following.

- Borukhov found that of 220 patients with **high cholesterol, all those treated with HBOT showed lower levels of cholesterol, and all ECGs in the 220 patients normalized.**

- Zhumanov showed that **liver function and fat metabolism improved through HBOT**.

OXYGEN AND THE IMMUNE SYSTEM

I pointed out earlier that antibiotics have had a rather short-lived period of glory. They have now been shown to devastate our normal intestinal flora—leaving us with overgrowths of Candida yeast and *Clostridium difficile*, as well as gradually creating a wide range of antibiotic-resistant bacteria.

We have survived in this dangerous world of microbes because we are allied with bacterial buddies, but we are also armed to the teeth with a powerful immune system.

Your immune system consists of fierce and devoted microscopic characters, equipped with a withering range of weapons against which few bacteria, viruses, or fungi can survive. One of the keys to your immune system's proper functioning is oxygen. Can oxygen be used as an antibiotic? Let's take a look at history and research.

"As for the person with a leprous affection, his clothes shall be rent, his head shall be left bare, and he shall cover his upper lip; and he shall call out, 'Unclean! Unclean!' He shall be unclean as long as the disease is on him. Being unclean, he shall dwell apart, his dwelling shall be outside the camp."

Leviticus, 13:45

For thousands of years, millions of people have been afflicted with leprosy. They have been cast out to the edge of society, in poverty and shame, with only rags to cover the sight of their ears and noses rotting off their faces, as the insidious disease marches along its deadly course. The bone under the damaged skin is slowly destroyed, as well.

In another type of leprosy, lumps form around the nerves—particularly in the fingers and toes—so that the nerves can't signal when the digits are being burned or injured.

Roman soldiers returning to Italy from Egypt in the first century BC brought leprosy to Europe, where it became known as "the Living Death." Isolation was again the rule, though burning at the stake was also known to occur. Those stricken with leprosy would often wear frocks to cover their shame.

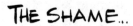

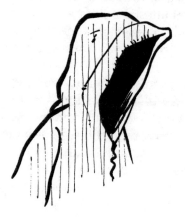

Spanish Conquistadors and African slaves brought leprosy to the Americas. In 1873, it was found that *Mycobacterium leprae*, a very close relative to *Mycobacterium tuberculosis*, was the bacteria responsible for both types of leprosy.

Most people's immune systems are capable of dealing with tuberculosis and leprosy mycobacteria, though this whole family has a trick up its sleeve. When gobbled up by your macrophages, these mycobacteria should be promptly digested by enzymes produced by the macrophages—but as I outlined earlier, the mycobacteria have the ability to block the enzymes from completing their digestion, leaving the mycobacteria free to live a comfortable life, protected from harm *inside* the macrophages.

One of the substances that macrophages secrete is **tumour necrosis factor**, the cause of much of the damage associated with leprosy, tuberculosis, atherosclerosis, and many other autoimmune diseases. This secretion of tumour necrosis factor results in severe destruction of the skin and bones in that area; this is called **lepromatous leprosy**.

It leads to deposits of granulomas around nerves, which causes the loss of nerve sensation and paralysis associated with **tuberculoid leprosy**. In both cases, it is the immune system response to the leprosy bacteria, rather than the bacteria itself, that causes the damage.

"One of the miraculous healings of a leper was by Jesus. A man with leprosy came to him and begged him on his knees, 'If you are willing, you can make me clean.' Filled with compassion, Jesus reached out his hand and touched the man. 'I am willing,' he said. 'Be clean!' Immediately the leprosy left him and he was cured. Jesus sent him away at once with a strong warning, 'See that you don't tell this to anyone. But go, show yourself to the priest and offer the sacrifices that Moses commanded for your cleansing, as a testimony to them.' Instead he went out and began to talk freely, spreading the news. As a result, Jesus could no longer enter a town openly, but stayed outside in lonely places."

Mark, 1:40-45

In Medieval Europe, if someone were accused of being a leper, he or she would be investigated by the community's leading citizens or priests and, if found to have the symptoms of leprosy, would be given one last chance at redemption. A funeral would be held. Holding a candle, the person would stand in the grave that had been dug for him or her. While the priest threw in three shovels of dirt, the accused would pray to Jesus to be healed. If the leprosy didn't disappear within seconds, the man or woman would be declared a leper.

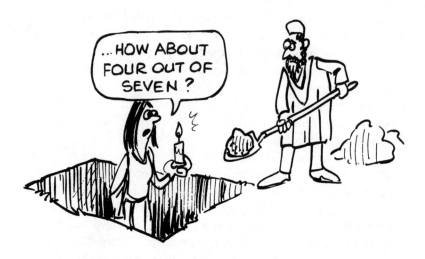

A leper would be cast out of the community to become one of the living dead—a beggar in the streets. No more attending church. No physical contact with other human beings. No drinking from public wells. This was the fate for hundreds of thousands of people over thousands of years.

In Brazil in 1938, Almeida and Costa treated nine leprosy sufferers with hyperbaric oxygen therapy for ten hours each, over three days. Six had a complete disappearance of the leprosy mycobacteria, and the rest showed marked improvement. Why didn't this dramatic breakthrough result in the world sweeping itself clean of this horrible plague?

In the 1940s, an antibiotic called Dapsone appeared that gave dramatic results against the leprosy bacteria. Soon, India alone was using 50 tons of Dapsone per year. The antibiotic had the side-effect of damaging the patients' red blood cells—but it was cheap, and became the primary treatment for leprosy world-wide.

By the 1980s, however, the leprosy bacteria, like the tuberculosis bacteria, was developing resistance to antibiotics. Dapsone was then combined with two other antibiotics, Rifampicin and Clofazimine, which are given for six to 24 months.

In the US in the 1970s, in a study done by Wilkinson, 45 leprosy patients were treated with four 30-minute hyperbaric oxygen therapy treatments. More than 50 percent showed major improvement, 40 percent moderate improvement, and the rest slight improvement.

In another study, by Rosasco, 200 people with leprosy discontinued their antibiotic therapy, which was replaced by two one-hour hyperbaric oxygen treatments per day, for three days. Ten patients were contacted five years later. None showed any recurrence of the disease.

A similar study was done by Mokashi in Bombay in 1979: 20 leprosy patients discontinued drug therapy. The patients were divided into two groups of ten: one group received no treatment and the other group received six one-hour hyperbaric oxygen treatments, over three days. Within eight months, those patients who had received hyperbaric treatments tested negative for leprosy, while the control group still had the disease.

These few studies indicate that the immune deficiencies that underlie the scourge of leprosy (and therefore probably tuberculosis) have been corrected with three days of treatment, using hyperbaric oxygen therapy. **Oxygen, nature's greatest gift to mankind, has subverted homeostasis' most primal adversary—a stubborn, chronic mycobacterial infection—without side-effects or development of resistant strains.**

Since it is believed that the leprosy bacteria is most likely picked up when the victim is a child—and leprosy takes two to ten years to develop—it's likely that these people will not acquire leprosy again. If they did, a few more days of hyperbaric oxygen therapy should get rid of it.

However, 500,000 new cases of leprosy are diagnosed each year—5,000 of them in North America. Most of these people will never receive antibiotic treatment, and it's unlikely that many of them will ever have hyperbaric oxygen therapy. It's still a treatment for the rich, though *soon* it may be affordable for the middle class—and in the future, some day, for the poor.

So, as you can see from the research, six leprosy patients were cured with hyperbaric oxygen therapy in 1938. More cases were successfully treated with oxygen in the 1970s—yet no crowds of lepers stormed the hyperbaric chambers begging for treatment. (Okay, so it took three days of treatment instead of three milliseconds, but beggars for miracles shouldn't be choosers.) Perhaps part of the reason is because people today have surrendered the treatment of their diseases to the medical profession, and few medical doctors are aware of the spectacular results that have been achieved using hyperbaric oxygen therapy.

Or, could it be that the medical profession, whose education is so strongly influenced by the pharmaceutical companies, has willingly turned a blind eye to something that could so effectively replace pharmaceuticals?

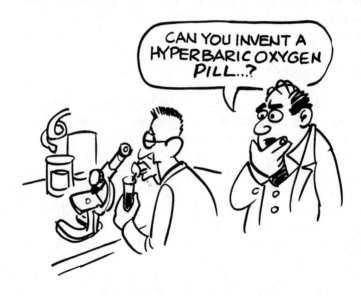

The next question is: will hyperbaric oxygen therapy be effective against leprosy's close cousin, tuberculosis, which is again rearing its ugly head as it acquires resistance to more and more antibiotics? An educated hunch says HBOT will be just as effective, but no trials have yet been done.

HBOT has been shown to aid in destroying the mycobacteria that triggers the delayed-type hypersensitivity reaction in leprosy—thus ending the tissue destruction associated with tumour necrosis factor. Will the same results occur when treating delayed-type hypersensitivity reactions triggered by fungal toxins, such as those of Candida yeast?

Certainly atherosclerosis-caused heart and brain problems—such as angina, heart attacks, and strokes—have been shown to benefit dramatically from the increased oxygen supplied by HBOT. Animal studies have shown that increased oxygen decreases atherosclerosis, although human studies outside of Russia have yet to be done.

The Russian studies have shown that the increased oxygen supplied by HBOT improved liver function, which in turn, improved fat metabolism. Some fungi such as *Rhizopus oryza*, *Schizosaccharomyces pombe*, and *Pneumocystis carnii* have been killed by HBOT; Candida yeast, however, is merely *inhibited* at the typical times and pressures used in HBOT.

Many stubborn bacteria, in addition to mycobacteria, plague mankind. One such bacteria is *Borrelia burgdorferi*, which can be transmitted from a tick bite. Extremely small and shaped like a corkscrew, *Borrelia burgdorferi* is a member of the **spirochete** family—the same family as syphilis. Like syphilis, *Borrelia burgdorferi* can quietly ravage the brain and organs of an individual who is carrying it, long after it first arrives in that person's body.

Over a two-year period, a tick goes through three life stages. It needs a single meal of blood from three separate warm-blooded hosts to complete its life cycle. The white-footed mouse is a host preferred by the nymph and larval stages of the tick. It is from this mouse that the tick most often picks up the bacteria *Borrelia burgdorferi*, although the bacteria can also come from voles, racoons, dogs, or chipmunks.

Adult ticks grow to about the size of sesame seeds, and prefer to get their blood meal from white-tailed deer. These industrious ticks have also learned to travel great distances by attaching to birds; they have even been found in deer flies, horse flies, and mosquitoes.

When the tick bites into its host for a bit of blood to send it on its way to the next developmental stage, *Borrelia burgdorferi* bacteria can get into the host's blood.

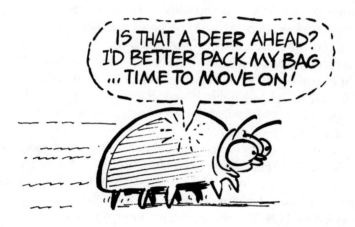

If you were the host who picked up this unwelcome bacterial guest, you might see an expanding rash around the site of the bite, a few days to a few weeks later. This might be accompanied by flu-like symptoms such as **fatigue, achiness, sore throat, headaches**, etc.

These are early-stage warnings that your immune system is struggling to deal with this invader; this is your chance to get antibiotics to kill it. Diagnosis of this spirochete bacteria, however, is difficult—it is often missed on blood tests.

The acute symptoms usually disappear, but may reappear as much more serious chronic problems, months to years later— and no two people manifest the same symptoms. **Muscle and joint pain,** especially of the larger joints such as the knees, are the most common symptoms.

Neurological symptoms can range from mild ones—such as **numbness, tingling, and burning in the extremities—to severe, debilitating pain, with fatigue and depression. Eye, heart, lung, and digestive disturbances** may or may not be present; symptoms may come and go. This is called **Lyme disease**.

When antibiotics are used in the later stages of this disease, they're often ineffective because the bacteria are safely hidden away inside your cells. At this point, the continued antibiotics will likely have ravaged the normal intestinal flora, leaving Candida yeast partying in its place—creating gas, bloating, bowel disturbances, fatigue, depression, and so on.

In 1998, at Texas A & M University, Fife conducted a study with 90 Lyme disease patients who hadn't responded to antibiotics for five years. They were treated with **two one-hour hyperbaric oxygen treatments per day at 2.36 atmospheres** (pressure equivalent to 14 metres or 45 feet below sea level). Within four days, they developed a skin rash and fever typical of dying spirochete bacteria—called a Jarisch-Herxheimer reaction—which passed after several weeks.

Some patients showed improvement during treatment; others improved after termination of the treatments. **All but four of the 90 patients showed significant improvement, such as relief of pain, fatigue, depression, and confusion.** Most maintained their improvement, but 30 percent required further treatments to regain the benefits.

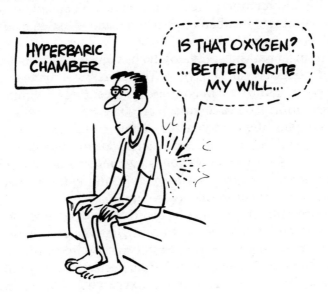

The obvious observation from this study is that **hyperbaric oxygen treatment begins to kill chronic *Borrelia burgdorferi*, the spirochete bacteria that causes Lyme disease, within four days.** Because it could achieve this—after years of intensive antibiotic therapy failed—then hyperbaric oxygen therapy is obviously the superior treatment for Lyme disease.

And anyone who has a tick-bite rash, or even the suspicion of a tick bite (since the rash doesn't always appear after a bite) should consider the treatment outlined at Texas A & M as the first treatment of choice: one-hour sessions, twice a day, for at least four days for acute symptoms—and more treatments for chronic symptoms. **Oxygen has again proven itself to be one of nature's greatest antibiotics.**

Another question to be asked is, will it work as well on its cousin, *Treponema pallidum*, the spirochete responsible for syphilis? It, too, is making a comeback, gaining resistance against antibiotics. I've not seen any studies done on it or on *Nisseria gonorrhea* (gonorrhea).

A sexually transmitted disease that is highly vulnerable to oxygen therapy is *Chlamydia trachomatis*, which can cause arthritis and blindness. Its cousin *Chlamydia pneumoniae* has been implicated in atherosclerosis, childhood asthma, adult emphysema, and Alzheimer Disease.

Like most parasites, Chlamydia has few antioxidant enzymes to defend itself against oxygen. Therefore, hyperbaric oxygen therapy should play a major role in preventing or eliminating diseases in which Chlamydia is involved.

Other parasites that have been shown to be oxygen-sensitive are *Plasmodium falciparum* (malaria), *Entamoeba histolytica* (amebic dysentery), *Trichomonas vaginalis*, *Giardia lamblia* (beaver fever), *Leishmania donovani* (sandfly fever), *Trichinella spiralis*, and *Schistosoma mansoni.*

Shistosomiasis is a parasitic blood-fluke disease found in one-third of the population in tropical countries. The immune system reaction against this worm consists largely of eosinophils, which are somewhat ineffective. The eggs of the worm are much more sensitive to oxygen than the adult, and are readily destroyed by oxygen.

How many thousands of soldiers have been knocked to the earth in the thick of battle by sword, arrow, bullet, or explosion—certain as they fell that their time on earth was done? What a relief to awake to find a medic wiping the mud from their wound, to smell flowers nearby, and see sunbeams breaking through the clouds—to still feel the breath of life in their lungs. The relief, the ecstasy to still be alive! Perhaps a short stay in the hospital, then home to family. Except for one little complication—there are bacteria called *Clostridium perfringens* in the dirt.

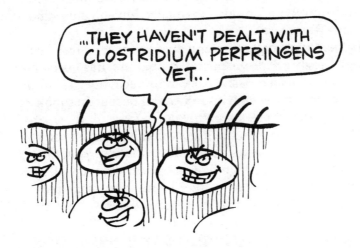

Clostridium perfringens normally wouldn't survive in a wound because they are anaerobic, which means they can't stand oxygen. If these bacteria—which are usually harmless—get trapped within a wall of inflammation through which your red blood cells can't deliver oxygen, they can thrive and multiply. *Clostridium perfringens* bacteria can produce more than a dozen toxins that can seep out through your defensive wall of inflammation, where they can do you great harm.

Alpha toxin can destroy membranes anywhere in your body. **Theta toxin** can destroy your heart tissue. Other toxins destroy your collagen, your fibrin—even your DNA. The disease these bacterial toxins cause is called **gas gangrene**.

If the bacteria aren't destroyed—or their toxins neutralized—then amputation of the affected limb is the next step, or death will ensue within hours. How many soldiers were thankful to have survived the battlefield, only to lose the war to this deadly bacteria a few days later? Over the centuries, these individuals would be innumerable.

Broad-spectrum antibiotics are commonly used to treat gangrene, but they have trouble penetrating the destroyed tissue that protects the bacteria, making surgical removal of the destroyed tissue necessary. Within this putrid mess, it's difficult to determine which tissue is damaged but still alive, and which is dead.

Hyperbaric oxygen therapy, two times per day for 90 minutes each, at 3 atmospheres of pressure, **has been shown to bring the damaged tissue back to life, leaving a clean line of demarcation between it and the dead tissue.** This makes it much easier for the surgeon to know where to cut.

The **extra oxygen in the blood has also been shown to** inactivate the toxins made by *Clostridium perfringens.* Also, **any plasma oxygen that can penetrate the wall of inflammation will destroy the Clostridium on contact.**

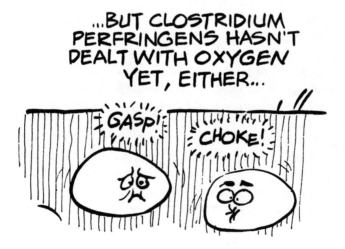

Antibiotics alone have a 50 percent success rate for stopping gangrene; the success rate climbs to 80 percent when surgery is used with the antibiotics, and to 95 percent when hyperbaric oxygen therapy is added to these two. With the use of hyperbaric oxygen therapy, 80 percent of survivors were able to avoid amputation, which is a dramatic improvement.

In modern society, gangrene is usually thought of as a rapidly progressing *sequela* to an acute injury infected by *Clostridium perfringens*. It is, however, more likely to be seen as a number of bacterial species taking advantage of decreased oxygenation of extremities, due to atherosclerosis of the arteries, especially in diabetics.

Hyperbaric oxygen therapy is usually only covered by insurance in the latest stages of these diseases—after all other treatments have failed. It is obvious that HBOT should be used at a much earlier stage for the best benefit.

We have seen that your intestinal flora are a critical part of you, and that their disruption by mercury fillings or antibiotics can weaken your immune system—by causing growth of organisms that are less friendly to your well-being, particularly Candida yeast.

The single-mindedness of wanting to use pharmaceutical antibiotics for every bacterial infection has overlooked the promise of oxygen as an antibiotic. Oxygen has already shown better results than antibiotics in treating leprosy and Lyme disease, and has been shown to be crucial in treating gangrene. Oxygen therapy needs to be studied further, to see if it will become the faster, more effective antibiotic of the future—without creating resistant strains of bacteria and fungus.

Letter from a Patient

Some years ago, I had the good fortune to be recommended to see Dr. Jonn Matsen. I was having a problem with Diverticulitus. My next course of action was to have some of my lower intestine removed and resected. I was not very happy with this solution, and was quick to take the suggestion that I see Dr. Jonn Matsen.

I had read his book *Eating Alive* and was quite impressed with the contents. My daughter had been seeing him for some serious allergy problems; she was the one who said that I should see him.

Dr. Matsen used muscle testing to detect problems with my digestive system and took a picture of my blood—which looked like a garbage dump.

We then did some food testing a few days later, and started me on a regime of herbs and vitamins. In four to five weeks, my blood was clear, and I had no further pain in my intestines.

Some years later, I had serious trouble with my liver as a result of taking ZOCOR for cholesterol. Dr. Matsen then took charge of my condition. I stopped the ZOCOR and went onto a natural product. I have never felt better in my life.

I truly believe in Naturopathic Medicine, and firmly believe that I owe my present good health to Dr. Matsen. I am truly grateful to have him as my Naturopathic Doctor, and also as a good friend.

Gino Gemma
Burnaby, BC

CHAPTER 6

Negative Ions: Positively Good

"The noblest question in the world is: What good can I do in it?'"

Benjamin Franklin, 1752

"The Doctor [Franklin], having published his method of verifying his hypothesis concerning the sameness of electricity with the matter of lightning, was waiting for the erection of a spire...when it occurred to him that by means of a common kite, he could have better access to the regions of thunder... ...just as he was beginning to despair of his contrivance, he observed some loose threads of the hempen string to stand erect.... Struck with this promising appearance, he immediately presented his knuckle to the key.... He perceived a very evident electric spark."

Joseph Priestley

Benjamin Franklin had just proven with his kite something that the electricity in his brain had already conjectured: that the lightning in the sky was electricity.

"In September 1752, I erected an Iron Rod to draw the Lightning down into my House, in order to make some

593

Experiments on it, with two Bells to give Notice when the rod should be electrified.

"I found the Bells rang sometimes when there was no Lightning or Thunder, but only a Dark Cloud over the Rod; that sometimes after a Flash of Lightning they would suddenly stop; and at other times, when they had not rang before, they would, after a Flash, suddenly begin to ring; that the Electricity was sometimes very faint, so that when a small Spark was obtained, another could not be got for sometime after, at other times the Spark would follow extremely quick, and once I had a continual Stream from Bell to Bell, the size of a Crow-Quill. Even during the same Gust there were considerable variations.

"...I was one night awakened by loud cracks on the staircase. Starting up and opening the door, I perceived that the brass ball instead of vibrating as usual between the bells, was repelled and kept at a distance from both; while the fire passed...whereby the whole staircase was inlightened as with sunshine, so that one might pick up a pin.

"Fire [electricity] only circulates. Hence have arisen some new items among us. We say B (and other Bodies alike ...) are electricised positively; A negatively; Or rather B is electricised plus or minus as we think proper. These terms we may use till philosophers give us better."

With a few simple experiments, Benjamin Franklin had shown that lightning was electricity, and that it had a **positive or plus (+) charge** that was attracted to the earth, which had a **negative or minus (-) charge**, and that it could be collected by an iron rod and passed safely through his house.

Being also a practical man, he designed and sold lightning rods that protected property and lives from the dangers of lightning strikes. He also observed that his bells sometimes would ring even when there was no lightning, indicating that these electrical charges were in the air in varying degrees without lightning present.

It would take another budding electrician, Guglielmo Marconi, to expose more of the riddle of atmospheric electricity. In 1898, Marconi successfully sent a message across the English Channel through the air without the use of wire. As astonishing as this feat was at the time, he proposed to send a similar message across the Atlantic.

Everyone thought this wouldn't work because you couldn't *see* across the Atlantic the way you could across the English Channel. The curvature of the earth would send the message off into space where it would never be heard from again.

In 1901, Marconi succeeded in sending a wireless message from Cornwall, England, to St. John's, Newfoundland; it became clear that further research needed to be done regarding the characteristics of the atmosphere. It was eventually discovered that there existed, far above our definition of breathable atmosphere, an **ionosphere** that had deflected Marconi's trans-Atlantic message back to earth.

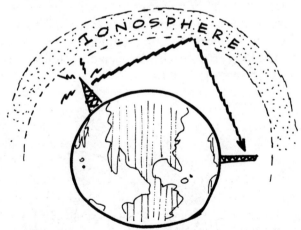

The atmosphere is 21 percent oxygen gas, and 78 percent nitrogen gas. **Oxygen has 8 protons (8+) and 8 electrons (8-)**, therefore the oxygen gas molecule (O_2) would have (16+) and (16-), giving the molecule an **overall neutral charge**. Nitrogen has one less proton and one less electron, therefore nitrogen gas (N_2) has (14+) and (14-)—again, a neutral charge.

As our twirling planet faces into the sun, the break of dawn sees our planet's face hit with a withering barrage of solar radiation—sometimes called the solar wind—crashing into our electromagnetic field at about a million miles per hour, bombarding our atmosphere with solar waves ranging from infrared to x-rays.

The sun's waves—shorter than the visible light spectrum, primarily the **ultraviolet** and **x-ray frequencies**—smash into the oxygen and nitrogen gas molecules in the upper atmosphere, knocking electrons off them in the process. The gas molecules that lose an electron become positively charged and are called **positive ions**, while the "free" electrons have a negative charge, making them **negative ions**.

Ions are very common during the day at elevations above 80 kilometres (50 miles); they peak at noon, and are highest in the longer days of summer. These ions interfere somewhat with radio waves during the day.

As the planet turns its back to the sun at dusk, the solar wind dies off, and many of the positive and negative ions join together to reform neutral gas molecules at night. Thus the ionosphere expands under the sun's influence during the day, and contracts in the earth's night-time shadow. Radio reception is usually much better at night because of the decreased ion activity.

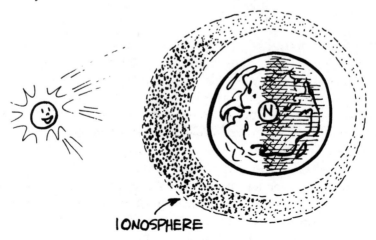

IONOSPHERE

Layers of ions reflect radio waves back to earth. The **F2 layer,** 200 to 1,000 kilometres (124 to 620 miles) above the earth's surface, is the part of the ionosphere that reflects the most radio waves back to earth. During the daytime, the F layer contains about 1,000,000,000 ions per cubic centimetre (cc)—about the size of a sugar cube—dropping overnight to about 500,000 ions per cc.

The **E layer,** closer to earth at 85 to 140 kilometres (53 to 87 miles) up, contains about 200,000 ions per cc during the day and 1,000 ions per cc at night. The **D layer,** the lowest layer, at 85 kilometres (53 miles) above the earth's surface, only exists in the daytime when ion formation is active.

While the daily cycles of dawn and dusk have the most dramatic effects on the ionosphere, the moon cycles play a role, too. The moon has a negative charge, like the earth, and therefore repels negatively charged ions. When the moon is full—on the opposite side of the earth from the sun—the moon's effect is to push the ionosphere closer to the earth's surface, increasing positive ion levels.

During the new moon, when the moon is on the same side of the earth as the sun, the effect is the opposite—to push the ionosphere away from the earth's surface, thus decreasing positive ion levels. The moon's net effect is to give a tidal flow to the ions of the atmosphere—not much different from the ebb and flow it causes on the oceans.

Every time an ultraviolet wave crashes into an atmospheric gas molecule, it loses a photon of energy. The farther down into the atmosphere the ultraviolet waves penetrate, the more gas molecules there are to absorb them. At 25 kilometres (16 miles) from earth, the oxygen molecules tend to recombine into threes rather than twos, to form **ozone** (O_3) rather than O_2.

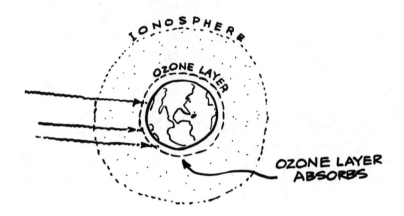

This **ozone layer** functions as a filter for deadly solar rays; the oxygen and nitrogen molecules absorb the photons, which split them into ions. This spares the gas molecules of the lower **troposphere**, and leaves us with the easy availability of O_2 for which we're designed. At the same time, the ozone layer helps provide a temperature stability that is conducive to us rather-delicate creatures.

The ozone layer allows only the weaker rays to penetrate through to the lower troposphere, where their photons are used by plants to generate power in the form of ATP, while releasing more oxygen. While the top of the troposphere—a little higher than Mt. Everest—may be -50° C (-58° F), at 39 kilometres (24 miles) higher, the temperature may be 30 to 40 degrees warmer, because of the ozone's ability to trap radiation.

Earth's atmosphere is 80 kilometres (50 miles) high. The lower 10 kilometres (six miles) is called the troposphere, which contains 75 percent of the atmosphere's air molecules. The word troposphere is taken from the Greek word *tropos*—to turn. Within the troposphere, weather is found. In the constant movement of air masses, we find the ions that put the spark in Ben Franklin's kite and the light in his staircase. While the O_2 levels in the troposphere are stable, its ions levels are highly variable.

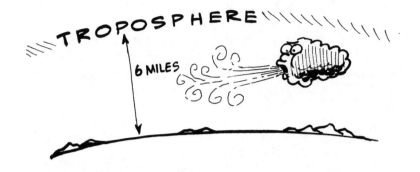

While ions from the ionosphere may spill down from on-high, they may also be produced in the lower levels by the friction created from the rolling and tumbling of weather fronts against each other, thus splitting molecules of oxygen into positive and negative ions.

Because the earth has a negative charge, it attracts positive ions to it so that the average ratio near the earth's surface is 5 positive ions to 4 negative ions. Lightning occurs when tumbling air fronts build up a massive positive charge that eventually finds release, slashing down toward the negatively charged earth.

Mineral deposits, especially those with high levels of radioactive substances, can create locally high levels of ions; some caves on the planet are examples of this. Falling water, such as waterfalls or surf crashing on the beach, can generate negative ion levels from 30,000 to 70,000 per cubic centimetre.

Plants, especially coniferous trees and ferns, give off copious quantities of negative ions. While sunny, open country might have 500 to 4,000 negative ions per cc, higher mountains— especially if forested with conifers—could have double that number.

The number of O_2 molecules breathed in per breath is in the trillions, so a few thousand ions would seem insignificant. People, however, intuitively seek out places that are high in negative ions because these places make them feel good.

A yogi in training must learn to absorb *prana* (the life force of the universe) from the atmosphere. The yogi might be advised to sit in a cave to meditate; if that cave is behind a waterfall, all the better to advance one toward enlightenment. Honeymooners go to Niagara Falls, everyone likes to walk the beaches of Hawaii, and mountain hiking has been popular for centuries.

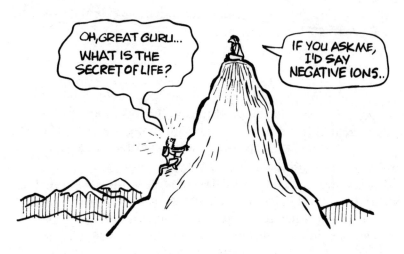

In the 1800s, Dr. George Bodington noticed that country people were far less susceptible to **Mycobacterium tuberculosis** (TB) than those who lived in the big cities of England. He speculated this was likely due to the cleaner and fresher air. Thus began the era of sanatoriums for the treatment of tuberculosis, with fresh country air and good food as the most common treatments.

In the US, Dr. Edward Trudeau had contracted TB that was considered terminal, so he went to the Adirondack Mountains of New York to die. Instead of dying, he fully recovered. In 1884, he built a sanatorium at Flower Lake, which treated approximately 12,500 patients in a span of over 70 years; many were cured.

The mountains of Davos, Switzerland, were decreed by many to have the best air, and a number of sanatoriums were also built there.

In the previous chapter, you read that hyperbaric oxygen therapy can kill the leprosy bacteria in a few days of treatment by increasing the amount of O_2 in the blood, and that success would likely apply to its cousin, the tuberculosis bacteria. But, going up into the mountains would actually decrease the amount of available O_2 because oxygen levels decrease with altitude.

What was it about this fresh mountain air that lent its healing properties to these sanatoriums?

Numerous studies have shown that the growth of plants can be increased by 50 percent when they are exposed to 10,000 positive *or* negative ions per cc. The depletion of all ions from the air *greatly reduced* the growth of plants. (See *The Ion Effect*, by Fred Soyka, listed in the Suggested Reading List on pages 633 to 636.)

Other studies have shown that both **positive and negative ions directly inhibit the growth of bacteria and fungi,** although *negative* **ions were more effective.** Bacteria die in the open air at a known rate; adding a low dose of negative ions increased the death rate of bacteria more than three-fold, while **increasing the negative ions to 10,000 per cc killed virtually all disease-causing bacteria.**

Mice infected with fungus, bacteria, or flu virus died sooner when exposed to positive ions, and lived longer when exposed to negative ions.

The Russian scientist Tchijewsky did research on ions, starting in the 1920s; he found that raising animals in **totally de-ionized air resulted in their deaths within a few weeks** from liver, kidney, and heart disease. From this he concluded, **"the real cause of death was the animals' inability to utilize oxygen properly. An organism receiving the cleanest type of air for breathing is condemned to serious illness if the air does not contain at least a small quantity of air ions."**

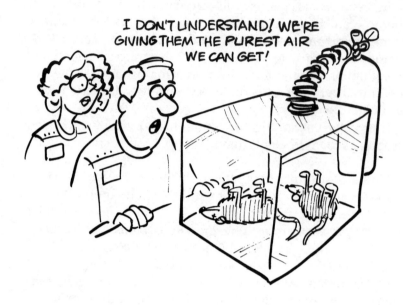

American researchers Windsor and Beckett found that breathing positive ions decreased breathing capacity by 30 percent, while breathing negative ions didn't affect breathing capacity in healthy men.

Other studies have shown that **positive ions decrease the activity of the cilia that line the respiratory passage** so that the cilias' ability to expel pollution is decreased, and **negative ions increased the cilias' detoxification ability**.

An Oxford University study found that people suffering from asthma, bronchitis, hay fever, and nasal catarrh reported an improvement in their symptoms when using a negative ion generator. Another study showed that **fibroblasts decreased their activity under the influence of positive ions, and increased their activity with negative ions**.

From these few studies (and there are many more), it can be seen that **micro-organisms are not designed to thrive in a world of ionized oxygen—but we are**. Both positive and negative ions are bad for the "Bad Guys," while *we* need ions—especially negative ions—to retain our health.

The intuitive or empirical **placement of sanatoriums up in the mountain air** wasn't a search for more oxygen to gain health; **it was a search for more negative ions**. The cities of the industrialized countries had paved over the vegetation and polluted the waters that produced negative ions and—by burning coal—added particles that further depleted the air of negative ions. The result: susceptibility to tuberculosis.

It is obvious that negative ions improved the function of patients' respiratory function and, likely, their immune systems. While it is well known that **your red blood cells pick up the oxygen from your lungs**, it has been proposed that **your white blood cells pick up the ions from your lungs**.

The normal charge of a white blood cell is negative, so it could be imperative to the function of your immune cells that they receive a sufficient number of negative ions **to remain "fully charged"** in their battles against shrewd would-be invaders.

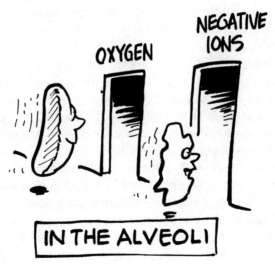

OXYGEN

NEGATIVE IONS

IN THE ALVEOLI

MEANWHILE, BACK TO BART

Bart Barnum is so impressed with the success he has seen with his star player's healing last season, he buys the hyperbaric oxygen chamber from his brother-in-law, and insists that all of his players use it regularly. By the time the season starts, all his players have healed their minor training-camp injuries; they continue to use the hyperbaric chamber at every opportunity.

The season starts with success, just as the previous season had finished, with win after win. A third of the way through the season, Bart Barnum is already planning where to put his second championship trophy . . . when things begin to unravel.

They lose a few home games—unheard of, the year before—though they still win most of their road games. As the season progresses, they have the worst record in the league for home losses, but still manage to win a few games on the road. In fact, the longer the road trip, the more games they seem to win. The sports writers give them the moniker "Team Schizophrenia."

Gradually a tension—unseen but clearly felt—builds between the players and the coach. The coach feels the players have tuned him out, that they aren't even doing the game basics correctly, never mind the intricate plays they'd mastered last year.

The players have different opinions, but generally don't see what the fuss is about. It is just a little slump they'll have to go through. They go through a streak of injuries where it seems like the whole team is on the injured list, or just coming off it. They lose 256 man-games to injuries, far more than the other teams—and the season is far from over.

It seems to the trainer that the players' reactions to relatively small injuries are exaggerated. Several players become injured when they start a bar fight, and end up getting severely pummelled. When the home losses reach eight in a row, and the shrinking crowds start booing, Bart Barnum does the only thing an owner can do. He goes to Las Vegas on holiday and has the manager fire the coach.

The assistant coach takes over, and the team responds with a home win; things look bright again in Springfield. It doesn't last long. Ten straight losses follow. A lot of yelling is heard in the locker room, with no result on the playing field. Trades are made, players are put on waivers, the general manager is also fired, and the crowds disappear.

Bart Barnum knows it is time to cut his losses, so he puts the team up for sale. No one wants to buy it.

If only he had studied ions.

EVIL WINDS

Hippocrates knew in 400 BC that winds that blow over mountain ranges, onto plains, tend to fall. Falling air compresses, losing moisture and gaining heat. These winds are bad for the health. The **Chinook wind** is like this; it falls off the east side of the Rocky Mountains, giving unseasonably warm weather to the Foothills country, but exacerbating migraines and increasing the incidence of colds. The friction of the fall creates a positive ion build-up, which creates the symptoms.

At the Hebrew University in Jerusalem, Sulman and others studied an even worse wind: the **Sharav wind** in Israel. The Arabs call it the **Hamsin**. It blows about 50 days a year.

It starts off as a falling wind. As it falls, its moisture content *decreases* and its positive ion levels *increase*. Then, the wind blows over an area of hot sand, which *further decreases* its moisture content and *further increases* its positive ion build-up. The lack of moisture prevents the positive ions from being conducted into the negatively charged earth, so a strong surge of positive ions rides ahead of the storm, like the waves at the bow of a ship.

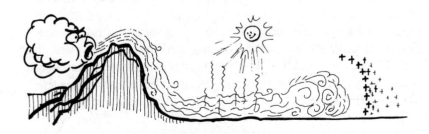

Weather-sensitive people (25 to 50 percent of the population, to varying degrees) reported that, a day or two **before** the arrival of a Sharav wind, they experienced irritability, anxiousness, migraines, heart symptoms, shortness of breath, tension, edema—especially swelling of the feet—and/or joint pain, etc.

When the Sharav wind blew, the frequency of car accidents would double, and wife beatings would soar. Tests showed that weather-sensitive individuals reacted with an increase of the stress hormones produced by the **adrenal glands, thyroid gland, and/or pineal gland.**

A study of one group of weather-sensitive people found that their blood levels of the pineal hormone **serotonin** had shot up, although other blood values were normal. Treatment with a negative ion generator brought their serotonin levels to normal and relieved their symptoms, while the serotonin levels and symptoms of the control group, who received no treatment, remained high. It is believed that the **hypothalamus**—the sensor of heat stress—is what releases the serotonin from the pineal gland.

We have seen that negative ions play a key role in respiratory health, immune function, oxygen utilization, and now, stress responses.

Unlike oxygen, **negative ions aren't spread evenly over the surface of the planet.** While atmospheric air normally has sufficient ions for survival, there are **ebbs and flows** tied into daily, monthly, and seasonal cycles, as well as regional geological variations and air-front turbulence. **These ebbs and flows can strongly affect physical, mental, and emotional health.**

A modern component has greatly aggravated the situation. The stripping away and covering over of natural vegetation has eliminated much of the negative ion production in urban areas. The air pollution from automobile exhaust and industry has caused the binding-up and neutralization of many negative ions.

Some of the lowest negative ion readings ever recorded have been taken in the Los Angeles and San Francisco areas during rush-hour traffic—in fact, negative ions were virtually non-existent. **Without negative ions, serotonin will rise— is this the root of road rage?**

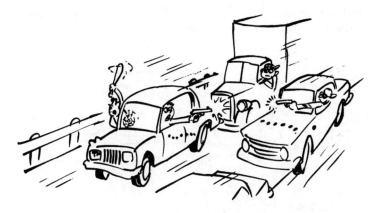

ANOTHER LOW NEGATIVE ION DAY
ON THE CALIFORNIA FREEWAY...

In our desire to control temperature, we have locked out natural air. We have airtight buildings with heating systems for the winter and air conditioning for the summer. In 1933, C. P. Yagoun published studies showing that the metal ducts of heating and air conditioning units can affect ion levels in housing.

Further studies have shown that the **metal ducts strip negative ions out of the air,** leaving people prone to more respiratory infections, as well as stress-hormone responses. Thus is born the sick-housing syndrome—our man-made version of Hippocrates' "bad wind."

Winter cold and flu season seems to match exactly the period when people are running their forced-air systems in homes, schools, offices, and automobiles. The weakening of the respiratory membranes with winter heating systems allows cold and flu viruses to gain entry into our bodies.

Most of us have been on an airplane where one person has been coughing and hacking and sneezing throughout the flight. When you get off, you have the feeling that all the people on the plane are now carrying that virus firmly entrenched in their upper respiratory system. In fact, it has been shown that on one flight from Chicago to Honolulu in 1994, one TB carrier spread the disease to four other passengers—thanks to the endless stream of conditioned air flowing out of the overhead vents, with nary a trace of a negative ion to be found.

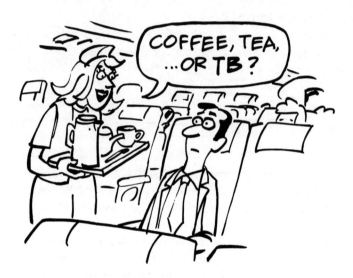

Following bicentennial celebrations in Philadelphia in 1976, 34 Legionnaires died from pneumonia caused by an unknown agent. Subsequent investigation found a new bacteria, *Legionella pneumophila*, in the air conditioning system of the hotel. In 1994, on a luxury cruiseship in the Caribbean, three passengers also died from *Legionella pneumophila*.

This bacteria was later found world-wide, but only seemed to be a problem in the industrialized world—and not normally hazardous to those with a strong immune system. Of course, it wasn't considered that the use of air conditioning systems may have contributed to weakened immune systems.

NEGATIVE IONS IMPROVE HEALTH

In a study done at a Swiss bank, 671 employees were divided into two groups: one group worked in regular office air, and the second group worked in air that had negative ions added. After several months, it was found that **for each single day lost to colds, flus, and sore throats in the negative ion group, the untreated group lost 16 days.**

A study done using negative ions with burn victims showed that within ten minutes, they felt decreased pain and restlessness, followed by decreased incidence of infection.

Man-made air tends to be depleted of ions—that is especially true of pure bottled oxygen, which is ion-free. As precious as oxygen is, it is not complete without its accompanying ions, especially negative ions.

The use of pure oxygen for extended periods of time could lead to complications. In my hypothetical story, Bart Barnum's hyperbaric oxygen treatment of his sports team is a perfect example.

The Israeli studies showed that when young, healthy people—especially males—are first exposed to high positive-ion weather fronts, their adrenals respond by producing hormones that give a sense of excitement, confidence, and euphoria.

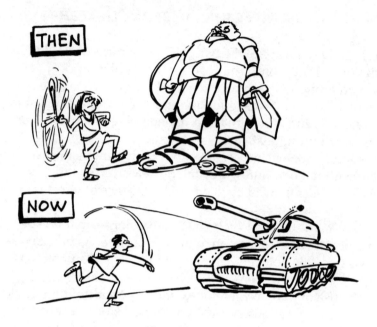

This would correlate with how well Bart Barnum's team did while regularly using the hyperbaric oxygen chambers at the beginning of the season—it kept their winning streak alive.

Gradually, as their adrenals weakened, fatigue would set in. Playing games at home would allow regular use of the chamber, which could aggravate the problem of ion stress. Road trips would take them away from the hyperbaric chamber, which would allow their young bodies to quickly bounce back and regain their winning spirit.

Prolonged ion-deficiency stress could gradually lead to total exhaustion, which means "end of season"—and for some, "end of career."

Older people and less-healthy people would be more likely to react to the stress of high positive ions with serotonin hormone or hyperthyroid response. In one Israeli study of 500 hyperthyroid patients, 45 percent recovered just with the addition of negative ions to their air.

NEGATIVE IONS IMPROVE ATHLETIC PERFORMANCE

Is it possible for negative ions to improve athletic ability? Look to the Russians for the answer. They've long been leaders in the study of negative ions, and it's no coincidence that during this period, they also were dominant in international athletics.

A study published in 1961 gave the results of experiments with 24 female gymnasts and 18 female track-and-field athletes. Each of these two groups was divided into a negative ion-treated group and a control group. The things measured were:

- **muscle strength;**
- **endurance to static work** (holding a sustained pressure);
- **endurance to dynamic work** (running in place or bicycling till exhaustion); and
- **speed of reaction time,** also known as quickness.

The track-and-field groups were also tested for **equilibrium** or balance. The results with the gymnasts and track-and-field athletes showed no changes in pulse rate, respiration, or blood pressure, and a slight increase in muscle strength in the negative ion group over the control group, after 25 days.

Static endurance
Gymnast control group: showed decreased endurance after 25 days
Gymnast negative ion group: improved by 46 percent

Track-and-field control group: endurance improved 40 percent after 25 days
Track-and-field negative ion group: improved by 192 percent

Dynamic endurance
Gymnasts: no control group
Gymnast negative ion group: improved by 87 percent over
25 days

Track-and-field control group: improved 24 percent after 25
days
Track-and-field negative ion group: improved 240 percent

Reaction time
Gymnast control group: shortened reaction time by 11
milliseconds
Gymnast negative ion group: shortened by 22 milliseconds

Track-and-field control group: shortened by 4.5 percent at the
end of 25 days
Track-and-field negative ion group: shortened by 16 percent

Equilibrium results
Track-and-field control group: improved 80 to 82 percent
after 25 days
**Track-and-field negative ion group: improved by 145 to 333
percent**

One of the pertinent observations made during this study
was that **the negative ion groups' cheerfulness and vitality
increased notably; they also showed improvement in sleep
and appetite.** Studies showed that the negative ion groups also
utilized vitamins B and C more effectively.

Studies done with male swimmers and boxers also showed
no increase in muscle strength by using negative ions, but
endurance and quickness dramatically improved.

This improvement in quickness (reaction time of the nervous
system) also includes **mental sharpness**, as shown by a study
done in a bank in South Africa. During two years of **using
negative ion generators, the error rate dropped from 2.5
percent to 0.5 percent.**

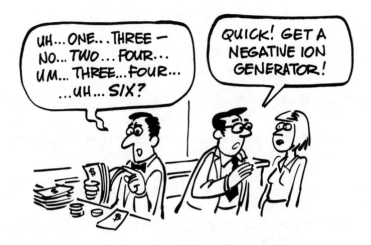

If Bart Barnum had known how important negative ions were to health, stamina, and stress-hormone reduction, he surely would have installed a negative ion generator in his hyperbaric oxygen chamber. He would have saved his athletes and himself a lot of grief, not to mention millions of dollars.

The problem is that oxygen can increase the potential for combustion and create a highly flammable situation—and generators create negative ions with the use of a spark. No one could run a negative ion generator in a hyperbaric oxygen chamber without blowing it up—that is, until **Guy Cramer invented his sparkless negative-ion generator.**

Guy Cramer is a little shy and very quiet—until you get him talking about ions. Then he will release a torrent of information that will swamp and overwhelm your merely mortal brain cells within minutes.

Ions are his passion; he has studied them fervently. Perhaps some of this is genetic. His grandfather, Donald Hings, was the creator of the Walkie-Talkie, used during World War II; he also invented the electric piano.

Guy Cramer has long been aware of the need to develop a negative ion generator that can work safely in a high-oxygen environment; he has studied and experimented with this problem for years. One of his breakthroughs came from studies on **zeolite** by NASA, when they were looking for a molecular sieve. Zeolite is a naturally occurring mineral that formed millions of years ago, when volcanic ash landed in an alkaline lake, forming repetitive layers of crystals of aluminum, oxygen, and silica.

These repetitive crystals give it the property of being a **universal** *adsorber*—that is, things are attracted to and stick to the outside of zeolite without actually changing its structure. Zeolite is used to adsorb oil from floors, to pull ammonia from kitty litter, and was even used to draw radioactive waste from cattle at Chernobyl.

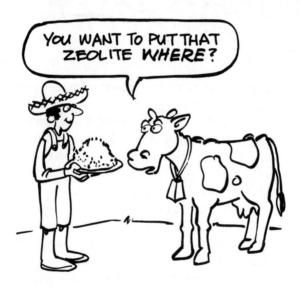

Guy Cramer's insight was to apply a negatively charged polymer backing (patented) to zeolite, to turn it from a universal adsorber into a **universal emitter—of negative ions**. No batteries necessary and no spark produced, therefore perfectly safe to use in a high-oxygen environment.

Now, **for the first time, people can get all the bacterial infection-fighting and injury-healing properties of hyperbaric oxygen therapy—along with the anti-pain, anti-stress, anti-viral, and pro-endurance benefits of negative ion therapy.**

Guy is also working on a way to convert forced-air heating and air conditioning into generators of negative ions. He has already produced a calendar that predicts monthly ion variations and their likely effects on some sports stars, as well as the stock market.

Of course, the wealthy are the first to benefit. At this time, his negative-ion-generating hat is mainly found on the golf courses of Carmel, California; a few leading-edge Hollywood stars are trying to knock a few strokes off their game.

Guy Cramer has joined with Gino Gemma to produce negative ion generators and hyperbaric oxygen chambers through their company, Hyperstealth (www.hyperstealth.com). I look forward to working with them to see how the combination of hyperbaric oxygen and negative ion therapy works on tough cases.

While the immediate benefits of this combination-treatment of HBOT and negative ions are obvious, there are future potentials to be explored here.

You know that your blood, skin, and intestinal cells are constantly being replaced as they die of old age or injury. These new cells originate from stem cells, the "universal mother" cells that can develop into any cell. It was thought that the stem cells for the human nervous system were used up during development of fetal nerves, and therefore it was impossible to grow new neurons to replace damaged ones—even though "lower" animals, like lizards and canaries, can grow new neurons.

Recent research has shown that the adult nervous system actually does have stem cells left after all. Cells lining the cavities of the **ventricles** of the brain—once considered the "most boring" cells of the brain because they didn't appear to *do* anything—are actually differentiated stem cells. Once they are differentiated, it means they have already chosen their "career," and can't take up a new vocation, such as replace your damaged nerve cells. Their offspring, however, are undifferentiated, which means they're open to career choices.

Injury to the nervous system gets them multiplying in earnest. Unfortunately, at this point, it seems that rather than become neurons, they are more likely to become **glial cells**, the support cells to the neurons.

As glial cells, they tend to make up much of the scar tissue in spinal cord injuries. It has been found that **epidermal growth factor** encourages the new cells to become glial cells, and **fibroblast growth factor** stimulates the new cells to become neurons.

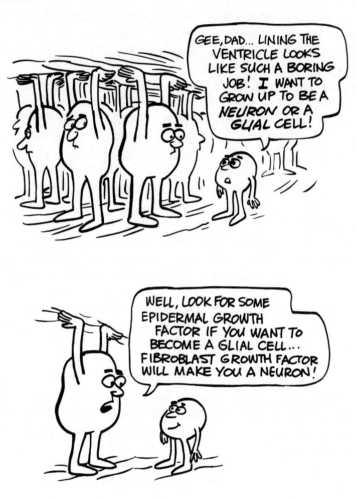

Since **fibroblast growth factor is made by your macrophages under the influence of oxygen, it may be that hyperbaric oxygen therapy is promoting improvement in stroke, cerebral palsy, and brain injury by activating stem cell production of**

new neurons. I don't know of any studies that have been done yet to investigate this.

The **hippocampus** is a receiving, sorting, and filing area of your brain. It takes information from other brain regions, helps sort the info into memories, and then sends them to other parts of your brain for storage. Damage to the hippocampus results in difficulty forming new memories, although recall of previous memories may be unaffected.

In 1998, a new type of medical research marker demonstrated that in the five human brains studied, all five **showed development of new neurons in the hippocampus.** These new brain neurons had to have originated from stem cells; animal studies found stem cells inside the hippocampus.

These stem cells divide constantly; some become identical daughter cells, while some migrate and become nerve cells. Exercise, creative play, and learning help increase the growth and survival rate of these new nerve cells. Injury such as stroke or epilepsy can dramatically increase their replication rate.

Stress neurotransmitters, like serotonin and stress adrenal hormones, inhibit stem cell proliferation in the hippocampus. This is where negative ion therapy—by reducing the production of stress hormones—may assist in the development of new neurons, in conjunction with hyperbaric oxygen stimulation of fibroblast growth factor.

The development of new neurons in humans is a brand new field; the use of negative ions with hyperbaric oxygen is an even newer treatment that has yet to be evaluated. This combination may turn out to play a key role in regenerating new brain tissue and spinal cord tissue.

Letter from a Patient

At the age of 20, I was diagnosed with Ankylosing Spondylitis (AS), a form of arthritis distinctive in that it is hereditary and takes many years before the telltale "hunchback" is apparent.

At 46, I was fed up with the roller-coaster good days/bad days syndrome, and scared of the future. Besides the constant ache from the arthritis, the list was long: headaches (often migraines), untimely and painful periods, fatigue, numbness in my feet, and rotation bouts of diarrhea and constipation. Talking about it felt ridiculous—like I was a hypochondriac.

On the advice of a friend, I saw a naturopathic doctor (Dr. Jonn Matsen), and began his program. Within six months, I felt 80 percent better than I had in my life. The next stage will be slower. Frankly, I didn't care how long it took since the quality of my life has changed so dramatically. The change I happily made to my lifestyle and eating is lifelong. For example, never one much for exercise (I was too tired), I now have energy to spare. Instead of dragging myself off to ski, run, or cycle, I plan these "now fun" activities into my day.

The added bonus is that since I started the program, I've not had any significant AS pain. I no longer take any exorbitantly expensive anti-inflammatories. Has the AS gone away forever? Probably not, but it is now manageable and for that, I am very grateful.

Roberta Beck
Port Moody, BC

CHAPTER 7

Stress

Our adrenal glands normally secrete hormones that help maintain sugar and mineral levels in the body. In emergencies, however, the adrenals secrete a powerful hormone called adrenalin—or epinephrine—that acts on the skeletal muscles so that we can either fight or flee from danger. This **fight or flight response** is obviously very important when we are in physical danger.

Real physical danger is a rarity in our society. Instead, many of us allow our own thoughts to create stress. Rather than living in the present moment, we are often feeling guilty about past events or worrying about the future and all the things we need to do; we create pictures in our minds of potential problems.

The trouble is that when you create a mental picture of a potential problem, your body doesn't know it is *not* a real problem—that it's merely an imaginary potential problem. Therefore, the body reacts exactly as if you were in extreme physical danger.

If you are constantly thinking about it, rather that doing something constructive to resolve it, a small *real* problem can turn into a major health problem. Instead of trying to avoid your problems by choosing unhealthy habits—drugs, alcohol, gambling, unhealthy eating habits, watching too much TV, sleeping too much, being too busy, etc.—deal with your problems quickly and decisively, or put them consciously aside until you can do so.

Talking about a problem with a good friend, a family member, or a counsellor often helps put it in its proper perspective, after a runaway mind has exaggerated it out of proportion.

When you are stressed, your body is shunting energy into the skeletal muscle system for fight or flight—so why not follow through with some vigorous exercise? Brisk walking, running, cycling, swimming, martial arts, and other aerobic activities are good ways to burn up accumulated stress and help decrease the sense of powerlessness that often accompanies it.

You can also reduce your stress through Tai Chi, yoga, Qi Gong, meditation, and breathing exercises, or by taking relaxation classes or listening to relaxation tapes. All of these methods can help re-balance the mind and body.

Here's a simple technique to prevent stressful thoughts from having a negative impact on your body. Place the three middle fingers of each hand on your forehead above your eyes and then pull the skin lightly apart so the skin in the centre of your forehead is slightly stretched. Holding these points for a few minutes helps to effectively disengage mental activity from the physical body, and takes the "sharper edge" off the problem for hours.

Creative visualization and positive thinking are other effective tools for changing the pictures we place in our minds. If having a negative picture in the mind has a negative effect on the body—even if the picture is not real—then holding a positive picture in the mind should have a positive effect on the body.

There are countless how-to books on the market for managing stress. *Making the Brain Body Connection*, by Sharon Promislow, contains simple yet effective strategies for reducing stress and improving how you feel and perform.

These are just some of the ways we can deal with stress. We all have potentially stressful situations in our lives; it's our response to these situations that can affect our health. Respond to stress with positive actions and take time to relax, on a daily basis.

Letter from a Patient

Since I've been to Dr. Matsen and been on THE EATING ALIVE PROGRAM, I have no more stomach pain due to ulcers. My sneezing and wheezing have quit, and my rash has never been back to haunt me.

This program has taken all three chronic illnesses out of my life, so now I am free to travel the world!

Beverly Pellegrin
Vancouver, BC

PART IV

HELPFUL
RESOURCES

Suggested Reading

THE FOOD SECTION

Sahelian, R. MD, and Gates, D., *The Stevia Cookbook*, 1999
    ISBN 0-89529-926-7
    Avery Publishing Group
    120 Old Broadway
    Garden City Park, NY 11040
    1-800-548-5757

Gittleman, A. L., *Get the Sugar Out – 501 Simple Ways to Cut the Sugar Out of Any Diet*, 1996
    ISBN 0-517-88653-7
    Three Rivers Press
    201 East 50th Street, New York, NY 10022

Chapter 1: Mercury: The Missing Link

Jerome, F. J., DDS, *The Tooth Truth*, 1995
    ISBN 1-887314-08-3
    ProMotion Publishing
    3368 F Governor Drive, Suite 144
    San Diego, CA 92122
    1-800-231-1776

Brown, E. H. and Hansen, R. T., DMD, *The Key to Ultimate Health*, 1998
    ISBN 1-879854-25-2
    Advanced Health Research Publishing
    1943 Sunnycrest Drive, Suite 183
    Fullerton, CA 92835
    1-888-792-1102

Chapter 2: Vaccines: Unanswered Questions

Coulter, H. L. and Fisher, B. L., *A Shot In the Dark*, 1991
    ISBN 0-89529-463-X
    Avery Publishing Group Inc.
    Garden City Park, NY 11040
    1-800-548-5757

Scheibner, Viera, PhD, *VACCINATION: 100 Years of Orthodox Research Shows that Vaccines Represent a Medical Assault on the Immune System*, 1993
    ISBN 0-646-15124-X
    Australian Print Group
    Maryborough, Victoria, Australia

Fisher, B. L., *The Consumer's Guide to Childhood Vaccines*, 1997
    ISBN 1-889204-01-3
    National Vaccine Information Center
    512 W. Maple Avenue, Suite 206
    Vienna, VA 22180
    1-800-909-7468

Hallaway, N., RN, and Strauts, Z., MD, *Turning Lead into Gold*
    ISBN 0-921586-51-5
    New Star Books
    2504 York Avenue
    Vancouver, BC Canada

Obomsawin, R., *Universal Immunization: Medical Miracle or Masterful Mirage?* 2000
    Health Action Network Society (HANS)
    202 – 5262 Rumble Street
    Burnaby, BC Canada V5J 2B6
    (604) 435-0512
    Fax: (604) 435-1561
    www.hans.org

Chapter 3: The Liver Connection

O'Regan, B. and Hirshberg, C., *Spontaneous Remissions*, 1993
ISBN 0-943951-17-8
Institute of Noetic Sciences
475 Gate Five Road, Suite 300
Sausalito, CA 94965

Horowitz, L. G., DMD, *Emerging Viruses*, 1996
ISBN 0-923550-12-7
Tetrahedron Publishing
20 Drumlin Road
Rockport, Mass 01966

Chapter 4: The Yeast Are Back

Vanderhaeghe, L. R. and Bouic, J. D., PhD, *The Immune System Cure*
ISBN 0-13-013074-5
Prentice-Hall Publishing 1999

Price, W. A., DDS, *Nutrition and Physical Degeneration*, 1945
ISBN 0-916-764-00-1
Price-Pottenger Nutrition Foundation
7890 Broadway
Lemon Grove, CA 91946
(619) 462-7600

Truss, C. O., MD, *The Missing Diagnosis*, 1983
ISBN 0-9615758-0-8
PO Box 26508
Birmingham, AL 35226

Crook, W. G., MD, *The Yeast Connection*, 1983
ISBN 0-394-74700-3
Random House Books
NY

Mendelsohn, R. S., MD, *Confessions of a Medical Heretic*, 1979
ISBN 0-8092-7726-3
Contemporary Books
180 N. Michigan Avenue
Chicago, Illinois 60601

Chapter 5: Oxygen: Nature's Best Cure

Neubauer, R. A., MD, and Walker, M.,DPM, *Hyperbaric Oxygen Therapy*, 1998
    ISBN 0-89529-759-0
    Avery Publishing
    Garden City Park, NY 11040
    1-800-548-5757

Jain, K. K., *Textbook of Hyperbaric Medicine*, 1999
    ISBN 0-88937-203-9
    Hogrefe and Huber Publishers

Chapter 6: Negative Ions: Positively Good

Soyka, F., and Edwards, A., *The Ion Effect*, 1977
    ISBN 0-7704-1512-5
    Seal Books
    www.hyperstealth.com

Chapter 7: Stress

Promislow, S., *Making the Brain Body Connection*, 1998
    ISBN 0-9681066-2-5
    Kinetic Publishing Corporation
    #713 1489 Marine Drive
    West Vancouver, BC V7T 1B8

References

INTRODUCTION

1. *JAMA*, 276:1473–9, 1996

CHAPTER 1

2. "WHO Environmental Health Criteria 118. Inorganic Mercury," World Health Organization (WHO), Geneva, 1991 ISBN 92 4 1571187
3. Sehnert, K. W., *et al.*, *Townsend Letter for Doctors & Patients*, 134–7, October 1995
4. *ADA News*, January 2, 1984
5. Stock, A., *Z Angew Chemie*, 39:461–88, 1926; *Arch Gewerbepath Gewerbehyg*, 7:388–413, 1936; *Zahnarztl Rundschau*, 10:403–7, 1939; *Biochem Z*, 304:73–80, 1940; *Ber Deutsch Chem Gesellschaft*, 75:1530, 1942; *Biochem Z*, 316:108–22, 1943
6. Störtebecker, P., *Mercury Poisoning from Dental Amalgam*, Störtebecker Foundation for Research, Stockholm, Sweden, 1985; also available from Bio-Probe, Inc., Orlando, Florida
7. *Deutsche Medizinische Wochenschrift*, 8, 1928
8. Crinnion, W. J., *Alternative Medicine Review*, 5(3):209–23, 2000
9. Koos, B. J., and Longo, L., *Am J Obstet Gynecol*, 126:390–409, 1976, taken from *Goodman and Gilman's The Pharmacological Basis of Therapeutics*, MacMillan Publishing Co., Ltd., 1980, Chapter 69: "Heavy Metals and Heavy-Metal Antagonists"
10. Crinnion, W. J., *Alternative Medicine Review*, 5(3):209–23, 2000
11. Ganther, H. E., *Science*, 175:1122, 1972, and Svensson, B. G., *et al.*, *Sci Total Envir*, 126:61–74, 1992
12. Ganther, H. E., *Environmental Health Perspectives*, 25:71–6, 1978
13. Dencker, L., *et al.*, *Project Catalogue* 1993/1994, The Swedish Medical Council, 1994. ISBN 91-85546-90-9
14. Gerhard, I., *Klinisches Labor*, 38:404–11, 1992
15. Aposhian, H. V., *Environmental Health Perspectives*, 106(4):1017–25, 1998

16.   Crinnion, W. J., *Alternative Medicine Review*, 5(3):209–23, 2000;
      Störtebecker, P., *Mercury Poisoning from Dental Amalgam*,
      Störtebecker Foundation for Research, Stockholm, Sweden,
      1985; also available from Bio-Probe, Inc., Orlando, Florida;
      Null, G., *Townsend Letter for Doctors & Patients*, 760–70,
      Aug/Sept 1992
17.   Levenson, J., *What Doctors Don't Tell You*, Vol. 11, No. 1, 2000
18.   Crinnion, W. J., *Alternative Medicine Review*, 5(3):209–23, 2000;
      Goodman and Gilman's The Pharmacological Basis of Therapeutics,
      MacMillan Publishing Co., Ltd., 1980
19.   Canadian Dental Association Dental Amalgam Patient
      Information Sheet, p. 4
20.   *ibid.*, p. 4
21.   *ibid.*, p. 1
22.   Null, G., *Townsend Letter for Doctors & Patients*, 760–70,
      August/September 1992
23.   Störtebecker, P., *Mercury Poisoning from Dental Amalgam*,
      Störtebecker Foundation for Research, Stockholm, Sweden,
      1985; also available from Bio-Probe, Inc., Orlando, Florida
24.   Aposhian, H. V., *Environmental Health Perspectives*,
      106(4):1017–25, 1998
25.   Siblerud, R. L., *Toxic Substances Journal*, 10:425–44, 1990b
26.   Clarkson, 1977, taken from *Goodman and Gilman's The
      Pharmacological Basis of Therapeutics*, MacMillan Publishing Co.,
      Ltd., 1980, Chapter 69: "Heavy Metals and Heavy-Metal
      Antagonists"
27.   Mantyla, D. G. and Wright, O. D., *Journal of the American Dental
      Association*, 92:1189–94, 1976
28.   *SRI Total Environ*, 99:23–35, 1990
29.   *Am J Physiol*, 229:8–12, 1975; *Proc Soc Exper Biol Med*, 120:805–8,
      1965; *Proc Soc Exper Biol Med*, 124:485–90, 1967; *Am J Physiol*,
      219:755–61, 1970; *Am J Physiol*, 220:808–11, 1971
30.   Hanson, M., *Orthomolecular Psychiatry*, Vol. 12 (3):194–201, 1983
31.   *Journal of the American Dental Association*, Vol. 122:54, 1991
32.   Hanson, M., *Orthomolecular Psychiatry*, Vol. 12 (3):194–201, 1983
33.   Eggleston, D., *J Prost Dent*, 51:617–23, 1984
34.   Stejskal, V., Presentation Given to the American Academy of
      Environmental Medicine 33rd Annual Meeting – November,
      1998, Baltimore, Maryland USA. See www.melisa.org
      (MELISA® is the registered trademark of MELISA® MEDICA
      FOUNDATION)

35. *ibid.*; and Stejskal, V., *et al.*, *Neuroendocrinology Letters*, 20:289–98, 1999
36. Sterzl, I., *et al.*, *Neuroendocrinology Letters*, 20:221–8, 1999
37. Stejskal, V., *et al.*, *Journal of Clinical Immunology*, 16(1):31–40, 1996
38. Tibbling, L., *et al.*, *International Journal of Occupational Medicine and Toxicology*, Vol. 4, No. 2, 1995
39. *Neuroepidemiology*, 8:128–141, 1989
40. 6th MELISA® Study Group—résumé. See www.melisa.org
41. *ibid.*
42. Stejskal, V., *Drug Information Journal*, Vol. 31:1379–82, 1997
43. Störtebecker, P., *Mercury Poisoning from Dental Amalgam*, Störtebecker Foundation for Research, Stockholm, Sweden, 1985; also available from Bio-Probe, Inc., Orlando, Florida
44. *ibid.*
45. Gustafsson, E., *Water, Air, and Soil Pollution*, 80:99–102, 1995
46. al-Hiyasat, A. S., *et al.*, *J Dent*, 26(5–6):487–95, 1998
47. Chen, H. Y., *et al.*, *J Prosthet Dent*, 82(4):468–75, 1999
48. Hibberd, A. R., *J Nutr Environ Med*, 8:219–31, 1998
49. www.mercola.com
50. Warren, T., *Townsend Letter for Doctors & Patients*, 50–60, April 1997
51. Swedish Medical Research Council, *Medicinska Forskningsradet*, 1992
52. www.geocities.com/Athens/9313/dent.html
53. *ibid.*
54. See Health Canada Information Letters, No. 608, 625, 638, 696; CDA Dental Materials & Devices Document; from Dr. D. W. Jones, May 17, 1985, to the Health Protection Branch; and the CDA Journal, January 1986 News Update, p. 6—This information is from www.geocities.com/Athens/9313/dent.html

CHAPTER 2

55. Schulte, A., *Schweiz Monatsschr Zahnmed*, 104(11):1336–40, 1994, or *J Dent Res*, 73(4):980, A–334
56. Canadian Dental Association Dental Amalgam Patient Information Sheet, p. 1
57. *Journal of the American Medical Association (JAMA)*, 280(8):701–7, 1998
58. Coulter, H. L. and Fisher, B. L., *A Shot In the Dark*, 1991, ISBN 0-89529-463-X, Avery Publishing, Garden City Park, NY 11040, 1-800-548-5757
59. *ibid.*
60. Wilson, G. S., *The Hazards of Immunization*, The University of London, Athlone Press, London, UK, 1967
61. *Townsend Letter for Doctors & Patients*, 205/206:148–50, 2000
62. Smith, L., *Townsend Letter for Doctors & Patients*, 205/206:50–4 & 126–30, 2000
63. Scheibner, V., *VACCINATION: 100 Years of Orthodox Research Shows that Vaccines Represent a Medical Assault on the Immune System*, Australian Print Group, Victoria, Australia, 1993
64. *ibid.*
65. Dettman, G., *Blackmores Communicator—The Professional Services Newsbrief of Blackmore Laboratories*, Vol. 6, Sydney, Australia, and Auckland, New Zealand, May 1983
66. Kalokerinos, A., *Every Second Child*, Thomas Nelson, Australia, 1981; and Kalokerinos, A., Dettman, G., *The Australasian Nurses Journal*, August 1980
67. Madsen, T., *JAMA*, 101(3):187–8, 1933
68. *JAMA*, 131(9):730–5, 1946
69. *Journal of Pediatrics*, 101(5):419–21, 1982
70. Torch, W. C., *Neurology*, 32(4):A169, 1982
71. *Pediatric Infection Dis*, 2:7, 1983
72. *American Journal of Epidemiology*, 1992
73. Storsaeter, J., et al., *Pediatrics Infectious Disease Journal*, 78:637–45, 1988
74. Sutter, R. W., et al., *Journal of Infectious Diseases*, 165:444–9, 1992
75. Odent, M. R., et al., *JAMA*, Aug. 24/31, 1994
76. Kemp, T., et al., *Epidemiology*, 8:678–80, 1997
77. *Pediatrics*, 68(5):650–9, 1981; United States Department of Health and Human Services, *Immunization: Survey of Recent Research*, April 1983

78. *New Zealand Medical Journal,* May 24, 1996; *Infectious Diseases in Clinical Practice,* October 22,1997
79. Herroelen, L., *et al., Lancet,* 338:1174–5, 1991
80. Ribera, E. F., Dutka, A.. J., *New England Journal of Medicine,* 309:614–5, 1983
81. Poullin, P., Gabriel, B., *Lancet,* 334:1293, 1994
82. Lilic, D., Ghosh, S. K., *Lancet,* 334:1292–3, 1994
83. Trevisani, F., *et al., Journal of Hepatology,* 19:317–8, 1993
84. Gross, K., *et al., Scandinavian Journal of Rheumatology* 24:50–2, 1995; Vautier, G., Carter, J. E., *British Journal of Rheumatology,* 33:991, 1995; Hachulla, E., *et al., Journal of Rheumatology,* 17:1250–1, 1990
85. Martinez, E., Domingo, P., *Clinical Infectious Diseases,* 15:1051, 1992
86. Benjamin, C. M., *et al., British Medical Journal,* 1075–78, April 25, 1992
87. Thompson, N. P., *et al., Lancet,* 1071–4, April 29, 1995
88. Wakefield, A. J., *et al., Lancet,* 637–41, February 28, 1998
89. www.Mercola.com: Why Japan Banned MMR Vaccine, February 21, 2001
90. Mendelsohn, R., "The Medical Time Bomb of Immunization Against Disease," *East West Journal,* November 1984
91. Pichichero, M. E., *et al., Pediatrics,* 256–60, February 1979
92. Halperin, S. A., *et al., Journal of Pediatrics,* 686–93, November 1989
93. Christie, D. C., *et al., New England Journal of Medicine,* 16–20, July 7,1994
94. Nkowane, B., *et al., American Journal of Public Health,* 77:434–8, 1987
95. Gustafson, T., *et al., New England Journal of Medicine,* 316:771–4, 1987
96. Edmondson, M., *et al., Journal of the American Medical Association,* 263:2467–71, 1990
97. Chen, R., *et al., American Journal of Epidemiology,* 129:173–82, 1989
98. "Immunization Public Health Protector?" Issued under NIB National Office of Health Development, Ottawa, Canada, 1979
99. *The Vancouver Sun,* Feb. 9, 2001
100. *WHO Chronicle* 22:8:354–362, 1968; 22:12:523–7, 1968; 23:10:465–476, 1969; 25:6:249–255, 1971; 29:134–139, 1975
101. Kalokerinos, A., Dettman, G., *The Australasian Nurses Journal,* August 1980

102. *JAMA*, 282(18):1763–6, 1999
103. www.iVillage/allHealth.com Vaccines: Vaccination Issues: Mercury to Be Removed from Vaccines
104. Uchida, T., *et al.*, *Int Arch Allergy Immunol*, 104(3):296–301, 1994
105. Manzini, B. M., *et al.*, *Pediatric Dermatology*, 15(1):12–17, 1998
106. *Pediatrics*, 104(3):570–4, 1999
107. www.iVillage/allHealth.com Vaccines: Vaccination Issues: Mercury to Be Removed from Vaccines
108. Healy, J. M., *Endangered Minds: Why Children Can't Think—and What We Can Do About It*, Touchstone, New York, New York, 1990
109. Shoenfeld, Y., Aron-Maor, A., *Journal of Autoimmunity*, 14(1):1–10, 2000
110. *Journal of the American Dental Association*, 130:191–9, 1999; *Journal of Neural Transmission*, 105:59–68, 1998
111. www.mercola.com Leading Mercury Scientist, Dr. Haley, Refutes ADA in Congressional Testimony, 6/9/01
112. www.autism-society.org/autism.html
113. *Lancet*, 351:611–2, 1998
114. *Digestive Diseases and Sciences* 45(4):723–9, 2000
115. www.mercola.com "Autism and Mercury" by Tim O'Shea, DC
116. www.edelsoncenter.com/autism.htm
117. Edelson, S. B., Cantor, D. S., *Toxicology and Industrial Health*, 14(4):553–63, 1998
118. Hallaway, N., Strauts, Z., *Turning Lead Into Gold*, New Star Books, Vancouver, BC, Canada
119. Obomsawin, R., *Universal Immunization: Medical Miracle or Masterful Mirage?*, Health Action Network Society, Burnaby, BC, Canada
120. www.mercola.com Doctor's Group Opposes Vaccine Mandates, 11/19/00
121. Obomsawin, R., *Universal Immunization: Medical Miracle or Masterful Mirage?* Health Action Network Society, Burnaby, BC, Canada

CHAPTER 3

122. Dalton, R. H., *Journal of the American Medical Association*, 20:599–600, 1893
123. *Smart Drug News*, 2(10), 1994; 4(10), 1996; see www.ceri.com
124. O'Regan and Hirshberg, *Spontaneous Remissions*, 1993, Institute of Noetic Sciences
125. Lewison, E. F., *National Cancer Institute Monographs*, 44:23–26, 1976
126. *Gynecologic Oncology*, 78(2):123–9, 2000
127. *Br J Urology*, 66(4):398–404, 1990; *Zuckerschwerdt Verlag*,154–60, 1986; *Therpiewoche* 36:1686–96, 1986; *Clin Ther*, 17(1):82–7, 1995
128. *Pharmacometrics* 31(1):1–11, 1986; *Acta Physiol Pol*, 39(3):188–94, 1988
129. *Prostate*, 26(3):133–9, 1995; *J Med Chem*, 38(4):735–8, 1995; *Prostate*, 34(2):92–9, 1998; *J Nat Prod*, 60(4):356–60, 1997
130. *Atherosclerosis*, 62(1):39–45, 1986; *Arch Immunol Ther Exp*, 35(5):725–9, 1987
131. Horowitz, L. G., DMD, *Emerging Viruses* 1996, ISBN 0-923550-12-7, Tetrahedron Publishing, 20 Drumlin Road, Rockport, Mass 01966
132. *Science*, 313, October 20, 1967
133. James, W., *Immunization—The Reality Behind The Myth*, Bergin & Garvey Publishers Inc., S. Hadley, Massachusetts, 1988
134. Crinnion, W., *Alt Med Review*, 5(1):52–63, 2000

CHAPTER 4

135. www.epa.gov/swercepp/ehs/firstaid/7487947.txt
136. Truss, C. O., MD, *The Missing Diagnosis*, 1983,
ISBN 0-9615758-0-8, PO Box 26508, Birmingham, AL 35226
137. *Alternatives*, 16(4), 1997
138. *Townsend Letter for Doctors & Patients*, 205/206:22, 2000
139. Patrick, L., Uzick, M., *Alternative Medicine Review*, 6(3):248–271,
2001
140. *ibid.*
141. *Environmental Health Perspectives*, 103(7):103–8, 1995
142. *Journal of the American Dental Association*, 28:548–58, 1941
143. Price, W. A., DDS, *Nutrition and Physical Degeneration*, 1945,
ISBN 0-916-764-00-1, Price-Pottenger Nutritional Foundation,
PO Box 2614, La Mesa, CA 92041, (714) 582-4168
144. *Science*, 275:41–2, 1997; *Clin Exp Allergy*, 29:766–71, 1999
145. *Canadian Medical Association Journal*, No. 37, p. 134 and p. 268,
1937
146. *Southern Medicine and Surgery (SMAS)*, Vol. 111:209–14, 1949;
SMAS, 113:101–7, 1951; *J of Applied Nutrition*, 6:224–78, 1953;
J of Applied Nutrition, 23(3 and 4):60–89, 1971
147. Mendelsohn, R. S., MD, *Confessions of a Medical Heretic*, 1979,
ISBN 0-8092-7726-3, Contemporary Books, 180 N. Michigan
Avenue, Chicago, Illinois 60601
148. Gandhi, M., *The Health Guide*, Shri Anand T. Hingorani,
Navajivan Trust, Ahmedabad, India, 1965
149. *New England Journal of Medicine*, 342(20):1516–18, 2000
150. www.abcnews.go.com/sections/living/DailyNews/
fda_interests0000925.html
151. *Journal of the American Medical Association*, 279(15):1200–5, 1998
152. *ibid.*
153. *ibid.*
154. *ibid.*
155. *Lancet*, 351:643–4
156. *Ann Rev Pub Health*, 13:363–83
157. *JAMA*, 276:1473–9, 1996
158. www.heall.com/body/altmed/treatment/disease/cancer/
hoxsey.html
159. *Accountability in Research*, 6:259–310
160. www.geocities.com/Athens/9313/fluor.html
161. *ibid.*

162. *Townsend Letter for Doctors & Patients*, 207:66–73, 2000
163. Sahelian, R., and Gates, D., *The Stevia Cookbook*, Avery Publishing Group, 1999; Rona, Z. P., *Health Naturally*, August/September 1996, p. 4–7

Bernard Windham's References

Each of the index numbers—in bold type and underlined, as cited in Part III—correlates with one or more reference numbers (shown in parentheses) from Bernard Windham's articles. This list of index numbers is followed by the actual references. Only references that are cited are listed. The articles themselves, including all references, can be found on the Eating Alive Website at www.eatingalive.com.

1: (51), (81), (98), (182), (225)

2: (35), (222), (228b), (256)

3: (60), (222), (225), (226), (234), (235), (265), (293), (313), (314), (342), (368), (369), (404)

4: (34), (35), (182), (204)

5: (14), (16), (17), (19), (36), (57), (61), (77 to 83), (94), (129), (130), (138), (161), (167), (183), (191), (196), (211), (216), (273), (292), (303), (332)

6: (18), (77), (83), (85), (93), (138), (183), (199), (211), (292), (315), (335)

7: (2), (36), (83), (89), (93), (183), (199), (209), (217), (261), (292), (335)

8: (199), (292), (315), (318)

9: (15), (35)

10: (240), (400)

11: (219), (247)

12: (B4), (B5), (B11), (B15), (B19), (B22), (B23), (B25), (B30 to 35)

13: (335), (348), (349), (363)

14: (35), (332)

15: (370)

16: (17), (40), (45), (59), (129), (131), (251), (296), (350)

17: (53), (116), (117), (161), (258), (389)

18: (311)

19: (14), (20), (25), (85), (99), (175), (262), (273), (274), (301)

20:   (1), (14), (16), (19), (20), (25), (34), (38), (61), (85), (99), (162), (211), (273), (274), (287), (327), (348), (360), (366), (369)

21:   (34), (158), (207)

22:   (20), (34), (35), (38), (85)

23:   (19), (27), (28), (29), (30), (35), (100), (192), (194)

24:   (192)

25:   (19), (25), (27), (29), (30), (35), (47), (48), (100), (182), (192), (292), (348), (349), (390)

26:   (25), (30), (35), (48)

27:   (B3), (B23), (B24)

28:   (B16 to 21)

29:   (38), (99), (363)

30:   (171), (172), (173), (253), (303), (362)

31:   (74), (156), (247)

32:   (10), (38), (275), (401)

33:   (10), (24), (38), (121)

34:   (10), (31), (38), (277), (433)

35:   (32), (245), (246), (247), (248)

36:   (14), (34), (99), (143), (283)

37:   (277)

38:   (69), (70), (123), (249), (290), (395)

39:   (68), (69), (70), (249), (290), (395)

40:   (70), (249), (290), (395)

41:   (68), (70), (249), (290), (395)

42:   (1), (34), (68 to 74), (99)

43:   (14), (34), (99)

44:   (1)

45:   (15)

46:   (284)

47:   (63)

48:   (156)

49:   (362), (408)

50:   (35), (139), (163)

51:   (271)

52:   (34), (35), (94), (95), (102), (170), (212), (222), (229), (271), (291), (302)

53:   (222), (302)

54:   (8), (26), (35), (40), (46), (94), (95), (97), (165), (212), (222), (228), (229), (233), (271), (317), (322), (349), (376)

55:   (35), (97), (229), (405), (423)

56:   (35), (204)

57:   (35), (102), (212), (233)

58: (35), (57), (94), (212), (222), (229), (233), (271), (317), (322), (440), (453)

59: (35), (95), (103), (212), (222), (271), (313), (322), (358)

60: (8), (75), (97), (222), (228), (271), (322)

61: (35), (95), (212), (222), (232), (233), (271)

62: (35), (38), (94), (180)

63: (26), (35), (95), (115), (222), (229), (232), (233), (313), (320), (368)

64: (222), (229)

65: (35), (40), (94), (107), (212), (222), (229), (233), (271), (285e), (317), (320), (322), (376), (453)

66: (40), (95), (212), (222), (271), (322), (376),(453)

67: (60), (94), (212), (222), (271), (313), (317), (323), (341), (376), (459)

68: (5), (35), (229), (309)

69: (35), (222), (271), (322)

70: (8), (35), (60), (212), (222), (229), (232), (233), (271), (293), (313), (317), (323), (368), (369), (375), (376), (440)

71: (35), (94), (222), (293), (317), (322), (369), (440)

72: (40), (187), (271), (317), (322), (349)

73: (5), (34), (35), (95), (115), (212), (222), (229), (233), (271), (317), (322), (349), (354), (376), (440), (453)

74: (35), (59), (94), (115), (205), (212), (222), (232), (233), (271), (306), (310)

75: (8), (35), (60), (91), (212), (222), (229), (270), (271), (291), (313), (323), (368)

76: (9), (35), (38), (229), (367)

77: (35), (94), (212), (222), (271), (317), (322), (376)

78: (35), (40), (222), (251), (317), (349), (350)

79: (12), (35), (113), (222), (229), (233), (323)

80: (35), (94), (212), (222), (440), (453)

81: (87), (251)

82: (35), (94), (212), (222), (322)

83: (35), (94), (98), (212), (222), (229), (248), (271)

84: (35), (40), (46), (57), (60), (75), (78), (82), (86), (87), (90), (94), (95), (100), (101), (115), (133), (168), (212), (222), (233), (271), (313), (317), (321), (322), (376)

85: (6), (35)

86: (212), (222), (323), (375), (385), (408), (459)

87: (34), (35), (294)

88: (35), (40), (94), (222), (271), (322)

89: (35), (95), (212), (222), (228), (229), (233), (271), (317), (322), (440)

90: (35), (94), (222), (271), (349), (376)

91: (212), (222)

92: (35), (212), (271), (322)
93: (233)
94: (120), (153), (397)
95: (57), (79), (82), (89), (93), (115), (196), (303)
96: (222), (271), (359)
97: (164)
98: (61)
99: (183), (189), (208), (238)
100: (209)
101: (282)
102: (20), (22), (23), (31), (36), (61), (162), (186), (281), (348), (366)
103: (281), (287)
104: (20), (49), (119c), (264), (287), (304), (338)
105: (43), (96), (198), (263), (264), (338), (339), (347), (427)
106: (35), (50), (91), (212), (222), (369), (382), (459)
107: (1), (3), (38), (39), (110), (160), (263), (264), (285c)
108: (23), (35), (37), (38), (110), (142), (241)
109: (10), (23), (38), (287), (338c)
110: (19), (20), (22), (23), (61), (112), (186), (210), (287), (304)
111: (20), (112), (186), (304), (339)
112: (112), (304), (391)
113: (20), (22), (23), (61), (304)
114: (19), (20), (38), (112), (304)
115: (61)
116: (3), (160)
117: (D34 to 36)
118: (D33), (D36), (D37), (D43)
119: (C2c), (C2d), (C23), (C30), (C40)
120: (C22), (C39), (C47), (C50)
121: (C15 to 23), (C36), (C47), (C51)
122: (C15 to 17), (C19), (C20), (C22)
123: (C24), (C25), (C27)
124: (C24), (C26)
125: (C24), (C25)
126: (C14), (C21), (C25c)
127: (C26)
128: (C11), (C12), (C30), (C35), (C40), (C48)
129: (C14 to 22), (C35), (C50)
130: (C29)
131: (C22), (C37), (C38), (C50)
132: (13), (33), (54), (96), (111), (126), (194), (252), (338), (410 to 412)
133: (33), (35), (56), (330), (331)

MAIN ARTICLE

Facts about Mercury and Dental Amalgam (with Medical Study References). Bernard Windham, Editor- Chemical Engineer

(1)   Denton, S. (MD), Butler, J., Dept. Of Psychology, Univ. Of North Texas, Proceedings of the First International Conference on Biocompatibility, Life Sciences Press, Oct 1990, p. 133–45

(2)   U.S. Environmental Protection Agency (EPA), 1999, "Integrated Risk Information System," National Center for Environmental Assessment, Cincinnati, Ohio, http://www.epa.gov/ncea/iris.htm

(3)   Marlowe, M., *et al.*, "Main and interactive effects of metallic toxins on classroom behavior," *J Abnormal Child Psychol*, 13(2):185–98, 1985; & Moon, C., *et al.*, "Main and interactive effect of metallic pollutants on cognitive functioning," *Journal of Learning Disabilities*, Apr 1985; & Pihl, R. O., *et al.*, "Hair element content in learning disabled children," *Science*, 198:204–6, 1977; & Gowdy, J. M., *et al.*, "Whole blood mercury in mental hospital patients," *Am J Psychiatry*, 135(1):115–7, 1978

(5)   D. Klinghardt (MD), "Migraines, Seizures, and Mercury Toxicity," Future Medicine Publishing, 1997

(6)   T. M. Schulein, *et al.*, "Survey of Des Moines area dental offices for mercury vapour," *Iowa Dent J*, 70(1):35–6, 1984; & D. W. Jones, *et al.*, "Survey of mercury vapour in dental offices in Atlantic Canada," *Can Dent Assoc J*, 4906:378–95, 1983; & R. W. Miller, *et al.*, "Report on independent survey taken of Austin dental offices for mercury contamination," *Texas Dent J*, 100(1):6–9, 1983; & A. Skuba, "Survey for mercury vapour in Manitoba dental offices," *J Can Dent Assoc*, 50(7):517–22, 1984; & R. H. Roydhouse, *et al.*, "Mercury in dental offices," *J Can Dent Assoc*, 51(2):156–8, 1985; & R. T. McNerney, *et al.*, "Mercury contamination in the dental office: a review," *NYS Dental Journal*, p. 457–8, Nov 1979

(8)   Redhe, O., *Sick From Amalgam*, R-Dental Ab, Frejavagen 33, S-79133 Falun, Sweden (100 cases) Olle Redhe: [olle.redhe@telia.com]

(9)   Dr. I. Gerhard, Dr. E. Roller, *et al.*, Tubingen Univ. Gynecological Clinic, Heidelberg, 1996; & "Heavy metals and fertility," *J of Toxicology and Environmental Health*, Part A, 54(8):593–611, 1998; & "Impact of heavy metals on hormonal and immunological factors in women with repeated miscarriages," & I. Gerhard, "Ganzheitiche diagnostik un therapie bie infertilitat," *Erfahrungsheilkunde*, 42(3):100–6, 1993; & "Unfruchtbarkeit bei frauen durch umweltgifte," in *Pravention, Diagnose und Therapie von Umwelterkrankungen*, J. D. Kruse-Jarres (Ed.), 1993, p. 51–68; & Gerhard, I., Waldbrenner, P., Thuro, H., Runnebaum, B., "Diagnosis of heavy metal loading by the oral DMPS and chewing gum tests," *Klinisches Labor*, 38:404–1, 1992

(10)   Editorial, *J California Dental Assoc*, 12:37, 1984; & Proceedings of Intl. Conference on Mercury Hazards in Dental Practice, Sept 2–4, 1981, Glasgow, Scot, Dept. of Clinical Physics and Bio-Engineering, (Gordon—Pregnancy in Female Dentists— a Mercury Hazard) & (several survey studies comparing level of mercury in hair of dental staff vs. controls); & Gordon H. P., Cordon L. D., "Reduction in mercury vapour levels in Seattle dental offices," *J Dent Res*, Abstract 1092, 57A:347, 1981

(12)   Dimaval Scientific monograph, sixth ed., Jan 1997, Dr Johann Ruprecht, Heyl Corporation

(13)   S. Hussain, *et al.*, "Mercuric chloride-induced reactive oxygen species and its effect on antioxidant enzymes in different regions of rat brain," *J Environ Sci Health*, 32(3):395–409 B May 1997; & S. Tan, *et al.*, "Oxidative stress induces programmed cell death in neuronal cells," *J Neurochem*, 71(1):95–105, 1998; & J. S. Bains, *et al.*, "Neurodegenerative disorders in humans and role of glutathione in oxidative stress mediated neuronal death," *Brain Res Rev*, 25(3):335–8, 199?; & P. Bulat, "Activity of Gpx and SOD in workers occupationally exposed to mercury," *Arch Occup Environ Health*, 71 Suppl:S37–9, Sep 1998; & Stohs, S. J., Bagchi, D., "Oxidative mechanisms in the toxicity of metal ions," *Free Radic Biol Med*, 18(2):321–6, 1995

(14)   (a) Magnus Nylander, "Mercury concentrations in the human brain and kidneys in relation to exposure from dental amalgam fillings," Proceedings, ICBM 1988; & M. Nylander, *et al.*, "Mercury concentrations in the human brain and kidneys and

exposure from amalgam fillings," *Swed Dent J*, 11:179–87, 1987; & *Prosth Dent*, 58:704–7, 1987; & (b) Schupp, Riedel, *et al.*, "Amalgamfullungen auf die quecksilberkonzentration in menschlichen," *Organen Dt Zahnarztl Z*, 47:490–6, 1992; & (c) Barregard, L., Svalander, C., Schutz, A., Westberg, G., Sallsten, G., Blohm, Molne, J., Attman, P. O., Haglind, P., "Cadmium, mercury, and lead in kidney cortex of the general Swedish population: a study of biopsies from living kidney donors," *Environ Health Perspect*, 107(11):867–71, Nov 1999

(15)   Svare, C. W., *et al.*, Univ. of Iowa, "The effects of dental amalgam on mercury levels in expired air," *J Dent Res*, 60(9):1668–71, 1981; & Patterson, J. E., "Mercury in human breath from dental amalgams," *Bull Env Contam Toxicol*, 34:459, 1985

(16)   K. Ott, *et al.*, "Mercury burden due to amalgam fillings," *Dtsch Zahnarztl Z*, 39(9):199–205, 1984; & Lichtenberg H., "Mercury vapour in the oral cavity in relation to number of amalgam surfaces and the classic symptoms of chronic mercury poisoning," *J Orthomol Med*, 11(2):87–94, 1996

(17)   J. Abraham, C. Svare, *et al.*, "The effects of dental amalgam restorations on blood mercury levels," *J Dent Res*, 63(1):71–3, 1984; & Snapp, K. R., Boyer, D. B., Peterson, L. C., Svare, C. W., "The contribution of dental amalgam to mercury in blood," *J Dent Res*, 68(5):780–5, May 1989

(18)   M. J. Vimy, F. L. Lorscheider, "Intra oral mercury released from dental amalgams and estimation of daily dose," *J Dent Res*, 64(8):1069–75, 1985; & *Res*, 64(8):1072–5, 1985

(19)   Matts Hanson, Dept of Zoophysiology, University of Lund, Sweden. "Amalgam hazards in your teeth," *J Orthomolecular Psychiatry*, 2(3):194–201, 1983; & F. L. Lorscheider, *et al.*, "Evaluation of the safety issue of mercury release from amalgam fillings," *FASEB J*, 7:1432–3, 1993

(20)   Vimy, M. J., Takahashi, Y., Lorscheider, F. L., "Maternal–fetal distribution of mercury released from dental amalgam fillings," Dept of Medicine and Medical Physiology, Faculty of Medicine, Univ of Calgary, Calgary, Alberta Canada, 1990, & *Amer J*

Physiol, 258:R939–45, 1990; & N. D. Boyd, M. J. Vimy, *et al.*, "Mercury from dental silver tooth fillings impairs sheep kidney function," *Am J Physiol*, 261 (Regulatory Integrative Comp Physiol 30):R1010–R1014, 1991; & L. Hahn, *et al.*, "Distribution of mercury released from amalgam fillings into monkey tissues," *FASEB J*, 4:5536, 1990

(22)   P. Kuhnert, *et al.*, "Comparison of mercury levels in maternal blood fetal cord blood and placental tissue," *Am J Obstet and Gynecol*, 139:209–12, 1981; & Vahter, M., Akesson, A., Lind, B., Bjors, U., Schutz, A.., Berglund, M., "Longitudinal study of methylmercury and inorganic mercury in blood and urine of pregnant and lactating women, as well as in umbilical cord blood," *Environ Res*, 84(2):186–94, Oct 2000

(23)   W. D. Kuntz, "Maternal and cord blood mercury background levels; longitudinal surveillance," *Am J Obstet and Gynecol*, 143(4):440–3, 1982

(24)   J. B. Brodsky, "Occupational exposure to mercury in dentistry and pregnancy outcome," JADA, 111(11):779–80, 1985

(25)   C. Malmström, M. Hansson, M. Nylander, Conference on Trace Elements in Health and Disease, Stockholm, May 25, 1992; & C. Malmström, *et al.*, "Silver amalgam: an unstable material," Swedish paper translated in Bio-Probe Newsletter, 9(1):5–6, Jan 1993; & C. Malmström, "Amalgam derived mercury in feces," *Journal of Trace Elements in Experimental Medicine*, 5, (Abs 122), 1992; & Nylander, *et al.*, Fourth International Symposium Epidemiology in Occupational Health, Como, Italy, Sept 1985

(26)   A. F. Zamm, "Removal of dental mercury: often an effective treatment for very sensitive patients," *J Orthomolecular Med*, 5(53):138–142, 1990 (22 patients)

(27)   Matts Hanson," Why is mercury toxic?: basic chemical and biochemical properties of mercury/amalgam in relation to biological effects," ICBM conference, Colorado Springs, Co., 1988, Proceedings; & Hartman, D. E., "Missed diagnoses and misdiagnoses of environmental toxicant exposure MCS," *Psychiatr Clin North Am*, 21(3):659–70, 1998; & *Merritt's Textbook of Neurology*, 9th Ed., Williams and Wilkins, Baltimore, 1995,

p. 668–; & *Clinical Management of Poisoning*, 3rd Ed., Haddad, Shannon, and Winchester, W. B. Saunders and Company, Philadelphia, 1998, p. 753; & U.S. EPA, Office of Health and Environmental Assessment, Mercury Health Effects, Update Health Issue Assessment, Final Report, 1984, EOA–600/8–84f

(28)   F. Schmidt, *et al.*, "Mercury in urine of employees exposed to magnetic fields," *Tidsskr Nor Laegeforen*, 117(2):199–202, 1997; & Sheppard, A. R., Eisenbud, M., *Biological Effects of Electric and Magnetic Fields of Extremely Low Frequency*, New York University Press, 1977; & Ortendahl, T. W., Hogstedt, P., Holland, R. P., "Mercury vapor release from dental amalgam in vitro caused by magnetic fields generated by CRTs," *Swed Dent J*, p. 31, Abstract 22, 1991

(29)   Mareck and Hockman, "Simulated crevice corrosion experiment for pH and solution chemistry determinations," *Corrosion*, 23:1000–6, 1974

(30)   T. Till, *et al.*, "Mercury release from amalgam fillings and oral dysbacteriosis as a cause of resorption phenomena," *Zahnarztl Welt/Reform (ZWR)*, 87;1130–4, 1978; & S. Olsson, *et al.*, "Release of elements due to electrochemical corrosion of dental amalgam," *J Dental Research*, 73:33–43, 1994; & T. Fusayama, *et al.*, *J Dental Research*, 42:1183–97, 1963; & H. Freden, *et al.*, "Mercury in gingival tissues adjacent to amalgam fillings," *Odontal Revy*, 25(2):207–10, 1974; & H. Reden, *Odontal Revy*, 25:207–210, 1971

(31)   Langan, Fan, Hoos, "The use of mercury in dentistry: a critical review of the literature," *JADA*, 115: 867, December 1987, Donated by The ADA; & Health damage due to exposure to mercury vapour (Mercury) Szkody zdrowotne wywolane narazeniem na pary rteci (Mercury). Moszczynski-P Jr; Moszczynski-P Czas-Stomatol. 1989 Apr; 42(4): 233–81989, POLISH; & I. Mandel, Assoc Dean for Research, School of Dental and Oral Surgury, Columbia Univ., N.Y., *JADA*, Vol. 122, Aug 1991

(32)   T. A. Cook, *et al.*, "Fatal mercury intoxication in a dental surgery assistant," *British Dent Journal*, 127:533–55, 1969

(33) (a) S. C. Langley–Evans, *et al.*, "SO2: a potent glutathione depleting agent," *Comp Biochem Physiol Pharmocol Toxicol Endocrinol*, 114(2):89–98; & (b) P.E. Emory, *et al.*, "Increased prevalence of poor sulphoxidation in patients with rheumatoid arthritis," *Ann Rheum Dis*, 51(3):318–20, 1992; & (c) Markovich, *et al.*, "Heavy metals (Hg, Cd) inhibit the activity of the liver and kidney sulfate transporter Sat-1," *Toxicol Appl Pharmacol*, 154(2):181–7, 1999; & (d) S. A. McFadden, "Xenobiotic metabolism and adverse environmental response: sulfur-dependent detox pathways," *Toxicology*, 111(1–3):43–65, 1996; & (e) Alberti, A., Pirrone, P., Elia, M., Waring, R. H., Romano, C., "Sulphation deficit in 'low-functioning' autistic children," *Biol Psychiatry*, 46(3):420–4, 1999

(34) Patrick Störtebecker, Associate Professor of Neurology, Karolinska Institute, Stockholm, *Mercury Poisoning from Dental Amalgam—a Hazard to Human Brain*, ISBN: 0-941011001-1 & *Dental Caries as a Cause of Nervous Disorders*, Bio-Probe Inc., http://www.bioprobe.com; & *Neurology for Barefoot Doctors*, Störtebecker Foundation for Research, 1988; & *J Canadian Dental Assoc*, 33(6):300–

(35) Huggins, H. A., Levy, T. E., *Uniformed Consent: The Hidden Dangers in Dental Care*, 1999, Hampton Roads Publishing Company Inc; & Hal Huggins, *It's All in Your Head*, 1997; & Center for Progressive Medicine, 1999, http://www.hugnet.com

(36) Sam Queen, *Chronic Mercury Toxicity—New Hope Against an Endemic Disease*, http://www.bioprobe.com; & F. L. Lorscheider, *et al.*, "Mercury exposure from silver tooth fillings: emerging evidence questions a paradigm," *FASEB J*, 9:504–8, 1995

(37) A. Anttila, *et al.*, Finnish Inst. of Occupational Health, "Effects of paternal occupation exposure to lead or mercury on spontaneous abortion," *J Occup Environ Med*, 37(8):915–21, 1995; & Cordier, S., Deplan, F., Mandereau, L., Hemon, D., "Paternal exposure to mercury and spontaneous abortions," *Br J Ind Med*, 48(6):375–81, Jun 1991; & Savitz D. A., Sonnenfeld, N. L., Olshan, A. F., "Review of epidemiologic studies of paternal occupational exposure and spontaneous abortion," *Am J Ind Med*, 25(3):361–83, Mar 1994; & Mohamed, *et al.*,

"Lazer light scattering study of the toxic effects of methylmercury on sperm motility," *J Androl*, 7(1):11–15, 1986

(38) S. Ziff, M. Ziff, *Infertility and Birth Defects: Is Mercury from Dental Fillings a Hidden Cause?*, Bio-Probe, Inc., ISBN: 0-941011-03-8.1987

(39) M. Inouye, *et al.*, "Behavorial and neuropathological effects of prenatal methyl mercury exposure in mice," *Neurobehav Toxicol Teratol*, 7;227–32, 1985; & P. Grandjean, *et al.*, "MeHg and neurotoxicity in children," *Am J Epidemiol*, 150(3):301–5, 1999; & Z. Annau, *et al.*, Johns Hopkins Univ., School of Public Health, "Mechanisms of neurotoxicity and their relationships to behavioral changes," *Toxicology*, 49(2): 219–25, 1988; & S. D. Vanay, *et al.*, "CNS arylsulfatases inhibited by methyl mercury," *Pharmacol Toxicol*, 69(1):71–4, 1991

(40) F. Perger, Amalgamtherape, in *Kompendiu der Regulationspathologie und Therapie*, Sonntag-Verlag, 1990; & "Belastungen durch toxische Schwermetalle," 87(2):157–63, 1993; & K. H. Friese, "Homoopathische behandlung der amalgamvergiftung," *Allg Homoopathische Z*, 241(5):184–7, & *Erfahrungsheikunde*, (4):251–3, 1996; & "Amalgamvergiftung_moglicher," *Der Naturazt*, 135(8):13–15, 1995; & "Schnupfen–Was tun?," *Therapeutikon*, 8(3):62–8, 1994; & Homoopathische Behandlung de Amalgamvergiftung & "Polemik und Wirklichkeit," *Allgemeine Homoopathische zeitschrift*, 239(6):225–33, 1994; & "Amalgamtherapie fur Arzte und Zahnarzte," Panta 3, 1992, Haug-Verlag.; & *Natura Med*, 7(4):295–306, 1992; & M. Strassburg, *et al.*, "Generalized allergic reaction from silver amalgam fillings," *Dtsche Zahnarztliche Zeit*, 22:3–9, 1967 (total: over 1,200 cases)

(43) Knapp, L. T., Klann, E., "Superoxide-induced stimulation of protein kinase C via thiol modification and modulation of zinc content," *J Biol Chem*, May 22, 2000; & B. Rajanna, *et al.*, "Modulation of protein kinase C by heavy metals," *Toxicol Lett*, 81(2–3):197–203, 1995; & A. Badou, *et al.*, "HgCl2-induced IL-4 gene expression in T cells involves a protein kinase C-dependent calcium influx through L-type calcium channels," & D. B. Veprintsev, 1996, Institute for Biological

Instrumentation, Russian Academy of Sciences, "Pb2+ and Hg2+ binding to alpha-lactalbumin," *Biochem Mol Biol Int,* 39(6):1255–65, Aug 1996

(45)   L. Pelletier, *et al.,* "In-vivo self reactivity of mononuclear cells to T cells and macrophages exposed to HgC_{l2}," *Eur J Immun,* 460–5, 1985; & Pelletier, *et al.,* "Autoreactive T cells in mercury-induced autoimmune disease," *J Immunol,* 137(8):2548–54, 1986; & *Scand J Immunology,* 31:65–74, 1990; & M. Kubicka, *et al.,* "Autoimmune disease induced by mercuric chloride," *Int Arch Allergy Immunol,* 109(1):11–20, Jan 1996

(46)   Veron, *et al.,* "Amalgam dentaires et allergies," *J Biol Buccale,* 14:83–100, 1986 (41 cases); & D. E. Swartzendruber, *Med Hyptheses,* 41(1):31–34, 1993

(47)   A. Buchner, *et al.,* "Amalgam tattoo of the oral mucosa: a clinicopathologic study of 268 cases," *Surg Oral Med Oral Pathol,* 49(2):139–47, 1980; & M. Forsell, *et al.,* "Mercury content in amalgam tattoos of human oral mucosa and its relation to local tissue reactions," *Euro J Oral Sci,* 106(1):582–7, 1998; & J. D. Harrison, *et al.,* "Amalgam tattoos: light and microscopy and electron-probe micro-analysis"; & T. Kanzaki, *et al.,* "Electron microscopic X-ray microanalysis of metals deposited in oral mucosa," *J Dermatol,* 19(8):487–92, 1992; & K. Nilner, *et al.,* "In vitro testing of dental materials by means of macrophage cultures," *J Biomed Mater Res,* 20(8):1125–38, 1986

(48)   K. Arvidson, "Corrosion studies of dental gold alloy in contact with amalgam," *Swed Dent J,* 68:135–9, 1984; & Skinner, E. W., *The Science of Dental Materials,* 4th Ed. revised, W. B. Saunders Co., Philadelphia, p. 284–5, 1957

(49)   A. Kingman, *et al.,* National Institute of Dental Research, "Mercury concentrations in urine and blood associated with amalgam exposure in the U.S. military population," *Dent Res,* 77(3):461–71, 1998

(50)   J. Kawada, *et al.,* "Effects of inorganic and methyl mercury on thyroidal function," *J Pharmacobiodyn,* 3(3):149–59, 1980; &

Ghosh, N., "Thyrotoxicity of cadmium and mercury," *Biomed Environ Sci*, 5(3):236–40, 1992

(51) Heintze, *et al.*, "Methylation of mercury from dental amalgam and mercuric chloride by oral streptococci," *Scan J Dent Res*, 91:150–2, 1983; & Rowland, Grasso, Davies, "The methylation of mercuric chloride by human intestinal bacteria," *Experientia Basel*, 31:1064–5, 1975; & M. K. Hamdy, *et al.*, "Formation of methyl mercury by bacteria," *App Microbiol*, Sep 1975; & W. Forth, "Toxikologie von quecksilberverbindungen," in *Quecksilber in der Umwelt-Hearing zur Amalgamprolematik*, Niedersachsisches Umweltministerium, 1991

(53) C. Thornsberry, MRL Services, Franklin, Tenn, Proceedings of Infectious Diseases Soc. of America, San Francisco, Ca.; & *USA Today*, April 1997; & *Science News*, Vol. 155, p. 356, June 5, 1999

(54) M. E. Lund, *et al.*, "Treatment of acute MeHg poisoning by NAC," *J Toxicol Clin Toxicol*, 22(1):31–49, 1984; & Livardjani, F., Ledig, M., Kopp, P., Dahlet, M., Leroy, M., Jaeger, A., "Lung and blood superoxide dismutase activity in mercury vapor exposed rats: effect of N-acetylcysteine treatment," *Toxicology*, 66(3):289–95, Mar 11, 1991; & G. Ferrari, *et al.*, Dept. of Pathology, Columbia Univ., *J Neurosci*, 15(4):2857–66, 1995; & R. R. Ratan, *et al.*, Dept. of Neurology, Johns Hopkins Univ., *J Neurosci*, 14(7):4385–92, 1994; & Z. Gregus, *et al.*, "Effect of lipoic acid on biliary excretion of glutathione and metals," *Toxicol Appl Pharmacol*, 114(1):88–96, 1992; & J. F. Balch, *et al.*, *Prescription for Nutritional Healing*, 2nd Ed., 1997

(56) X. M. Shen, *et al.*, "Neurobehavioral effects of NAC conjugates of dopamine: possible relevance for Parkinson's Disease," *Chem Res Toxicol*, 9(7):1117–26, 1996; & *Chem Res Toxicol*, 11(7):824–37, 1998; & A. Nicole, *et al.*, "Direct evidence for glutathione as mediator of apoptsosis in neuronal cells," *Biomed Pharmacother*, 52(9):349–55, 1998; & J. P. Spencer, *et al.*, "Cysteine & GSH in PD," mechanisms involving ROS," *J Neurochem*, 71(5):2112–22, 1998; & P. Jenner, "Oxidative mechanisms in PD," *Mov Disord*, 13 (Supp1):24–34, 1998; & D. Offen, *et al.*, "Use of thiols in treatment of PD," *Exp Neurol*, 141(1):32–9, 1996; & A. D. Owen, *et al.*, *Ann NY Acad Sci*, 786:217–33, 1996; & J. J. Heales, *et al.*, *Neurochem Res*, 21(1):35–9, 1996

(57)   (a) N. Campbell, M. Godfrey, "Confirmation of mercury retention and toxicity using DMPS provocation," *J of Advancement in Medicine*, 7(1), 1994 (80 cases); & (b) D. Zander, *et al.*, "Mercury mobilization by DMPS in subjects with and without amalgams," *Zentralbl Hyg Umweltmed*, 192(5):447–54, 1992 (12 cases)

(59)   A. Frustaci, *et al.*, "Marked elevation of mycardial trace elements in Idiopathic Dilated Cardiomyopathy," *J of American College of Cardiology*, 33(6):1578–83, 1999; & Husten L., "Trace elements linked to cardiomyopathy," *Lancet*, 353(9164):1594, 1999; & D. V. Vassalo, "Effects of mercury on the isolated heart muscle are prevented by DTT and cysteine," *Toxicol Appl Pharmacol*, 156(2):113–8, Apr 15, 1999; & N. G. Ilblack, *et al.*, "New aspects of murine coxsackie B_3 myocarditis: focus on heavy metals," *European Heart J*, 16:supp O:20–4, 1995

(60)   V. D. M. Stejskal, Dept. of Clinical Chemistry, Karolinska Institute, Stockholm, Sweden LYMPHOCYTE IMMUNO-STIMULATION ASSAY—MELISA® & V. D. M. Stejskal, *et al.*, "MELISA®: tool for the study of metal allergy," *Toxicology in Vitro*, 8(5):991–1000, 1994

(61)   E. Lutz, *et al.*, "Concentrations of mercury in brain and kidney of fetuses and infants," *Journal of Trace Elements in Medicine and Biology*, 10:61–67, 1996; & G. Drasch, *et al.*, "Mercury burden of human fetal and infant tissues," *Eur J Pediatr*, 153:607–610, 1994

(63)   K. Peiper, *et al.*, "Study of mercury uptake in dental students," *Dtsch Zahnarzt Z*, 44(9):714–, 1989

(68)   K. A. Ritchie, *et al.*, Univ. of Glasgow, "Psychomotor testing of dentists with chronic low level mercury exposure," *J Dent Res*, 74:420, IADR Abstract 160 (1995); & *Occup Environ Med*, 52(12): 813–7, 1995

(69)   D. Gonzalez-Ramirez, *et al.*, "Urinary mercury, porphyrins, and neurobehavioral changes of dental workers in Monterrey, Mexico," *J Pharmocology and Experimental Therapeutics*, 272(1):264–74, 1995

(70)   D. Echeverria, *et al.*, Batelle Center for Public Health Research, Seattle, "Behavioral effects of low level exposure to Hg vapor among dentists," *Neurotoxicology & Teratology*, 17(2):161–8, 1995

(71)   S. C. Foo, *et al.*, "Neurobehavioral effects in occupational chemical exposure," *Environmental Research*, 60(2):267–73, 1993; D. G. Mantyla, *et al.*, "Mercury toxicity in the dental office: a neglected problem," *JADA*, 92:1189–94, 1976

(72)   D. L. Smith, "Mental effects of mercury poisoning," *South Med J*, 71:904–5, 1978

(73)   M. E. Cianciola, *et al.*, "Epidemiologic assessment of measures used to indicate exposure to mercury vapor," *Toxicol Eniviron Health*, 52(1):19–33, 1997

(74)   A. C. Bittner, *et al.*, "Behavior effects of low level mercury exposure among dental professionals," *Neurotoxicology & Teratology*, 20(4):429–39, 1998

(75)   Katsunuma, *et al.*, "Anaphylaxis improvement after removal of amalgam fillings," *Annals of Allergy*, 64(5):472–5, 1990; & Yoshida, S., Mikami, H., Nakagawa, H., Amayasu, H., "Amalgam allergy associated with exacerbation of aspirin-intolerant asthma," *Clin Exp Allergy*, 29(10):1412–4, 1999; & M. Drouet, *et al.*, "Is mercury a respiratory tract allergen?" *Allerg Immunol* (Paris), 22(3):81, 1990

(77)   I. Skare, "Mass balance and systemic uptake of mercury released from dental fillings," *Water, Air, and Soil Pollution*, 80(1–4):59–67, 1995

(78)   G. Drasch, *et al.*, "Silver concentrations in human tissues: the dependence on dental amalgam," *J Trace Elements in Medicine and Biology*, 9(2):82–7,1995; & L. J. Calsakis, *et al.*, "Allergy to silver amalgams," *Oral Surg*, 46:371–5, 1978

(79)   L. Bjorkman, *et al.*, "Mercury in saliva and feces after removal of amalgam fillings," *Toxicology and Applied Pharmacology*, 144(1):156–62, 1997; & (b) *J Dent Res*, 75:38–, IADR Abstract 165, 1996

(80)   M. Osterblad, *et al.*, "Antimicrobial and mercury resistance
among persons with and without amalgam fillings,"
Antimicrobial Agents and Chem, 39(11):2499, 1995

(81)   L. I. Liang, *et al.*, "Mercury reactions in the human mouth with
dental amalgams," *Water, Air, and Soil Pollution*, 80:103–7

(82)   J. Begerow, *et al.*, "Long-term mercury excretion in urine after
removal of amalgam fillings," *Int Arch Occup Health*, 66:209–12,
1994

(83)   I. Skare, *et al.*, Swedish National Board of Occupational Safety
and Health, "Human exposure to Hg and Ag released from
dental amalgam restorations," *Archives of Environmental Health*,
49(5):384–94, 1994

(85)   J. A. Weiner, *et al.*, "The relationship between mercury
concentration in human organs and predictor variables," *Sci Tot
Environ*, 138(1–3):101–15, 1993; & "An estimation of the uptake
of mercury from amalgam fillings in Swedish subjects," *Sci Tot
Environ*, 168(3):255–65, 1995

(86)   E. R. Smart, *et al.*, "Resolution of lichen planus following
removal of amalgam restorations," *Br Dent J*, 178(3):108–12,
1995 (12 cases); & H. Markow, "Regression from orticaria
following dental filling removal," *New York State J Med*,
1648–52, 1943; & G. Sasaki, *et al.*, "Three cases of oral lichenosis
caused by metallic fillings," *J Dermatol*, 12:890–2, Dec 23, 1996;
& J. Bratel, *et al.*, "Effect of replacement of dental amalgam on
OLR," *Journal of Dentistry*, 24(1–2):41–5, 1996 (161 cases)

(87)   A. Skoglund, *Scand J Dent Res*, 102(4):216–22, 1994; and
99(4):320–9, 1991 (40 cases); & P. O. Ostman, *et al.*, "Clinical and
histologic changes after removal of amalgam," *Oral Surgery,
Oral Medicine, and Endodontics*, 81(4):459–65, 1996; & S. H.
Ibbotson, *et al.*, "The relevance of amalgam replacement on oral
lichenoid reactions," *British Journal of Dermatology*, 134(3):420–3,
1996 (270 cases)

(89)   (a) Berglund, A., Molin, M., "Mercury levels in plasma and
urine after removal of all amalgam restorations: the effect of
using rubber dams," *Dent Mater*, 13(5):297–304, Sep 1997; &

M. Molin, *et al.*, "Kinetics of mercury in blood and urine after amalgam removal," *J Dent Res*, 74:420, IADR Abstract 159, 1995; & (b) M. Molin, *et al.*, "Mercury, selenium, and GPX before and after amalgam removal," *Acta Odontol Scand*, 48:189–202, 1990

(90)   P. Koch, *et al.*, "Oral lesions and symptoms related to metals," *Dermatol*, 41(3):422–30, 1999; & "Oral lichenoid lesions, mercury hypersensitivity, ...," *Contact Dermatitis*, 33(5): 323–8, 1995; & S. Freeman, *et al*, "Oral lichenoid lesions caused by allergy to mercury in amalgam," *Contact Dermatitis*, 33(6):423–7, Dec 1995 (Denmark); & H. Mobacken, *et al.*, *Contact Dermatitis*, 10:11–15, 1984; & M. Jolly, *et al.*, "Amalgam-related chronic ulceration of oral mucosa," *Br Dent J*, 160:434–7, 1986; & C. Camisa, *et al.*, "Contact hypersensitivity to mercury," *Cutis*, 63(3):189–, 1999

(91)   B. Lindqvist, *et al.*, "Effects of removing amalgam fillings from patients with diseases affecting the immune system," *Med Sci Res*, 24(5):355–6, 1996

(93)   L. Barregard, *et al.*, "People with high mercury uptake from their own dental amalgam fillings," *Occup Envir Med*, 52:124–8, 1995; & S. Langworth, *et al.*, "A case of high mercury exposure from dental amalgam," *European J Oral Sci*, 104(3):320–1, 1996; & R. Stromberg, *et al.*, "A case of unusually high mercury exposure from amalgam fillings," *Tandlakartidningen*, 88(10):570–2, 1996; & McCann, *et al.*, "Intravenous gamma globulin (IVIG) treatment of autoimmune kidney disease associated with mercury (Hg++) toxicity," *J Allergy Clin Immunol*, 95(1) (Pt 2):145

(94)   F. Berglund, *Case reports spanning 150 years on the adverse effects of dental amalgam*, Bio-Probe, Inc., Orlando, FL 1995, ISBN 0-9410011-14-3 (245 cured); & Tuthill, J. Y., "Mercurial neurosis resulting from amalgam fillings," *The Brooklyn Medical Journal*, 12(12):725–42, December 1898

(95)   Lichtenberg, H. J., "Elimination of symptoms by removal of dental amalgam from mercury poisoned patients," *J Orthomol Med*, 8:145–8, 1993; & Lichtenberg, H., "Symptoms before and after proper amalgam removal in relation to serum-globulin reaction to metals," *Journal of Orthomolecular Medicine*, 11(4):195–203, 1996 (119 cases)

(96) A. F. Goldberg, et al., "Effect of amalgam restorations on whole body potassium and bone mineral content in older men," *Gen Dent*, 44(3):246–8, 1996; & K. Schirrmacher, "Effects of lead, mercury, and methyl mercury on gap junctions and [Ca2+] in bone cells," *Calcif Tissue Int*, 63(2):134–9, Aug 1998

(97) Redhe, O., Pleva, J., "Recovery from ALS and from asthma after removal of dental amalgam fillings," *Int J Risk & Safety in Med*, 4:229–36, 1994; & Vanacore, N., Corsi, L., Fabrizio, E., Bonifati, V., Meco, G., "Relationship between exposure to environmental toxins and motor neuron disease: a case report," *Med Lav*, 86(6):522–33, Nov–Dec 1995

(98) A. Seidler, et al., "Possible environmental factors for Parkinson's disease," *Neurology*, 46(5):1275–84, 1996; & Vroom, F. O., Greer, M., "Mercury vapor intoxication," 95:305–18, 1972; & Ohlson, et al., "Parkinson's disease and occupational exposure to mercury," *Scand J. of Work Environment Health*, 7(4):252–6, 1981; L. G. Goleta, "Therapeutic properties of Unitihiol," *Farm Zh*, 1:18–22, 1980

(99) M. Nylander, et al., "Mercury accumulation in tissues from dental staff and controls," *Swedish Dental Journal*, 13:235–43, 1989; & M. Nylander, et al., *Br J Ind Med*, 48(11):729–34, 1991; & "Mercury in pituitary glands of dentists," *Lancet*, 442, Feb 26, 1986

(100) M. Hanson, et al., "The dental amalgam issue: a review," *Experientia*, 47:9–22, 1991; & J. A. Weiner, et al., "Does mercury from amalgam restorations constitute a health hazard," *Sci Total Environ*, 99(1–2):1–22, 1990; & R. Marxkors, "Korrosionserscheinungen an Amalgamf llungen und Deren Auswirkungen auf den Menschlichen Organismus," *Das Deutsche Zahn rztebl*, 24, 53, 117, and 170, 1970

(101) E. Henriksson, et al., "Healing of lichenoid reactions following removal of amalgam," *J Clinical Periodontol*, 22(4):287–94, 1995; & M. Forsbec, et al., *Journal of Clinical Immunology*, 16(1):31–40, Jan 1996; & A. Larsson, et al., "The histopathology of oral mucosal lesions associated with amalgam," *Oral Dis*, 1(3):152–8, 1995

(102) R. L. Siblerud, *et al.*, "Evidence that mercury from silver fillings may be an etiological factor in multiple sclerosis," *Sci Total Environ*, 142(3):191–, 1994; & "Mental health, amalgam fillings, and MS," *Psychol Rep*, 70(3 Pt2):1139–51, 1992; & T. Engalls, *Am J Forensic Med Pathol*, 4(1):55–61, Mar 1983; & Siblerud, R. L., and Kienholz, E., "Evidence that mercury from dental amalgam may cause hearing loss in multiple sclerosis patients," *J Orthomol Med*, 12(4):240–4, 1997

(103) A. P. Tanchyk, "Amalgam removal for treatment of arthritis," *Gen Dent*, 42(4):354–, July 1994

(107) R. L. Siblerud, *et al.*, "Psychometric evidence that mercury from dental fillings may be a factor in depression, anger, and anxiety," *Psychol Rep*, 74(1), 1994; & *Amer J of Psychotherapy*, 58:575–87, 1989; *Poisoning and Toxicology Compendium*, Leikin & Palouchek, Lexi–Comp,1998, p. 705

(110) N. Roeleveld, *et al.*, "Mental retardation and parental occupation," *Br J Ind Med*, 50(10):945–54, 1993

(111) T. W. Clarkson, *et al.*, "Biliary secretion of glutathione-metal complexes," *Fundam Appl Toxicol*, 5(5):816–31, 1985; & D. Quig, Doctors Data Lab, "Cysteine metabolism and metal toxicity," *Altern Med Rev*, 3(4):262–70, 1998; & J. de Ceaurriz, *et al.*, "Role of gamma-glutamyltraspeptidase (GGC) and extracellular glutathione in disposition of inorganic mercury," *J Appl Toxicol*, 14(3):201–, 1994; & W. O. Berndt, *et al.*, "Renal glutathione and mercury uptake," *Fundam Appl Toxicol*, 5(5):832–9, 1985; & R. K. Zulups, *et al.*, *J Toxicol Environ Health*, 44(4):385–99, 1995; & D. Jay, "Glutathione inhibits SOD activity of Hg," *Arch Inst Cardiol Mex*, 68(6):457–61, 1998

(112) A. Oskarsson, *et al.*, "Mercury in breast milk in relation to fish consumption and amalgam," *Arch Environ Health*, 51(3):234–41, 1996; & "Risk assessment in relation to neonatal metal exposure," *Analyst*, 123(1):19–23, 1998; & Drasch, *et al.*, "Mercury in human colostrum and early breast milk," *J Trace Elem Med Biol*, 12:23–7, 1998; & Grandjean, P., Jurgensen, P. J., Weihe, P., "Milk as a source of methylmercury exposure in infants," *Environ Health Perspect*, 102(1):74–7, Jan 1994

(113)   T. A. Glavinskiaia, *et al.*, "Complexons in the treatment of lupus erghematousus," *Dermatol Venerol*, 12:24–8, 1980; & A. F. Hall, *Arch Dermatol*, 47:610–1, 1943

(115)   G. Hall, V-TOX, Mercury levels excreted after vitamin C IV as chelator by number of fillings, Int Symposium "Status Quo and Perspectives of Amalgam and Other Dental Materials" European Academy, Ostzenhausen/Germany, April 29–May 1, 1994; & *Heavy Metal Bulletin*, Vol. 3, issue 1, p. 6–8, Apr 1996 (200 cured or significantly improved)

(116)   Liebert, C. A., Wireman, J., Smith, T., Summers, A. O., "The impact of mercury released from dental 'silver' fillings on antibiotic resistances in the primate oral and intestinal bacterial flora," *Met Ions Biol Syst*, 34:441–60, 1997; A. O. Summers, *et al.*, *Antimicrobial Agents and Chemotherapy*, 37(4):825–34, 1993; & *The Physiologist*, 33(4), A–116, 1990; & J. Wireman, *et al.*, *Appl Environ Microbiol*, 63(11):4494–503, 1997; & M. Vimy, *et al.*, "Silver dental fillings provoke an increase in mercury and antibiotic resistant bacteria in the mouth and intestines of primates," *APUA Newsletter*, Fall 1991

(117)   C. Edlund, *et al.*, "Resistance of the normal human microflora to mercury and antimicrobials," *Clin Infect Dis*, 22(6):944–50, 1996

(119)   L. Ronnback, *et al.*, "Chronic encephalopathies induced by low doses of mercury or lead," *Br J Ind Med*, 49:233–40, 1992; & H. Langauer-Lewowicka, "Changes in the nervous system due to occupational metallic mercury poisoning," *Neurol Neurochir Pol*, 31(5):905–13, Sep–Oct 1997; & Kim, P., Choi, B. H., "Selective inhibition of glutamate uptake by mercury in cultured mouse astrocytes," *Yonsei Med J*, 36(3):299–305, 1995; & Brookes, N., "In vitro evidence for the role of glutamate in the CNS toxicity of mercury," *Toxicology*, 76(3):245–56, 1992

(120)   L. Pohl, Dept. of Dental Materials Science, Umea Univ., Sweden, "The dentist's exposure to elemental mercury during clinical work," *Acta Odontol Scand*, 53(1):44–8, 1995

(121)   A. S. Rowland, *et al.*, "The effect of occupational exposure to mercury vapor on the fertility of female dental assistants," *Occupational & Environmental Medicine*, 55(1), 1994

(123) I. Skare, *et al.*, "Mercury exposure of different origins among dentists and dental nurses," *Scand J Work Environ Health*, 16:340–7, 1990

(126) K. R. Hoyt, *et al.*, "Mechanisms of dopamine–induced cell death and differences from glutamate-induced cell death," *Exp Neurol*, 143(2):269–81, 1997; & P. Froissard, *et al.*, Universite de Caen, "Role of glutathione metabolism in the glutamate-induced programmed cell death of neuronal cells," *Eur J Pharmacol*, 236(1): 93–9, 1997

(129) P. Hultman, *et al.*, Dept. Of Pathology, Linkoping Univ., Sweden, "Adverse immunological effects and immunity induced by dental amalgam," *FASEB J*, 8:1183–90, 1994; & *Toxicol Appl Pharmacol*, 113(2):199–208, 1992

(130) S. Enestrom, *et al.*, "Does amalgam affect the immune system?" *Int Arch Allergy Immunol*, 106:180–203, 1995

(131) Christensen, M. M., Ellermann–Eriksen, S., Mogensen, S. C., "Influence of mercury chloride on resistance to generalized infection with herpes simplex virus type 2 in mice," *Toxicology*, 114(1): 57–66, 1996; & S. Ellermann–Eriksen, *et al.*, "Effect of mercuric chloride on macrophage–mediated resistance mechanisms against infection," *Toxicology*, 93:269–97, 1994; & M. Kubicka-Muranyi, *et al.*, "Systemic autoimmune disease induced by mercuric chloride," *Int Arch Allergy Immunol*, 109(1):11–20, 1996; & M. M. Christensen *et al.*, Institute of Medical Microbiology, "Comparison of interaction of meHgCl2 and HgCl2 with murine macrophages," *Arch Toxicol*, 67(3):205–11, 1993

(133) M. Molin, *et al.*, "Mercury in plasma in patients allegedly subject to oral galvanism," *Scand J Dent Res*, 95:328–34, 1987

(138) D. Zander, *et al.*, "Studies on human exposure to mercury amalgam fillings," *Ubl Hyg*, 190:325–, 1990

(139) G. Sallsten, *et al.*, "Mercury in cerebrospinal fluid in subjects exposed to mercury vapor," *Environmental Research*, 65:195–206, 1994

(142) Ariza, M. E., Bijur, G.N., Williams, M.V., "Lead and mercury mutagenesis: role of H₂O₂, superoxide dismutase, and xanthine oxidase," *Environ Mol Mutagen*, 31(4):352–61, 1998; & M. E. Ariza, *et al.*, "Mercury mutagenisis," *Biochem Mol Toxicol*, 13(2):107–12, 1999; & M. E. Ariza, *et al.*, "Mutagenic effect of mercury," *In Vivo*, 8(4):559–63, 1994

(143) P. Boffetta, *et al.*, "Carciagenicity of mercury," *Scand J Work Environ Health*, 19(1):1–7, 1993; & "Study of workers compensated for mercury intoxication," *J Occup Med*, 36(11):1260–4, 1994; & *J Occup Med*, 36(11):1260–4, 1994

(153) International Academy of Oral Medicine and Toxicology, "A Scientific Response to the American Dental Association Special Report and Statement of Confidence in Dental Amalgam, IAOMT, POB 608531, Orlando, FL 32860–8531, http://emporium.turnpike.net/P/PDHA/mercury/asr.htm; & IAOMT, Protocol for Mercury/Silver Filling Removal, http://emporium.turnpike.net/P/PDHA/mercury/iaomt.htm

(156) E. G. Miller, *et al.*, "Prevalence of mercury hypersensitivity among dental students," *J Dent Res*, 64:Abstract 1472, p. 338,1985; & D. Kawahara, *et al.*, "Epidemiologic study of occupational contact dermatitis in the dental clinic," *Contact Dermatitis*, 28(2):114–5, 1993

(158) Wenstrup, *et al.*, "Trace element imbalances in the brains of Alzheimer's patients," *Research*, 533:125–31, 1990; & F. L. Lorscheider, B. Haley, *et al.*, "Mercury vapor inhibits tubulin binding...," *FASEB J*, 9(4):A-3485, 1995; & Vance, *et al.*, *Neurotoxicology*, 9:197–208, 1988; & l. de Saint-Georges, *et al.*, "Inhibition by mercuric chloride for the in vitro polymerization of microtubules," *CR Seances Soc Biol Fil*, 178(5):562–6, 1984

(160) B. Windham, "Health effects of toxic metals: an annotated bibliography," 1999; & B. Windham, "Cognitive and behavioral effects of toxic metals," 2000 (over 100 medical study references)

(161) F. L. Lorscheider, *et al.*, "Inorganic mercury and the CNS: genetic linkage of mercury and antibiotic resistance,"

Toxicology, 97(1):19–22, 1995; & M. C. Roberts, Dept. of Pathobiology, Univ. of Washington, "Antibiotic resistance in oral/respiratory bacteria," *Crit Rev Oral biol Med*, 9(4):522–, 1998

(162) N. K. Mottet, *et al.*, "Health risks from increases in methylmercury exposure," *Health Perspect*, 63:133–40, 1985; & M. K. Mohamed, *et al.*, "Effects of methyl mercury on testicular functions in monkeys," *Toxicol*, 60(1):29–36, 1987; & M. K. Mohamed, *et al.*, *Toxicol* (Copenhagen), 58(3):219–24, 1986; & N. F. Ivanitskaia, "Evaluation of effect of mercury on reproductive function of animals," *Gig Sanit*, 12:48–51, 1991

(163) Ahlrot-Westerlund, B., Multiple sclerosis and mercury in cerebrospinal fluid. Second Nordic Symposium on Trace Elements and Human Health, Odense, Denmark, Aug 1987; & *Nutrition Research*, 1985 Supplement

(164) Swedish National Dept. of Health, Mercury Amalgam Review Panel, 1987

(165) Anneroth, G., Ericson, T., Johansson, I., Mornstad, H., Skoglund, A., "Comprehensive medical examination of patients with alleged adverse effects from dental amalgams," *Acta Odontal Scand*, 50(2):101–11, 1992

(167) M. L. Olsted, *et al.*, "Correlation between amalgam restorations and mercury in urine," *J Dent Res*, 66(6):1179–82, 1987

(168) J. Laine, *et al.*, "Immunocompetent cells in amalgam-associated oral licheinoid contact lesions," *Oral Pathol Med*, 28(3):117–21, 1999; & "Contact allergy to dental restorative materials in patients with oral lichenoid lesions," *Contact Dermatitis*, 36(3):141–6, 1997; & "Resolution of OLL after replacement of amalgam restorations," *Br J Dermatol*, 126(1):10–15, 1992 (20 cases); & A. Adachi, *et al.*, "Efficacy of dental metal elimination in the management of atopic dermatitis," *J Dermatology*, 24(1):141–6, 1997

(170) R. L. Siblerud, "A comparison of mental health of multiple sclerosis patients with silver dental fillings and those with fillings removed," *Psychol Rep*, 70(3), Pt2:1139–51, 1992

(171) A. Jokstad, "Mercury excretion and occupational exposure of dental personnel," *Community Dent Oral Epidemiology*, 18(3):143–8, 1990

(172) B. Nilsson, *et al.*, Dept. of Environmental Medicine, Univ. of Umea, "Urinary mercury excretion in dental personnel," *Swed Dent J*, 10(6):221–32, 1986; & *Swed Dent J*, 10(1–2):1–14, 1986; & *Science of the Total Environment*, 94(3):179–85, 1990

(173) D. Zander, *et al.*, "Mercury exposure of male dentists, female dentists, and dental aides," *Zentralbl Hyg Umweltmed*, 193(4):318–28, 1992

(175) L. Larkfors, *et al.*, "Methylmercury induced alterations in the nerve growth factor level in the developing brain," *Res Dev Res*, 62(2):287–, 1991; & Soderstrom, S., Fredriksson, A., Dencker, L., Ebendal, T., "The effect of mercury vapor on cholinergic neurons in the fetal brain," *Brain Research & Developmental Brain Res*, 85:96–108, 1995; & *Toxicol Lett*, 75(1–3):133–44, 1995

(180) Pinto, O. F., *et al.*, *J Intl Acad Prev Med*, 3(2), 1976; & Huggins, H. A., "Proposed role of dental amalgam toxicity in leukemia and hemotopoietic dyscrasias," *International J of Biosocial and Medical Research*, 11:84–93, 1989; & Schimpff, S. C., Young, W. H., Greene W. H., "Origin of infections in acute nonlymphocytic leukemia," *Annals of International Medicine*, 77:707–11, 1972; & Y. Kinjo, *et al.*, "Cancer mortality in patients exposed to methylmercury through fish diet," *J Epidemiol*, 6(3):134–8, 1996

(182) Pleva, J., "Dental mercury – a public health hazard," *Rev Environ Health*, 10(1):1–7, 1994; & Pleva, J., "Mercury from dental amalgams: exposure and effects," *Int J Risk & Safety in Med*, 3:1–22, 1992; & "Mercury – a public health hazard," *Reviews on Environmental Health*, 10:1–27, 1994; & "Mercury poisoning from dental amalgam," *J. Of Orthomol. Medicine*, 4(3):141–8, 1989; & *J Orthomol Psych*, 12(3), 1983; & Emler & Cardone, Oral Roberts Univ., "An assessment of mercury in mouth air," *Journal of Dental Research*, March 1985; & Vimy and Lorschieder, University of Calgary, "Intra oral mercury released from dental amalgam," *Journal of Dental Research*, 64:1069–71,

1985; & "Serial measurements of intra oral mercury," *Journal Dental Research*, 64:1072–5, 1985

(183) World Health Organization (WHO), 1991, Environmental Health Criteria 118, Inorganic Mercury, WHO, Geneva; & Envir. H. Crit. 101, Methyl Mercury

(186) Yang, J., Wang, Y. 1., "Maternal–fetal transfer of metallic mercury via the placenta and milk," *Annals of Clin & Lab Sci*, 27(2):135–41, 1997; & C. N. Ong, *et al.*, "Concentrations of heavy metal in maternal and umbilical cord blood," *Biometals*, 6(1):61–6, 1993; & Y. K. Soong, *et al.*, *J of Formosa Medical Assoc*, 90(1):59–65, 1991; & T. Suzuki, *et al.*, Dept. Of Human Ecology, Univ. Of Tokyo, "Mercury in human amniotic fluid," *Scand J Work Environ & Health*, 3:32–5, 1977; & D. A. Spencer, *et al.*, "Mercury concentration in cord blood," *Arch Dis Child*, 63(2):202–3, 1988; & S. Sugiyama, *et al.*, "Comparison of heavy metal concentrations in human umbilical cord blood in 1980 and 1990," Kinki Univ. School of Medicine, Osaka, Japan; & R. Sikorski, *et al.*, "The intrapartum content of toxic metals in maternal and umbilical cord blood," *Ginekol Pol*, 60(3):151–5, 1989

(187) Klobusch, J., Rabe, T., Gerhard, I., Runnebaum, B., "Alopecia and environmental pollution," *Klinisches Labor*, 38:469–76, 1992; & "Schwermetallbelastungen bei patientinnen mit alopezie," *Arch Gynecol Obstet*, 254(1–4):278–80, 1993; & G. Kunzel, *et al.*, *Arch Gynecol Obstet*, 254:277–8, 1993

(189) U.S. CDC, Toxicology Division, Atlanta, GA, and WHO, Environmental Health Criteria 101,1990

(191) D. Brune, *et al.*, "Gastrointestinal and in vitro release of metals from conventional and copper-rich amalgams," *Scand J Dent Res*, 91:66–71, 1983; & *Sci Tot Envir*, 44:..., 1985; & "Metal release from dental materials," *Biomaterials*, 7:163–75, 1986

(192) N. Nogi, "Electric current around dental metals as a factor producing allergic metal ions in the oral cavity," *Nippon Hifuka Gakkai Zasshi*, 99(12):1243–54, 1989; & M. D. Rose, *et al.*, Eastman Dental Institute, "The tarnished history of a posteria

restoration," *Br Dent J*, 185(9):436, 1998; & J. Bergdahl, A. J. Certosimo, *et al.*, National Naval Dental Center, "Oral electricity," *Gen Dent*, 44(4):324–6, 1996; & R. H. Ogletree, *et al.*, School of Materials Science, GIT, Atlanta, "Effect of mercury on corrosion of eta' Cu-Sn phase in dental amalgams," *Dent Mater*, 11(5):332–6, 1995; & R. D. Meyer, *et al.*, "Intraoral galvanic corrosion," *Prosthet Dent*, 69(2):141–3, 1993; & B. M. Owens, *et al.*, "Localized galvanic shock after insertion of an amalgam restoration," *Compenium*, 14(10):1302–4, 1306–7, 1993; & Johansson, E., Liliefors, T., "Heavy elements in root tips from teeth with amalgam fillings," Department of Radiation Sciences, Division of Physical Biology, Box 535, 751 21 Uppsala, Sweden

(194) Lu, S. C., "Regulation of hepatic glutathione synthesis: current concepts and controversies," *FASEB J*, 13(10):1169–83, 1999; & R. B. Parsons, *J Hepatol*, 1998, 29(4):595–602; & R. K. Zalups, *et al.*, "Nephrotoxicity of inorganic mercury co-administered with L-cysteine," *Toxicology*, 109(1):15–29, 1996; & T. L. Perry, *et al.*, "Hallevorden-Spatz Disease: cysteine accumulation and cysteine dioxygenase deficiency," *Ann Neural*, 18(4):482–9, 1985

(196) G. Sandborgh-Englund, "Pharmakinetics of mercury from dental amalgam," Medical School Dissertation, Dept. of Basal Oral Sciences, Karolinska Institute, (Stockholm), 1998, 1–49; & G. Sandborgh-Englund, *et al.*, "Mercury in biological fluids after amalgam removal," *J Dental Res*, 77(4):615–24, 1998

(198) E. S. West, *et al.*, *Textbook of Biochemistry*, MacMillan Co, 1957, p. 853; & B. R. G. Danielsson, *et al.*, "Ferotoxicity of inorganic mercury: distribution and effects of nutrient uptake by placenta and fetus," *Biol Res Preg Perinatal*, 5(3):102–9, 1984; & Danielsson, *et al.*, *Neurotoxicol Teratol*, 18:129–134, ?

(199) Dr. P. Kraub, M. Deyhle, Universitat Tubingen - Institut fur Organische Chemie, "Field study on the mercury content of saliva," 1997, http://www.uni-tuebingen.de/KRAUSS/amalgam.html; (20,000 people tested for mercury level in saliva and health status/symptoms compiled)

(204) Tom Warren, *Beating Alzheimer's*, Avery Publishing Group, 1991

(205) M. F. Ziff, *et al.*, *A Persuasive New Look at Heart Disease As It Relates to Mercury*, Bio- Probe, Inc., ISBN 0-941011-08-9; & *J of American College of Cardiology*, 33(6):1578–83, 1999

(207) Pendergrass, J. C., Haley, B. E., Univ. of Kentucky Dept. of Chemistry, "The toxic effects of mercury on CNS proteins: similarity to observations in Alzheimer's Disease," IAOMT Symposium paper, March 1997; & "Mercury vapor inhalation inhibits binding of GTP ...—similarity to lesions in Alzheimer's Diseased brains," *Neurotoxicology*, 18(2):315–24, 1997; & *Met Ions Biol Syst*, 34:461–, 1997

(208) L. T. Friberg, "Status quo and perspectives of amalgam and other dental materials," International Symposium Proceedings, G. Thieme Verlag Struttgart, 1995

(209) Mark Richardson, Environmental Health Directorate, Health Canada, *Assessment of Mercury Exposure and Risks from Dental Amalgam*, 1995, Final Report; & G. M. Richardson, *et al.*, "A Monte Carlo assessment of mercury exposure and risks from dental amalgam," *Human and Ecological Risk Assessment*, 2(4):709–61

(210) Mats Berlin, "Is amalgam in dental fillings hazardous to health?," *Lakartidningen*, 89(37):2918–23, 1992; & "Prenatal exposure to mercury vapor: effects on brain development," *Fundamental and Applied Toxicology*, 1,112, 1: 7(?); & M. Berlin, "Mercury in dental filling materials – environmental medicine risk analysis," paper for the Swedish Council for Coordinating and Planning Research, 1998

(211) M. J. Vimy, F. L. Lorscheider, Faculty of Medicine, Univ. of Calgary, July 1991. (Study findings) & *J Trace Elem Exper Med*, 3:111–123, 1990

(212) Ziff, M. F., "Documented clinical side effects to dental amalgams," *ADV. Dent Res*, 1(6):131–4, 1992; & S. Ziff, *Dentistry Without Mercury*, 8th Edition, 1996, Bio-Probe, Inc., ISBN 0-941011-04-6; & *Dental Mercury Detox*, Bio-Probe, Inc. http://www.bioprobe.com. (cases: FDA Patient Adverse Reaction Reports—762; Dr. M. Hanson—Swedish patients—519

(includes many MS); Dr. H. Lichtenberg—100 Danish patients; Dr. P.Larose—80 Canadian patients; Dr. R. Siblerud—86 Colorado patients; Dr. A. V. Zamm—22 patients (see (26))

(216) T. W. Clarkson, et al., in *Biological Monitoring of Toxic Metals*, 1988, Plenum Press, N.Y., "The prediction of intake of mercury vapor from amalgams," p. 199–246 & p. 247–260; & *Environmental Health Perspective*, 100:31–8, April 1993; & F. L. Lorscheider, et al., *Lancet*, 337:1103, 1991

(217) Agency for Toxic Substances and Disease Registry, U.S. Public Health Service, *Toxicological Profile for Mercury*, 1999; & Apr 19, 1999, Media Advisory, New MRLs for toxic substances, MRL: elemental mercury vapor/inhalation/chronic & MRL: methyl mercury/ oral/acute; & http://www.atsdr.cdc.gov/mrls.html

(219) D. E. Cutright, et al., Dept. of Prosthodontics, Temple Univ., "Systemic mercury levels caused by inhaling mist during high-speed amalgam grinding," *J Oral Med*, 28(4):100–4,1973; & A. Nimmo, et al., "Inhalation during removal of amalgam restorations," *J Prosthet Dent*, 63(2):228–33, Feb 1990

(222) M. Daunderer, *Handbuch der Amalgamvergiftung*, Ecomed Verlag, Landsberg, 1998, ISBN 3-609-71750-5 (in German); & "Improvement of nerve and immunological damages after amalgam removal," *Amer J of Probiotic Dentistry and Medicine*, Jan 1991; & Toxicologische erfahrungen am menchen; quecksilber in der umwelf-hearing zum amalgamproblem," *Niedersachsiscles Umweltministerium*, 1991; & "Amalgam," Ecomed Verlag, Landsberg, 1995; & "Amalgamtest," *Forum Prakt Allgen Arzt*, 29(8):213–4, 1990; & "Besserung von Nerven – und Immunschaden nach Amalgamsanierung," *Dtsch Aschr F Biologische Zahnmedzin*, 6(4):152–7, 1990 (amalgam removal & DMPS, over 3,000 cases)

(225) S. Yannai, et al., "Transformations of inorganic mercury by Candida albicans and saccharomyces cerevisiae," *Applied Envir Microbiology*, 7:245–7, 1991; & N. E. Zorn, et al., "A relationship between Vitamin B_{12}, mercury uptake, and methylation," *Life Sci*, 47(2):167–73, 1990; & W. P. Ridley, et al., *Environ Health Perspectives*, 43–6, Aug 19, 1977; & R. E. DeSimone, et al., *Biochem Biophys Acta*, May 28, 1973; & Yamada, Tonomura,

"Formation of methyl mercury compounds from inorganic mercury by Clostridium cochlearium," *J Ferment Technol*, 50:159–1660, 1972

(226) (a) B. J. Shenker, *et al.*, Dept. of Pathology, Univ. of Penn. School of Dental Med., "Immunotoxic effects of mercuric compounds on human lymphocytes and monocytes: alterations in cell viability," *Immunopharmacol Immunotoxicol*, 14(3):555–77, 1992; & M. A. Miller, *et al.*, "Mercuric chloride induces apoptosis in human T lymphocytes," *Toxicol Appl Pharmacol*, 153(2):250–7, 1998; & Rossi, A. D., Viviani, B., Vahter, M., "Inorganic mercury modifies Ca2+ signals, triggers apoptosis, and potentiates NMDA toxicity in cerebral granule neurons," *Cell Death and Differentiation*, 4(4):317–24, 1997; & Goering, P. L., Thomas, D., Rojko, J. L., Lucas, A. D., "Mercuric chloride-induced apoptosis is dependent on protein synthesis," *Toxicol Lett*, 105(3):183–95, 1999; & (b) B. J. Shenker, *et al.*, "Immune suppression of human T-cell activation," *Immunopharmacol Immunotoxicol*, 14(3):555–77, 1992; & 14(3):539–53; & 15(2–3):273–90, 1993

(228) Dr. T. Rau, Paracelsus Allergy Clinic, Lustmuhle, Switzerland, 1996 (www); & Dr. B. Shelton, Director, The Allergy Center, Phoenix, Arizona, in (293); & E. Cutler, *Winning the War against Asthma & Allergies*, DAMS (1-800-311-6265)

(229) M. Davis, editor, *Defense Against Mystery Syndromes*, Chek Printing Co., March, 1994 (case histories documented); & Kantarjian, A., "A syndrome clinically resembling amyotrophic lateral sclerosis following chronic mercurialism," *Neurology*, 11:639–44, 1961

(232) Adolph Coors Foundation, "Coors Amalgam Study: Effects of placement and removal of amalgam fillings," 1995. (www) & *Internations DAMS Newsletter*, p. 17, Vol. VII, Issue 2, Spring 1997 (31 cases)

(233) Sven Langworth, *et al.*, "Amalgamnews and Amalgamkadefonden," 1997 and Svenska Dogbladet, 1997 (286 cases); & F. Berglund, Bjerner/Helm, Klock, Ripa, Lindforss, Mornstad, Ostlin, "Improved health after removal of dental amalgam fillings," Swedish Assoc. of Dental Mercury Patients, 1998. (www.tf.nu) (over 1,000 cases), (Sweden has banned

amalgam fillings and Gov't maintains health records on all citizens); & Heavy Metal Bulletin, no.3, 1996 and no.1, 1999, p. 7,8; & Klock, B., Blomgren, J., Ripa, U., Andrup, B., "Effekt av amalgamavlägsnande på patienter som misstänker att de lider eller har lidit av amalgamförgiftning," *Tandläkartidn*, 81(23):1297–1302, 1989

(234) P. E. Bigazzi, "Autoimmunity and heavy metals," *Lupus*, 3:449–53, 1994; & Pollard, K. M., Pearson, D. l., Hultman, P., "Lupus-prone mice as model to study xenobiotic-induced autoimmunity," *Environ Health Perspect*, 107(Suppl 5):729–35, 1999; & Nielsen, J. B., Hultman, P., "Experimental studies on genetically determined susceptibility to mercury-induced autoimmune response," *Ren Fail*, 21(3–4):343–8, May–Jul 1999; & Hultman, P., Enestrom, S., "Mercury induced antinuclear antibodies in mice," *Clinical and Exper Immunology*, 71(2):269–74, 1988

(235) H. J. Hamre, "Mercury from dental amalgam and chronic fatigue syndrome," *The CFIDS Chronicle*, p. 44–7, Fall 1994

(238) World Health Organization Scientific Panel Members (Dr. Lars Friburg—chairman; Dr. Fritz Lorscheider, Professor of Medical Physiology, Univ. of Calgary; Dr. Murray Vimy, Professor of Oral Biology and Dental Medicine, Univ. of Calgary Medical School; Dr. Vasken Aposhian, Dept. Head, Molecular and Cellular Biology, Univ. of Arizona; Dr. David Eggleston, Univ. of California, researcher on mercury in the brain; Dr. Boyd Haley, Univ. of Kentucky, researcher on mercury in the brain and Alzheimer's Disease (http://www.altcorp.com/); Dr. Gustav Drasch, Univ. of Munich, researcher on mercury in brains of dead infants and fetuses; Dr. D. Echeverria, Neuro-Toxicologist, researcher on reproductive problems and birth defects in dental workers; BBC Panorama Program on Dental Amalgam: "The Poison in Your Mouth," June 1994)

(240) K. W. Hinkleman, *et al.*, "Mercury release during ultrasonic scaling of amalgam," *J Dent Res*, 74(SE):131, Abstract 960, 1995; & Haikel, Y., Gasser, P., Salek, P., Voegel, J. C., "Exposure to mercury vapor during setting, removing, and polishing amalgam restorations," *J Biomed Mater Res*, 24(11):1551–8, Nov 1990

(241) R. Schoeny, U.S. EPA, "Use of genetic toxicology data in U.S. EPA risk assessment: the mercury study," *Environ Health Perspect*, 104, Supp 3:663–73, 1996; & C. H. Lee, *et al.*, "Genotoxicity of phenylHg acetate in humans as compared to other mercury compounds," 392(3):269–76

(245) P. Lokken, "Lethal mercury poisoning in a dental assistant," *Nor Tannlaegeforen Tid*, 81(4):275–88, Apr 1971; & R. Wronski, *et al.*, "A case of panarteritis nodoa associated with chronic mercury poisoning," *Dtsch Med Wohenschr*, 102(9):323–5, Mar 1977

(246) K. Lyer, *et al.*, "Mercury poisoning in a dentist," *Arch Neurol*, 33:788–90, 1976

(247) E. C. Lonnroth, *et al.*, "Adverse health reactions in skin, eyes, and respiratory tract among dental personnel in Sweden," *Swed Dent J*, 22(1–2):33–45, 1998; & L. Kanerva, *et al.*, "Occupational contact urticaria," *Contact Dermatitis*, 35(4):229–33, 1996

(248) Y. Finkelstein, "The enigma of parkinsonism in chronic borderline mercury intoxication, resolved by challenge with penicillamine," *Neurotoxicology*, 17(1):291–5, Spring 1996

(249) C. H. Ngim, *et al.*, Dept. of Occupational Medicine, Univ. of Singapore, "Chronic neurobehavioral effects of elemental mercury in dentists," *British Journal of Industrial Medicine*, 49(11):782–90, 1992

(251) Y. Omura, *et al.*, Heart Disease Research Foundation, NY, NY, "Role of mercury in resistant infections and recovery after Hg detox with cilantro," *Acupuncture & Electro-Therapeutics Research*, 20(3):195–229, 1995; & "Mercury exposure from silver fillings," *Acupuncture & Electrotherapy Res*, 133–, 1996

(252) B. J. Shenker, *et al.*, Dept. of Pathology, Univ. of Pennsylvania, "Immunotoxic effects of mercuric compounds on human lymphocytes and monocytes: alterations in cellular glutathione content," *Immunopharmacol Immunotoxicol*, 15(2–3):273–90, 1993

(253) S. Langworth, *et al.*, "Exposure to mercury vapor and impact on health in the dental profession in Sweden," *J Dent Res*, 76(7):1397–404, 1997

(256) D. B. Alymbaeva, *et al.*, *Med Tr Prom Ekol*, 6:13–15, 1995 (Russian)

(258) J. M. Aguiar, *et al.*, "Heavy metals and antibiotic resistance in Escherichia coli isolates from ambulatory patients," *Chemother*, 2(4):238–40, 1990

(261) New Scientist: This Week, Nov 22, 1997, p. 4 (and editorial), and Jan 10, 1998; & *Neurotoxicology and Teratology*, 19:417, Jan 1998

(262) Chang, L. W., "The neurotoxicology and pathology of organomercury, organolead, and organotin," *J Toxicol Sci*, 15 Suppl 4:125–51, 1990; & "Latent effects of methyl mercury on the nervous system after prenatal exposure," *Environ Res*, 13(2):171–85, 1977

(263) H. Iioka, *et al.*, "The effect of inorganic mercury on placental amino acid transport," *Nippon sanka Fujinka Gakkai Zasshi*, 39(2):202–6, 1987

(264) B. R. Danielsson, *et al.*, "Behavioral effects of prenatal metallic mercury inhalation exposure in rats," *Neurotoxicol Teratol*, 15(6):391–6, 1993; & A. Fredriksson, *et al.*, "Prenatal exposure to metallic mercury vapour and methylmercury produce interactive behavioral changes in adult rats," *Neurotoxicol Teratol*, 18(2):129–34, 1996; & "Behavioral effects of neonatal metallic mercury exposure in rats," *Toxicology*, 74(2–3):151–60, 1992

(265) K. Lohmann, *et al.*, "Multiple chemical sensitivity disorder in patients with neurotoxic illnesses," *Gesundheitswesen*, 58(6):322–31, 1996

(270) D. W. Eggleston, "Effect of dental amalgam and nickel alloys on T-lympocytes," *J Prosthet Dent*, 51(5):617–623, 1984; & D. W. Eggleston, *et al.*, *J Prosthet Dent*, 58(6):704–7, 1987; & *J of the*

American Medical Assoc, Sept 96; & Tan, X. X., Tang, C., Castoldi, A. F., Costa, L., "Effects of inorganic and organic mercury on intracellular calcium levels in rat T lymphocytes," *J Toxicol Environ Health*, 38(2):159–70, 1993

(271) (a) B. A. Weber, "The Marburg Amalgam Study," *Arzt und Umwelt*, Apr 1995 (266 cases); & (b) "Amalgam and Allergy," Institute for Naturopathic Medicine, 1994; & (c) "Conuctivitis sicca (dry eye study)," Institute for Naturopathic Medicine, 1994; & "Alternative treatment of multiple sclerosis, tumor, or cancer," Institute for Naturopathic Medicine, 1997

(273) R. Schiele, *et al.*, Institute of Occupational Medicine, Univ. of Erlamgem - Nurnberg, "Studies of organ mercury content related to number of amalgam fillings," Symposium paper, March 12, 1984, Cologne, Germany; & (38); & "Quecksilber-mobiliztion durch DMPS bei personen mit und ohne amalgamfullungen," *Zahnarztl Mitt*, 79(17):1866–8, 1989; & J. J. Kleber, "Quecksilberverkonzen-tration im urin nach DMPS," in *Status Quo and Perspectives of Amalgam*, L. T. Friberg (ed.), Georg-Thieme Verlag, Stuttgart, New York, 1005, p. 61–9

(274) L. Friberg, *et al.*, "Mercury in the brain and CNS in relation to amalgam fillings," *Lakartidningen*, 83(7):519–21, 1986 (Swedish Medical Journal); & T. Suzuki, *et al.*, *Ind Health*, 4:69–75, 1966

(275) L. M. Mikhailova, *et al.*, "Influence of occupational factors on disease of reproductive organs," *Pediatriya Akusherstvoi Ginekologiya*, 33(6):56–8, 1971

(281) T. W. Clarkson, *et al.*, "Transport of elemental mercury into fetal tissues," *Biol Neonate*, 21:239–44, 1972; & M. R. Greenwood, *et al.*, "Transfer of metallic mercury into the fetus," *Experientia*, 28:1455–6, 1972

(282) Press Release, Swedish Council for Planning and Coordinating Research (FRN), Stockholm, February 19, 1998

(283) A. Ahlbom, *et al.*, "Dentists, dental nurses, and brain tumors," *British Medical Journal*, 292:262, Mar 8, 1986

(284) R. Glass, "Mortality of New England Dentists," U.S. Dept. of
       Health, Public Health Service, Washington, DC, 1966; & R.
       Simpson, *et al.*, "Suicide rates of Iowa dentists," J Amer Dental
       Assoc, 107:441–, 1983; & B. B. Arnetz, *et al.*, "Suicide among
       Swedish dentists," *Scand J Soc Med*, 15(4):243–6, 1987

(285) (c) L. Soleo, *et al.*, "Effects of low exposure to inorganic mercury
       on pyschological performance," *Br J Ind Med*, 47(2):105–9, 1990;
       & (e) M. S. Hua, *et al.*, "Chronic elemental mercury
       intoxication," *Brain Inj*, 10(5):377–84, 1996; & (f) Gunther, W.,
       et al., "Repeated neurobehavioral investigations in workers ...,"
       Neurotoxicology, 17(3–4):605–14, 1996; & (g) Levine, S. P.,
       Cavender, G. D., Langolf, G. D., Albers, J. W., "Elemental
       mercury exposure: peripheral neurotoxicity," *Br J Ind Med*,
       39(2):136–9, May 1982

(287) M. C. Newland, *et al.*, "Behavioral consequences of in utero
       exposure to mercury vapor in squirrel monkeys," *Toxicology
       Applied Pharmacology*, 139:374–86, 1996; & "Prolonged
       behavioral effects of in utero exposure to methyl mercury or
       lead," *Toxicol Appl Pharmacol*, 126(1):6–15, 1994; & K. Warfvinge,
       et al., "Mercury distribution in neonatal cortical areas...after
       exposure to mercury vapor," *Environmental Research*,
       67:196–208, 1994

(290) D. Echeverria, *et al.*, "Neurobehavioral effects from exposure to
       dental amalgam: new distinctions between recent exposure and
       Hg body burden," *FASEB J*, 12(11):971–80, Aug 1998; &
       Amalgam and Health, Swedish Council for Planning and
       Coordination of Research, 1999, p. 297–307

(291) H. A. Huggins, T. E. Levy, "Cerebrospinal fluid protein changes
       in MS after dental amalgam removal," *Alternative Med Rev*,
       3(4):295–300, Aug 1998

(292) M. Daunderer, H. Schiwara, *et al.*, "Quecksilber,
       Methylquecksilber, ... in Korpermaterial von Amalgamtrager,"
       Klin Lab, 38:391–403, 1992; & M. Gradl, *et al.*, in *Akute und
       chronische Toxizitat von Spurenelemente*, Wissenschaftliche
       Verlagsgesellschaft nbH, Stuttgart, 1993, p. 65–71; &
       A. Gebhardt, "Ermittlung der Quecksilberbelastung aus
       Amalgamfullurngen," *Labormedizin*, 16:384–86, 1992; &

R. Mayer, *et al.*, "Zur Ermittlung de Quecksilberfreisetzung aus Amalgamfullungen," *Die Quintessenz*, 45:1143–52, 1994; & K. Mayer, "Risikobestimmung der Amalgambelastung," *ZWR*, 105(4):213–18 & 105(5):280–3; & "Amalgam: zeitbombe in mund?," *ZWR*, 104(3):209–214, 1995; & J. G. D. Birkmayer, *et al.*, "Quecksilberdepots im Organismus korrelieren mit der Anzahl der Amalgamfullungen," *Biol Zahnmedizin*, 6(2):57–61, 1990

(293) H. Huggins, Burton Goldberg, & Editors of Alternative Medicine Digest, *Chronic Fatigue, Fibromyalgia & Environmental Illness*, Future Medicine Publishing, Inc, 1998, p. 197–; & U. Dorffer, "Anorexia Hydragyra: ...," *Monatsschr Kinderheilkd*, 137(8):472, 1989

(294) "Do amalgam fillings influence manic depression?," *Journal of Orthomolecular Medicine*, 1998, http://www.depression.com/news/news_981116.htm.

(296) L. Bucio, *et al.*, "Uptake, cellular distribution and DNA damage produced by mercuric chloride in a human fetal hepatic cell line," *Mutat Res*, 423(1–2):65–72, Jan 25, 1999; & L. Verschaeve, *et al.*, "Comparative in vitro cytogenetic studies in mercury-exposed human lymphocytes," *Mutat Res*, 157(2–3):221–6, 1985; & L. Verschaeve, "Genetic damage induced by low-level mercury exposure," *Envir Res*, 12:306–10, 1976

(301) Chang, L. W., "Neurotoxic effects of mercury," *Environ Res*, 14(3):329–73, 1977; & "Histochemical study on the localization and distribution of mercury in the nervous system after mercury intoxication," *Exp Neurol*, 35(1):122–37, 1972; & "Ultrastructural studies of the nervous system after mercury intoxication," *Acta Neuropathol* (Berlin), 20(2):122–38 and 20(4):316–34, 1972

(302) D. Klinghardt, IAOMT Conference & tape, 1998, "Large study by M. Daunderer (Germany) of MS patients after amalgam removal"

(303) H. V. Aposhian, *et al.*, "Mobilization of mercury in humans by DMPS," *Envir Health Perspectives*, Vol. 106, Supp. 4, Aug 1998; & *Toxicology*, 97(1–3):23–38, 1995; & "Urinary mercury after administration DMPS," *FASEB J*, 6:2472–6, 1992

(304) M. J. Vimy, *et al.*, "Mercury from maternal silver tooth fillings: a source of neonatal exposure," *Biological Trace Element Research*, 56:143–52, 1997

(306) E. M. Oliveira, *et al.*, "Mercury effects on the contractile activity of the heart muscle," *Toxicol Appl Pharmacol*, 1:86–91, 1994

(309) *The Tribune*, Mesa, Az., Apr 13, 1998 (Paul Mills, Apalachee Junction); & Kyle, B. P., *Nordic J of Biological Med*, 2000

(310) R. L. Siblerud, "The relationship between mercury from dental amalgam and the cardiovascular system," *Science of the Total Envir*, 99(1–2):23–35, 1990

(311) Chang, L. W., Hartmann, H. A., "Blood-brain barrier dysfunction in experimental mercury intoxication," *Acta Neuropathol* (Berlin), 21(3):179–84, 1972; & Ware, R. A., Chang, L.,W., Burkholder, P. M., "An ultrastructural study on the blood-brain barrier disfunction following mercury intoxication," *Acta Neurolpathol* (Berlin), 30(3):211–14, 1974; & "Prenatal and neonatal toxicology and pathology of heavy metals," *Adv Pharmacol Chemother*, 17:195–231, 1980

(313) V. D. M. Stejskal, *et al.*, "Mercury-specific lymphocytes: an indication of mercury allergy in man," *J of Clinical Immunology*, 16(1);31–40, 1996

(314) M. Goldman, *et al.*, "Chemically induced autoimmunity ...," *Immunology Today*, 12:223–, 1991; & K. Wearying, *et al.*, "Systemic autoimmunity due to mercury vapor exposure in genetically susceptible mice," *Toxicol Appl Pharmacol*, 132(2):299–309, 1995; & L. M. Bagentose, *et al.*, "Mercury-induced autoimmunity in humans," *Immunol Res*, 20(1): 67–78, 1999; & "Mercury-induced autoimmunity," *Clin Exp Immunol*, 114(1):9–12, 1998

(315) B. Engin-Deniz, *et al.*, "Die queckssilberkonzentration im spichel zehnjariger kinder in korrelation zur anzahl und Grobe iher amalgamfullungen," *Zeitschrift fur Stomatologie*, 89:471–179, 1992

(317) S. Zinecker, "Amalgam: Quecksilberdamfe bis ins Gehirn," *der Kassenarzt*, 32(4):23, 1992; "Praxiproblem Amalgam," *Der Allgermeinarzt*, 17(11):1215–21, 1995 (1,800 patients)

(318) V. Schneider, "Untersuchungen ...," Dissertation, Frankfurt, a>M.,1976

(320) U. F. Malt, *et al.*, "Physical and mental problems attributed to dental amalgam fillings," *Psychosomatic Medicine*, 59:32–4, 1997 (99 cured)

(321) R. L. Siblerud, "Relationship between dental amalgam and health," *Toxic Substances Journal*, 10:425–44, 1990b; & "Effects on health following removal of dental amalgams," *J Orthomolecular Med*, 5(2):95–106; & "Relationship between amalgam fillings and oral cavity health," *Ann Dent*, 49(2):6–10, 1990 (86 cured)

(322) P. Engel, "Beobachtungen uber die gesundheit vor und nach amalgamentfernug," *Separatdruck aus Schweiz. Monatsschr Zahnm*, 108(8), 1998 (75 cases amalgam removal) http://soho.globalpoint.ch/paul-engel (89% significant improvement)

(323) Dr. Kohdera, Faculty of Dentistry, Osaka Univ., International Congress of Allergology and Clinical Immunology, EAACI, Stockholm, June 1994; & *Heavy Metal Bulletin*, 1(2), Oct 1994 (160 cases cured-eczema); Tsunetoshi Kohdera, MD, dermatology, allergology, 31 Higashitakada-cho Mibu Nakagyo-ku Schimazu Clinics Kyoto 604 Japan email:smc-inet@mbox.kyoto-inet.or.jp; & P. Dallmann, "Kon nen durch Quecksilber entstehen?" PeDa_Eigenverisg, 1995; & G. Ionescu, *Biol Med*, 2:65–8, 1996; S. S. Tsyganok, "Unithiol in treatment of dermatoses," *Vestn Dermatol Venerol*, (9):67–9, 1978; & (these clinics use MELISA test for diagnosis of immune reactivity) Neukirchen (clinic)(Germany, near Czech border). Director; Gruia Ionescu, owns two Clinics, cases paid by insurance companies in Germany. email: Spezialklinik-Neukirchen@toolpool.de fax: 0049 9947 10 51 11

(327) Danscher, G., *et al.*, "Localization of mercury in the CNS," *Environ Res*, 41:29–43, 1986; & Danscher, G., Horsted-Bindslev, P., Rungby, J., "Traces of mercury in organs from primates with

amalgam fillings," *Exp Mol Pathol*, 52(3):291–9, 1990; & "Ultrastructural localization of mercury after exposure to mercury vapor," *Prog Histochem Cytochem*, 23:249–55, 1991; & R. Pamphlett, *et al.*, "Entry of low doses of mercury vapor into the nervous system," *Neurotoxicology*, 19(1):39–47, 1998; & Pamphlett, *et al.*, "Oxidative damage to nucleic acids in motor neurons containing Hg," *J Neurol Sci*, 159(2):121–6, 1998 (rats & primates); & Pamphlett, R., Waley, P., "Motor neuron uptake of low dose inorganic mercury," *J Neurological Sciences*, 135:63–7, 1996; & Schionning, J. D., Danscher, G., "Autometallographic inorganic mercury correlates with degenerative changes in dorsal root ganglia of rats intoxicated with organic mercury," *APMIS*, 107(3):303–10, Mar 1999

(330)   C. M. Tanner, *et al.*, "Abnormal liver enzyme metabolism in Parkinson's," *Neurology*, 41(5):Suppl 2:89–92, 1991; & M. Watanabe, *et al.*, *Amino Acids*, 15(2):143–50, 1998; & M. T. Heafield, *et al.*, "Plasma cysteine and sulphate levels in patients with Motor neuron disease, Parkinson's Disease, and Alzheimer's Disease," *Neurosci Lett*, 110(1–2), 216–20, 1990; & A. Pean, *et al.*, "Pathways of cysteine metabolism in MND/ALS," *J Neurol Sci*, 124, Suppl:59–61, 1994

(331)   C. Gordon, *et al.*, "Abnormal sulphur oxidation in systemic lupus erythrmatosus (SLE)," *Lancet*, 339(8784):25–6, 1992; & P. Emory, *et al.*, "Poor sulphoxidation in patients with rheumatoid arthritis," *Ann Rheum Dis*, 51(3):318–20, 1992; & P. Emory, *et al.*, *Br J Rheumotol*, 31(7):449–51,1992

(332)   Trepka, M. J., Heinrich, J., Krause, C., Schulz, C., Wjst, M., Popescu, M., Wichmann, H. E., "Factors affecting internal mercury burdens among German children," *Arch Environ Health*, 52(2):134–8, 1997; & L. Soleo, *et al.*, "Influence of amalgam fillings on urinary mercury excretion," (S. Italy), *G Ital Med Lav Ergon*, 20(2):75–81, 1998

(335)   A. Engqvist, *et al.*, "Speciation of mercury excreted in feces from individuals with amalgam fillings," *Arch Environ Health*, 53(3):205–13, 1998; & Dept. of Toxicology & Chemistry, Stockholm Univ., National Institute for Working Life, 1998 (www.niwl.se/ah/1998-02.html)

(338) (a) W. Y. Boadi, *et al.*, Dept. Of Food Engineering and Biotechnology, T-I Inst of Tech., Haifa, Israel, "In vitro effect of mercury on enzyme activities and its accumulation in the first-trimester human placento," *Environ Res*, 57(1):96–106, 1992;& "In vitro exposure to mercury and cadmium alters term human placental membrane fluidity," *Pharmacol*, 116(1):17–23, 1992; & (b) J. Urbach, *et al.*, Dept. of Obstetrics & Gynecology, Rambam Medical Center, Haifa, Israel, "Effect of inorganic mercury on in vitro placental nutrient transfer and oxygen consumption," *Reprod Toxicol*, 6(1):69–75, 1992; & (c) Karp, W., Gale, T. F., *et al.*, Effect of mercuric acetate on selected enzymes of maternal and fetal hamsters," *Environmental Research*, 36:351–8; & W. B. Karp, *et al.*, "Correlation of human placental enzymatic activity with trace metal concentration in placenta," *Environ Res*, 13:470–7, 1977

(339) H. Drexler, *et al.*, "The mercury concentration in breast milk resulting from amalgam fillings and dietary habits," *Environ Res*, 77(2):124–9, 1998

(341) A. Tosti, *et al.*, "Contact stomatitis," *Semin Cutan Med Surg*, 16(4):314–9, 1997; & T. Nakada, *et al.*, "Patch test materials for mercury allergic contact dermatitis," *Dermatitis*, 36(5):237–9, 1997

(342) V. Stejskal, "MELISA®: A new technology for diagnosing and monitoring of metal sensitivity," Proceedings: 33rd Annual Meeting of American Academy of Environmental Medicine, Nov. 1998, Baltimore, Maryland

(347) G. Benga, "Water exchange through erythrocyte membranes," *Neurol Neurochir Pol*, 1997 Sep–Oct; 31(5):905–13

(348) A. Kistner, "Quecksilbervergiftung durch amalgam: diagnose und therapie," *ZWR*, 104(5):412–17, 1995; & Mass, C., Bruck, W., "Study on the significance of mercury accumulation in the brain from dental amalgam fillings through direct mouth-nose-brain transport," *Zentralbl Hyg Umweltmed*, 198(3): 275–91, 1996

678   Eating Alive II

(349) M. Schaeffer, et al., "Risikofaktor Amalgam-Ein Problemstoff,"
       Schriftenreihe mweltmedizin, Forum Medizin
       Verlagsgesellschaft, 1996; & (b) Nixon, D. E., Mussmann, G. V.,
       Moyer, T. P., "Inorganic, organic, and total mercury in blood
       and urine," J Anal Toxicol, 10(1):17–22, 1996

(350) F. Schweinsberg, "Risk estimation of mercury intake from
       different sources," Toxicol Lett, 72:45–51, 1994; & L. D.
       Pzheusskaia, "Disintoxication therapy of patients with
       nonspecific inflammatory diseases of the female genital
       organs," Akush Ginekol, (4):30–4, 1977

(354) W. Behnke, "Kopfschmerz un migrane: schon mal an amalgam
       gegcht?" Der Allgemeinarzt, 17(11):1222–3, 1995; & J. Lechner,
       "Quecksilberbelastung,...," Dtsch Z Biol Zahnmed, 8(1):8–14,
       1992

(358) N. I. Shtelmakh, et al., "Comparative treatments of rheumatoid
       arthritis," Vrasch Delo, 1:49–52, 1982

(359) G. Tapparo, "Toxische Untersunchungen zu Amalgam," Die
       Zahn Arztwoche, 1992

(360) Buchet, J. P., Lauwerys, R. R., "Influence of DMPS on the
       mobilization of mercury from tissues of rats pretreated with
       mercuric chloride, phenylmercury acetate, or mercury vapor,"
       Toxicology, 54(3):323–33, 1989

(362) G. Bohmer, et al., "Quecksilber-mobilisation mit dern DMPS bei
       arztlichem und zahnarztlichem personal im Vergleich," Der
       Artikulator, 30:11–12, 1989; & W. Legrum, "Wie problematisch
       ist der dentalwerkstoff amalgam?" Dtsch Med Wochenschr,
       115(39):1490–4, 1990; & M. Cikrt, et al., "Mobilization of
       mercury using DMPS," Plzen Lek Sborn, 68(Supp):119, 1993;
       & R. Hickel, et al., "Die Quecksilberbelastung von
       Zahnmedizinstudenten anch beruflicher Amalgaexposition,"
       Dtsch Zahnarztl Z, 50(7):506–10, 1995

(363) J. W. Reinhardt, Univ. of Iowa College of Dentistry, "Side
       effects: mercury contribution to body burden from dental
       amalgam," Adv Dent Res, 6:110–3, 1992

(366) "Zahnamalgam und Schwangerschaft," *Geburtshilfe Frauenheikd*, 55(6):M63–M65, 1995; & T. Zinke, "Gibt es neue Erkenntnisse zur Amalgamproblematic?" in *Status Quo and Perspectives of Amalgam and Other Dental Materials*, L. F. Friberg (Ed.), Georg=Thieme-Verlag, Stuttgart, New York, 1995, p.1–7

(367) I. Gerhard, "Amalgam aus gynakologischer Sicht," *Der Frauenarzt*, 36(6):627–8, 1995; & "Schdstoffe und Fertillitatsstorungen," *Schwermetalle und Mineralstoffe, Geburtshilfe Frauenheikd*, 52(7):383–96, 1992; & "Reproductive risks of heavy metal and pesticides in women," in: *Reproductive Toxicology*, M. Richardson (Ed.), VCH Weinhelm, 1993, 167–83; & *Unfruchtbarkeit bei Frauen durch Umwelterkrankungen*, J. D. Kruse-Jarres (Ed.), 1993, 51–68

(368) Stejskal, V. D. M., Danersund, A., Lindvall, A., Hudecek, R., Nordman, V., Yaqob, A., *et al.*, "Metal-specific memory lymphocytes: biomarkers of sensitivity in man," *Neuroendocrinology Letters*, 1999

(369) Sterzl, I., Prochazkova, J., Stejskal, V. D. M., *et al.*, "Mercury and nickel allergy: risk factors in fatigue and autoimmunity," *Neuroendocrinology Letters*, 20:221–8, 1999

(370) Magos, L., Clarkson, T. W., Hudson, A. R., "The effects of dose of elemental mercury and first pass circulation time on organ distribution of inorganic mercury in rats," *Biochim Biophys Acta*, 991(1):85–9, 1989

(375) Stejskal, V. D. M., Danersund, A., Lindvall, A., "Metal-specific memory lymphocytes: biomarkers of sensitivity in man, *Neuroendocrinology Letters*, 1999; & Stejskal, V., Hudecek, R., Mayer, W, "Metal-specific lymphocytes: risk factors in CFS and other related diseases," *Neuroendocrinology Letters*, 20:289–98, 1999

(376) Melchart, D., Wuhr, E., Weidenhammer, W., Kremers, L., "A multicenter survey of amalgam fillings and subjective complaints in non-selected patients in the dental practice," *Eur J Oral Sci*, 106:770–7, 1998 (6,744 patients in 34 clinics)

(382) Sterzl, I., Fucikova, T., Zamrazil, V., "The fatigue syndrome in autoimmune thyroiditis with polyglanular activation of autoimmunity," *Vnitrni Lekarstvi*, 44:456–60, 1998

(385) Kohdera, T., Koh, N., Koh, R., "Antigen-specific lymphocyte stimulation test on patients with psoriasis vulgaris," XVI International Congress of Allergology and Clinical Immunology, Oct 1997, Cancun, Mexico; & Ionescu, G., "Schwermetallbelastung bei atopischer dermatitis und psoriasis," *Biol Med*, 2:65–8, 1996

(389) Brunker, P., Rother, D., Sedlmeier, R., *J Mol Gen Genet*, 251(3), 1996; & Williams, M. V., *Environ Mol Mutagen*, 27(1):30–3, 1996

(390) Ellingsen, D. G., Nordhagen, H. P., Thomassen, Y., "Urinary selenium excretion in workers with low exposure to mercury vapour," *J Appl Toxicol*, 15(1):33–6, 1995

(391) Schumann, K., "The toxicological estimation of heavy metal content (Hg, Cd, Pb) in food for infants and small children," *Z Ernahrungswiss*, 29(1):54–73, 1990 (article in German with English abstract)

(395) Shapiro, I. M., Cornblath, D. R., Sumner, A. J., "Neurophysiological and neuropsychological function in mercury-exposed dentists," *Lancet*, 1:1147–50, 1982; & Szzell, B. P., and Oler, J., "Chronic low-level mercury exposure and neuropsychological functioning," *J of Clin and Exper Neuropsych*, 8:581–93, 1986

(397) Hudecek, R., Danersund, A., "Removal of incompatible dental material in patients with intolerance of dental materials," in *Amalgam and Health: The Swedish Council for Planning and Research Coordination*, 1999, p. 78–84

(400) Kim, D. E., Song, K. B., Kim, Y. J., "Mercury contents in hair of dental personnel and evaluation of various agents suppressing mercury vaporization," *Taehan Chikkwa Uisa Hyophoe Chi*, 27(7):649–59

(401) Sikorski, R., Juszkiewicz, T., "Women in dental surgeries: reproductive hazards in occupational exposure to mercury," *Int Arch Occup Environ Health*, 59(6):551–7, 1987

(404) M. E. Godfrey, "Candida, dysbiosis, and amalgam," *J Adv Med*, 9(2), 1996; & Romani, L., Immunity to Candida albicans: Th1, Th2 cells, and beyond," *Curr Opin Microbiol*, 2(4):363–7, 1999; & Alfred V. Zamm, "Candida albicans therapy: dental mercury removal, an effective adjunct," *J Orthmol Med*, 1(4):261–5, 1986

(405) Jenny Stejskal, Vera Stejskal, "The role of metals in autoimmune diseases and the link to neuroendocrinology," *Neuroendocrinology Letters*, 20:345–58, 1999 (see #218)

(408) Eedy, D. J., Burrows, D, Dlifford, T., Fay, A., "Elevated T cell subpopulations in dental students," *J Prosthet Dent*, 63(5):593–6, 1990; & Yonk, L. J., *et al.*, "CD+4 helper T-cell depression in autism." *Immunol Lett*, 25(4):341–5, 1990; & Jaffe, J. S., Strober, W., Sneller, M. C., "Functional abnormalities of CD8+ T cells define a unique subset of patients with common variable immunodeficiency," *Blood*, 82(1):192–, 1993

(410) J. R. Cade, *et al.*, "Autism and schizophrenia linked to malfunctioning enzyme for milk protein digestion," *Autism*, Mar 1999

(411) Puschel, G., Mentlein, R., Heymann, E., "Isolation and characterization of dipeptidyl peptidase IV from human placenta," *Eur J Biochem*, 126(2):359–65, Aug 1982; & Kar, N. C., Pearson, C. M., "Dipeptyl peptidases in human muscle disease," *Clin Chim Acta*, 82(1–2):185–92, 1978; & Seroussi, K., *Autism and Pervasive Developmental Disorders*, 1998, p. 174, etc.

(412) Moreno-Fuenmayor, H., Borjas, L., Arrieta, A, Valera, V., "Plasma excitatory amino acids in autism," *Invest Clin*, 37(2):113–28, 1996; & Rolf, L. H., Haarman, F. Y., Grotemeyer, K. H., Kehrer, H., "Serotonin and amino acid content in platelets of autistic children," *Acta Psychiatr Scand*, 87(5):312–6, 1993; & Naruse, H., Hayashi, T., Takesada, M., Yamazaki, K., "Metabolic changes in aromatic amino acids and monoamines in infantile autism and a new related treatment," *No To*

Hattatsu, 21(2):181–9, 1989; & Carlsson, M. L., "Is infantile autism a hypoglutamatergic disorder?" *J Neural Transm*, 105(4–5):525–35, 1998

(423)   C. R. Adams, *et al.*, "Mercury intoxication simulating ALS," *JAMA*, 250(5):642–5, 1983; & T. Barber, "Inorganic mercury intoxification similar to ALS," *J of Occup Med*, 20:667–9, 1978

(427)   Chetty, C. S., McBride, V., Sands, S., Rajanna, B., "Effects in vitro on rat brain Mg(++)-ATPase," *Arch Int Physiol Biochim*, 98(5):261–7, 1990; & M. Burk, *et al.*, *Magnesium*, 4(5-6):325–32, 1985?

(433)   Epidemiologisk undersokning av fosterkador hos 1.2 milj. barn, fodda sedan 1967; Norge yrkesmed. Avd. Haukelands sykehus. Aftenposton 6 mpv 1997

(440)   Kidd, R. F., "Results of dental amalgam removal and mercury detoxification," *Altern Ther Health Med*, 6(4):49–55, Jul 2000

(453)   Blumer, W., "Mercury toxicity and dental amalgam fillings," *Journal of Advancement in Medicine*, 11(3):219, Fall 1998

(459)   Isny Clinic (South Germany), Kurt Muller, MD, member of Editorial board for Ganzheitliches Medicine Journal. Wassertornstrasse 6 , Isny, BRD Fax: 0049 7562 550 52

ARTICLE B

Oral Galvanism and Electromagnetic Fields (EMF): factors along with mercury's negative vapor pressure and extreme toxicity in significant exposure levels and oral effects from amalgam fillings. B. Windham (Ed.)

(B3)   R. H. Ogletree, *et al.*, School of Materials Science, GIT, Atlanta, "Effect of mercury on corrosion of etaÆ Cu-Sn phase in dental amalgams," *Dent Mater*, 11(5):332–6, 1995

(B4)   R. D. Meyer, *et al.*, "Intraoral galvanic corrosion," *Prosthet Dent*, 69(2):141–3, 1993; & J. Pleva, *J Orthomol Psych*, 12(3), 1983; & *J Of Orthomol Medicine*, 4:141–8, 1989; & "Mercury – a public health hazard," *Reviews on Environmental Health*, 10:1–27, 1994

(B5)   A. Buchner, *et al.*, "Amalgam tattoo of the oral mucosa: a clinicopathologic study of 268 cases," *Surg Oral Med Oral Pathol*, 49(2):139–47, 1980; & M. Forsell, *et al.*, "Mercury content in amalgam tattoos of human oral mucosa and its relation to local tissue reactions," *Euro J Oral Sci*, 106(1):582–7, 1998; & J. D. Harrison, *et al.*, "Amalgam tattoos: light and microscopy and electron-probe micro-analysis"; & T. Kanzaki, *et al.*, "Electron microscopic X-ray microanalysis of metals deposited in oral mucosa," *J Dermatol*, 19(8):487–92, 1992; & K. Nilner, *et al.*, "In vitro testing of dental materials by means of macrophage cultures," *J Biomed Mater Res*, 20(8):1125–38, 1986

(B11) Hal Huggins, *Its All in Your Head*, 1997; & Proceedings: ICBM Conf. Colorado, 1988; & S. Ziff, *Dentistry Without Mercury*, 8th Edition, 1996, Bio-Probe, Inc., ISBN 0-941011-04-6

(B15) V. Nadarajah, *et al.*, "Localized cellular inflammatory response to subcutaneously implanted dental mercury," *J Toxicol Environ Health*, Oct 11: 49(2):113–25

(B16) D. Brune, *et al.*, *Scand J Dent Res*, 19:66–71, 1983; & *Sci Tot Envir*, 44:..., 1985; & "Metal release from dental materials," *Biomaterials*, 7:163–75, 1986

(B17) C. Toomvali, "Studies of mercury vapor emission from different dental amalgam alloys," LIU-IFM-Kemi-EX 150, 1988; & D. B. Boyer, "Mercury vaporization from corroded dental amalgam," *Dental Materials*, 4:89–93, 1988

(B18) A. Berglund, "A study of the release of mercury vapor from different types of amalgam alloys," *J Dent Res*, 72:939–46, 1993

(B19) H. Lichtenberg, "Mercury vapor in the oral cavity in relation to the number of amalgam fillings and chronic mercury poisoning," *Journal of Orthomolecular Medicine*, 11(2):87–94, 1996

(B20) V. Psarras, *et al.*, Effect of selenium on mercury vapour released from dental amalgams," *Swed Dent J*, 18:15–23, 1994

(B21) L. E. Moberg, "Long term corrosion studies of amalgams and casting alloys in contact," *Acta Odontal Scand*, 43:163–77, 1985;

& L. E. Moberg, "Corrosion products from dental alloys," Published Dissertation, Stockholm, 1985

(B22) T. Weaver, *et al.*, "An amalgam tattoo causing local and systemic disease," *Oral Surg Oral Med Oral Pathol*, 63(1):137–40, 1987; & J. P. McGinnis, *et al.*, "Amalgam tattoo: use of energy dispersive X-ray analysis as an aid in diagnosis," *J Amer Dent Assoc*, 110(1):52–4, 1985

(B23) J. Pleva, *J Orthomol Psych*, 12(3), 1983 & *J Orthomol Medicine*, 4:141–8, 1989

(B24) P. E. Schneider, *et al.*, "Mercury release from Dispersalloy amalgam," IADR Abstracts #630, 1982; & N. Sarkar, "Amalgamtion reaction of Dispersalloy re-examined," IADR Abstracts #217, 1991; & N. K. Sarkar, *et al.*, IADR Abstracts # 895, 1976; & R. S. Mateer, *et al.*, IADR Abstracts #240, 1977; & N. K. Sarkar, *et al.*, IADR Abstracts #358, 1978; & N. W. Rupp, *et al.*, IADR Abstracts # 356, 1979

(B25) H. J. Lichtenberg, "Elimination of symptoms by removal of dental amalgam from mercury poisoned patients," *J Orthomol Med*, 8:145–8, 1993; & "Symptoms before and after removal of amalgam," *J Orthomol Med*, 11(4):195–, 1996

(B30) Forsell, M., Larsson, B., *et al.*, "Reactions of the oral mucosa related to silver amalgam: a review," *Eur J Oral Sci*, 106(1):582–7, Feb 1998; & Fisher, *et al.*, *J Oral Rehab*,11:399–405, 1984; & Goldschmidt, *et al.*, *J Perio Res*, 11:108–15, 1976; & Zander, *JADA*, 55:11–15, 1957; & *App J Prosth Dent*, 11:522–32, 1961; & Trott and Sherkat, *JCDA*, 30:766-70, 1964; & Sanches, Sotres, *et al.*, *J Periodo*, 140:543–6, 1969; & Turgeon, *et al.*, *JCDA*, 37:255–6, 1972; & Trivedi and Talim, *J Prosth Dentistry*, 29:73–81, 1973

(B31) E. R. Smart, *et al.*, "Resolution of lichen planus following removal of amalgam restorations," *Br Dent J*, 178(3):108–12,1995 (12 cases); & H. Markow, "Regression from orticaria following dental filling removal," *New York State J Med*, 1648–52, 1943; & G. Sasaki, *et al.*, "Three cases of oral lichenosis caused by metallic fillings," *J Dermatol*, 12:890–2, Dec 23, 1996; & J. Bratel, *et al.,* "Effect of replacement of dental amalgam on OLR," *Journal of Dentistry,* 24(1-2):41–5, 1996 (161 cases)

(B32) A. Skoglund, *Scand J Dent Res,* 102(4):216–22, 1994; and 99(4):320–9,1991 (40 cases); & P. O. Ostman, *et al.,* "Clinical & histologic changes after removal of amalgam," *Oral Surgery, Oral Medicine, and Endodontics,* 81(4):459–65, 1996; & S. H. Ibbotson, *et al.,* "The relevance of amalgam replacement on oral lichenoid reactions," *British Journal of Dermatology,* 134(3):420–3, 1996 (270 cases)

(B33) Y. Omura, *et al.,* Heart Disease Research Foundation, NY, NY, "Role of mercury in resistant infections and recovery after Hg detox with cilantro," *Acupuncture & Electro-Therapeutics Research,* 20(3):195–229, 1995; & "Mercury exposure from silver fillings," *Acupuncture & Electrotherapy Res,* 133–, 1996

(B34) R. L. Siblerud, "Relationship between dental amalgam and health," *Toxic Substances Journal,* 10:425–44, 1990b; & "Effects on health following removal of dental amalgams," *J Orthomolecular Med,* 5(2):95–106; & "Relationship between amalgam fillings and oral cavity health," *Ann Dent,* 49(2):6–10, 1990 (86 cured)

(B35) Redhe, O., *Sick From Amalgam,* R-Dental Ab, Frejavagen 33, S-79133 Falun, Sweden (in Swedish) (100 cases)

ARTICLE C
Neurological and Immune Reactive Conditions Affecting Kids: The mercury connection to neurological pervasive developmental disorders (autism, schizophrenia, dyslexia, ADD, childhood depression, learning disabilities, OCD, etc.) and developmental immune conditions (eczema, asthma, and allergies). Bernard Windham – Chemical Engineer

(C2) (c) Gary Null, *Second Opinion: Vaccinations,* Gary Null and Associates, Inc. 2000, http://www.garynull.com/marketplace/documents.asp; & (d) "Advocacy Groups Call for Research to Investigate Link Between Autism Increase and Vaccination," April 16, 1999: Autism Research Institute, Cure Autism Now, Autism Autoimmunity Project, and National Vaccine Information Center

(C11) V. D. M. Stejskal, Dept. of Clinical Chemistry, Karolinska Institute, Stockholm, Sweden, "Lymphocyte immuno-stimulation assay - MELISA," & "Mercury-specific lymphocytes: an indication of mercury allergy in man," *J Clinical Immunology*, 16(1):31–40, 1996; & V. D. M. Stejskal, *et al.*, "MELISA: tool for the study of metal allergy," *Toxicology In Vitro*, 8(5):991–1000, 1994, see: http://www.melisa.org

(C12) Sterzl, I., Prochazkova, J., Stejaskal, V. D. M., *et al.*, "Mercury and nickel allergy: risk factors in fatigue and autoimmunity," *Neuroendocrinology Letters*, 20:221–8, 1999; & V. Stejskal, "MELISA: a new technology for diagnosing and monitoring of metal sensitivity," Proceedings: 33rd Annual Meeting of American Academy of Environmental Medicine, Nov 1998, Baltimore, Maryland

(C14) Kurek, M., Przybilla, B., Hermann, K., Ring, J., "An opioid peptide from cows milk, beta-casomorphine-7, is a direct histamine releaser in man," *Int Arch Allergy Immunol*, 97(2): 115–20, 1992

(C15) Tejwani, G. A., Hanissian, S. H., "Modulation of mu, delta, and kappa opioid receptors in rat brain by metal ions and histidine," *Neuropharmacology*, 29(5): 445–52, 1990

(C16) Mondal, M. S., Mitra, S., "Inhibition of bovine xanthine oxidase activity by $Hg2+$ and other metal ions," *J Inorg Biochem*, 62(4): 271–9, 1996

(C17) Sastry, K. V., Gupta, P. K., "In vitro inhibition of digestive enzymes by heavy metals and their reversal by chelating agents: Part 1, mercuric chloride intoxication," *Bull Environ Contam Toxicol*, 20(6):729–35, 1978; & W. Y. Boadi, *et al.*, Dept. of Food Engineering and Biotechnology, T-I Inst of Tech., Haifa, Israel, "In vitro effect of mercury on enzyme activities," *Environ Res*, 57(1):96–106, 1992; & Horvath, K., Papadimitriou, J. C., Rabsztyn, A., Drachenberg, C., Tildon, J. T., "Gastrointestinal abnormalities in children with autistic disorder," *J Pediatr*, 135:559–63, 1999

(C18) McFadden, S. A., "Phenotypic variation in xenobiotic metabolism and adverse environmental response: focus on sulfur-dependent detoxification pathways," *Toxicology*, 111(1–3):43–65, 1996; & Markovich, *et al.*, "Heavy metals (Hg, Cd) inhibit the activity of the liver and kidney sulfate transporter Sat-1," *Toxicol Appl Pharmacol*, 154(2):181–7, 1999; & Matts, R. L., Schatz, J. R., Hurst, R., Kagen, R., "Toxic heavy metal ions inhibit reduction of disulfide bonds," *J Biol Chem*, 266(19):12695–702, 1991; & T. L. Perry, *et al.*, "Hallevorden-Spatz Disease: cysteine accumulation and cysteine dioxygenase deficiency," *Ann Neurol*, 18(4):482–9, 1985; & Ceaurriz, *et al.*, "Role of gamma-glutamyltraspeptidase (GGC) and extracellular glutathione in disopition of inorganic mercury," *J Appl Toxicol*, 14(3):201–, 1994

(C19) Puschel, G., Mentlein, R., Heymann, E., "Isolation and characterization of dipeptidyl peptidase IV from human placenta," *Eur J Biochem*, 126(2):359–65, Aug 1982; & Kar, N. C., Pearson, C. M., "Dipeptyl peptidases in human muscle disease," *Clin Chim Acta*, 82(1–2):185–92, 1978; & Seroussi, K., *Autism and Pervasive Developmental Disorders*, 1998, p. 174, etc.

(C20) Stefanovic, V., *et al.*, "Kidney ectopeptidases in mercuric chloride-induced renal failure," *Cell Physiol Biochem*, 8(5): 278–84, 1998

(C21) Crinnion, W. J., "Environmental toxins and their common health effects," *Altern Med Rev*, 5(1):52–63, 2000

(C22) Windham, B., "Annotated Bibliography: Adverse health effects related to mercury and amalgam fillings and clinically documented recoveries after amalgam replacement," (over 1,500 peer-reviewed references); www.home.earthlink.net/ ~berniew1/amalg6.html

(C23) Autism: a unique form of mercury poisoning, www.autism.com/ari/mercurylong.html; & Dr. A. Holmes, Autism Treatment Center, Baton Rouge, LA, http://www.healing-arts.org/children/holmes.htm; & Jaquelyn McCandless, M.D., Autism Spectrum Treatment Center, Woodland Hills, CA; & L. Redwood, "Mercury and autism," *Vitamin Research News*, 15(5):1–12, May 2001

(C24) J. R. Cade, *et al.*, "Autism and schizophrenia linked to malfunctioning enzyme for milk protein digestion," *Autism*, Mar 1999, http://www.hsc.ufl.edu/post/post0399/post03_19/1.html; & Application of the Exorphin Hypothesis to Attention Deficit Hyperactivity Disorder: A Theoretical Framework by Ronald Hoggan, A Thesis Submitted to The Faculty of Graduate Studies in Partial Fulfilment of the Requirements for The Degree of Master of Arts, Graduate Division of Educational Research, Calgary, April, 1998, University of Calgary

(C25) Reichelt, K. L., "Biochemistry and psychophysiology of autistic syndromes," *Tidsskr Nor Laegeforen*, 114(12):1432–4, 1994; & Reichelt, K. L., *et al.*, "Biologically active peptide-containing fractions in schizophrenia and childhood autism," *Adv Biochem Psychopharmacol*, 28:627–43, 1981; Lucarelli, S., Cardi, E., *et al.*, "Food allergy and infantile autism," *Panminerva Med*, 37(3):137–41, 1995; & Shel, L., "Autistic disorder and the endogenous opioid system," *Med Hypotheses*, 48(5):413–4, 1997

(C26) Huebner, F. R., Lieberman, K. W., Rubino, R. P., Wall, J. S., Demonstration of high opioid-like activity in isolated peptides from wheat gluten hydrolysates," *Peptides*, 5(6):1139–47, 1984

(C27) Willemsen-Swinkels, S. H., Buitelaar, J. K., Weijnen, F. G., Thisjssen, J. H., Van Engeland, H., "Plasma beta-endorphin concentrations in people with learning disability and self-injurious and/or autistic behavior," *Br J Psychiatry*, 168(1):105–9, 1996; & Leboyer, M., Launay, J. M., *et al.*, "Difference between plasma N- and C-terminally directed beta-endorphin immunoreactivity in infantile autism," *Am J Psychiatry*, 151(12): 1797–1801, 1994

(C29) Eedy, D. J., Burrows, D., Dlifford, T., Fay, A., "Elevated T cell subpopulations in dental students," *J Prosthet Dent*, 63(5):593–6, 1990; & Yonk, L. J., *et al.*, "CD+4 helper T-cell depression in autism," *Immunol Lett*, 25(4):341–5, 1990

(C30) Edelson, S. B., Cantor, D. S., "Autism: xenobiotic influences," *Toxicol Ind Health*, 14(4): 553–63, 1998; & Liska, D. J., "The detoxification enzyme systems," *Altern Med Rev*, 3(3):187–98,

1998; & © HRI-Pfeiffer Center Autism Study; paper presented to Dan Conference, Jan 2001; www.hriptc.ort/Publish0900/index.html.

(C35) Stejskal, V. D. M., Danersund, A., Lindvall, A., Hudecek, R., Nordman, V., Yaqob, A., *et al.*, "Metal-specific memory lymphocytes: biomarkers of sensitivity in man," *Neuroendocrinology Letters*, 1999; & V. D. M. Stejskal, *et al.*, "Mercury-specific lymphocytes: an indication of mercury allergy in man," *J of Clinical Immunology*, 16(1):31–40, 1996; & V. Stejskal, "MELISA: a new technology for diagnosing and monitoring of metal sensitivity," Proceedings: 33rd Annual Meeting of American Academy of Environmental Medicine, Nov 1998, Baltimore, Maryland. See http://www.melisa.org

(C36) Alberti, A., Pirrone, P., Elia, M., Waring, R. H., Romano, C., "Sulphation deficit in 'low-functioning' autistic children," *Biol Psychiatry*, 46(3):420–4, 1999

(C37) Wakefield, A., *et al.*, "Ileal-lymphoid-nodular hyperplasia and pervasive developmental disorder in children," *Lancet*, 351(9103):637–41, 1998; & Kawashima, H., Mori, T., Kashiwagi, Y., Takekuma, K., Hoshika, A., Wakefield, A., "Detection and sequencing of measles virus from peripheral mononuclear cells from patients with inflammatory bowel and autism," *Dig Dis Sci*, 45(4):723–9, 2000; & Wakefield, A., *et al.*, "Inflammatory bowel disease syndrome and autism," *Lancet*, Feb 27, 2000; & (b) Singh, V. K., Lin, S. X., Yang, V. C., "Serological association of measles virus and human herpesvirus-6 with brain autoantibodies in autism," *Clin Immunol Immunopathol*, 89(1):105–8, Oct 1998

(C38) B. J. Shenker, *et al.*, "Immunotoxic effects of mercuric compounds on human lymphocytes and monocytes: alterations in B-cell function and viability," *Immunopharmacol Immunotoxicol*, 15(1):87–112, 1993; & J. R. Daum, "Immunotoxicology of mercury and cadmium on B-lymphocytes," *Int J Immunopharmacol*, 15(3):383–94, 1993

(C39) Pfieffer, S. I., Norton, J., Nelson, L., Shott, S., "Efficacy of vitamin B6 and magnesium in the treatment of autism," *J*

Autism Dev Disord, 25(5):481-93, Oct 1995; & Chuang, D., *et al.*, National Institute of Mental Health, *Science News*, 158:309, Nov 11, 2000; & "Lithium protects against neuron damage by glutamate," *Science News*, 3–14-98, p. 164; & Moore, G. J., *et al.*, *Lancet*, Oct 7, 2000; & *Science News*, 10–31–98, p. 276

(C40) Autism-Mercury@egroups.com, web group of parents with autistic kids and autism doctors and researchers; & (b) Dr. S. B. Edelson, http://www.edelsoncenter.com; & (c) Eppright, T. D., Sanfacon, J. A., Horwitz, E. A.., "ADHD, infantile autism, and elevated blood-lead: a possible relationship," (case study) *Mo Med*, 93(3):136–8, 1996

(C47) Moreno-Fuenmayor, H., Borjas, L., Arrieta, A., Valera, V., "Plasma excitatory amino acids in autism," *Invest Clin*, 37(2):113–28, 1996; & Rolf, L. H., Haarman, F. Y., Grotemeyer, K. H., Kehrer, H., "Serotonin and amino acid content in platelets of autistic children," *Acta Psychiatr Scand*, 87(5):312–6, 1993; & Naruse, H., Hayashi, T., Takesada, M., Yamazaki, K., "Metabolic changes in aromatic amino acids and monoamines in infantile autism and a new related treatment," *No To Hattatsu*, 21(2):181–9, 1989; & Carlsson, M. L., "Is infantile autism a hypoglutamatergic disorder?" *J Neural Transm*, 105(4–5):525–35, 1998

(C48) Reichrtova, E., *et al.*, "Cord serum immunoglobulin E related to environmental contamination of human placentas with oganochlorine compounds," *Envir Health Perspec*, 107(11):895–9, 1999; & Gavett, S. H., *et al.*, "Residual oil fly ash amplifies allergic cytokines, airway responsiveness, and inflammation in mice," *Am J Respir Crit Care Med*, 160(6):1897–1904, 1999; & Kramer, U., *et al.*, "Traffic-related air pollution is associated with atopy in children living in urban areas," *Epidemiology*, 11(1):64–70, 2000

(C50) B. Windham, Cognitive and Behavioral Effects of Toxic Metals (over 100 medical study references), berniew1@earthlink.net

(C51) Walsh, W. J., Health Research Institute, Autism and Metal Metabolism, http://www.hriptc.org/autism.htm, Oct 20, 2000; & Walsh, W. J., Pfeiffer Treatment Center, Metal-Metabolism and Human Functioning, 2000, http://www.hriptc.org/

mhfres.htm; & HRI-Pfeiffer Center Autism Study; paper
presented to Dan Conference, Jan 2001

ARTICLE D
Effects of Toxic Metals on Learning Ability and Behavior

(D33) T. Colburn, *et al.*, "Developmental effects of endocrine-
disrupting chemicals in wildlife and humans," *Environmental
Health Perspectives*, 101(5), Oct 1993; & "Mercury found in dead
Florida Bay cormorants," *Tallahassee Democrat*,1-15-95; & "Are
environmental hormones emasculating wildlife?" *Science News*,
145:25–27, 1994; & C. F. Facemire, *et al.*, "Reproductive
impairment in the Florida panther," *Health Perspect*, 103
(Supp4):79–86, 1995; & I. Gerhard, *et al.*, "The limits of
hormone substitution in pollutant exposure and fertility
disorders," *Zentralbl Gynakol*, 114:593–602, 1992

(D34) "Cadmium Hazards to Fish, Wildlife, and Invertebrates," U.S.
Fish & Wildlife Service, Contamination Hazard Biological
Report 85(1.2), 1987; & "Mercury bioaccumulation in lake
ecosystems," Electric Power Research Inst., *EPRI Journal*,
December, 1994, p. 5; & Bender, M. T., and Williams, J. M.,
Public Health Reports, 414:416–20, 1999

(D35) *Birth Defects Prevention News*, March 1986, p. 3; & Ryan, P. B.,
et al., "Exposure to arsenic, cadmium, and lead in drinking
water," *Environ Health Perspectives*, 108(8), Aug 2000

(D36) Florida Dept. of Environmental Protection, Florida Coastal
Sediment Contaminants Atlas: A Summary of Coastal Sediment
Quality Surveys, 1994; & Mac Donald Environmental Sciences
Ltd., Development of an Approach to the Assessment of
Sediment Quality in Florida Coastal Waters, FDEP, January
1993; & J. H. Trefry, *et al.*, Marine & Environmental Chemistry
Laboratories, Fla. Institute of Technology, Toxic Substances
Survey for the Indian River Lagoon System, Volume I: Trace
Metals in the Indian River Lagoon, SJWMD, Feb 1993; & D. C.
Heil, Fla. Dept. of Natural Resources, Division of Marine
Resources, Evaluation of Trace Metal Monitoring in Florida
Shellfish, March 1986; & U.S. EPA, Environmental Monitoring
and Assessment Program, Estuaries: Louisianian Province–1992
& 1991

(D37) H. R. Casdorph, *Toxic Metal Syndrome*, Avery Publishing Group, 1995; & S. E. Levick, Yale Univ. School of Medicine, *New England Journal of Medicine*, July 17, 1980; & Muldoon, S. B., *et al.*, "Effects of lead levels on cognitive function of older women," *Neuroepidemiology*, 15(2):62–72, 1996; & Neddleman, H. L., *et al.*, "The long-term effects of exposure to low doses of lead in childhood," *N Eng J Med*, 322(2):83-8, 1990; & Michael Smith, "Woman's poison fillings blamed for attack on mother," *The Daily Telegraph*, 9–26–1998, p. 14

(D43) B. Windham, "Annotated Bibliography: Health effects related to mercury from amalgam fillings and documented clinical results of replacement of amalgam fillings," 2001, (over 800 references & 60,000 clinical cases), www.home.earthlink.net/~berniew1/indexa.html); & (b) B. Windham, "Common exposure levels and developmental effects of mercury in infants," 2001, www.home.earthlink.net/~berniew1/indexk.html

Index

Macular degeneration: 438, 578
Manic depression: xii
Measles: 374, 376, 390, 391,
  394, 462, 505, 506
Melatonin: 455, 528, 529
MELISA® testing: 7, 327–331,
  336, 338, 381, 389, 396
Mercuric chloride: 3, 4, 296,
  308, 329, 474, 527
Mercury: v, vii, x, 3–8, 11–13,
  18, 19, 24, 40, 41, 43, 44, 49,
  50, 58, 59, 63–65, 85, 91,
  271, 275–360, 367, 372, 380,
  382–389, 391, 392, 394, 395,
  397, 400, 401, 449, 450, 465,
  467–470, 473–475, 527, 528,
  531, 548, 591
Mercury-amalgam fillings/
  mercury fillings: 3–6, 40,
  44, 65, 276, 277, 279, 281,
  286, 290, 291, 295, 296, 299,
  301–303, 305–308, 310–314,
  316, 318, 326–329, 331–336,
  338, 340–348, 356–358, 360,
  372, 382, 384, 389, 392, 400,
  470, 474, 475, 506, 512, 527,
  591
Mercury vapour: 3, 4, 6, 286,
  300–303, 307–312, 314, 317,
  357, 359, 465, 474
Methionine: 7, 285, 404, 408,
  442
Methylmercury: 4, 303–306,
  310, 318
Methyl-Sulfonyl-Methane
  (MSM): 7, 20, 59, 83, 283,
  285, 450, 541
Migraines: 45, 334, 337, 605,
  606, 618

Milk thistle: 20, 59, 83, 541,
  542
Multiple sclerosis (MS): xii,
  44, 46, 96, 290, 291, 329,
  332–334, 337, 341, 366, 374,
  390, 462, 494, 573
Mycobacteria: 487–489, 580,
  582, 583, 585, 600
Myopia: 578

N-acetylcysteine (NAC): 7,
  285, 449
NAD/NADP: 529–531
National Vaccine Information
  Center, The: 13, 14, 364, 365,
  626
Negative ions: x, 35–37, 596,
  599, 601–603, 606, 607,
  609–615, 617
Neutrophil: 321, 556, 557, 566
Nicotinic acid: 529

Organic: x, 27, 67, 82, 109–111,
  464, 466
Osteoblasts: 558, 559, 566
Osteoclasts: 558, 559, 566
Osteoporosis: 26, 539
Oxygen: 1, 17, 23, 31–33, 35,
  101, 102, 106, 108, 309, 357,
  406, 409, 410, 440, 444, 445,
  454, 467, 475–477, 489, 491,
  494, 496, 499, 545–591,
  595–599, 601–604, 606, 609,
  610, 613–617
Ozone layer: 465, 598

p53: 47, 434, 435, 438, 451
Parkinson's disease: xii, 4, 44,
  329, 331, 334, 415, 462

List of Naturopathic Associations

**To find a Naturopathic Physician in your area,
please contact the association nearest you.**

British Columbia Naturopathic Association
2238 Pine Street
Vancouver, BC   V6J 5G4
(604) 736-6646   Fax: (604) 736-6048
Toll-free in Canada: 1-800-277-1128
Website: www.bcna.ca

Ontario Association of Naturopathic Doctors
344 Bloor Street West, Suite 602
Toronto, Ontario   M5S 3A7
(416) 233-2001   Fax: (416) 233-2924
Website: www.oand.com

Canadian Association of Naturopathic Doctors
1255 Sheppard Ave. East
North York, Ontario   M2K 1E2
(416) 496-8633   Fax: (416) 496-8634
Toll-free: 1-800-551-4381
Website: www.naturopathicassoc.ca

American Association of Naturopathic Physicians
3201 New Mexico Avenue, NW Suite 350
Washington, DC   20016
(202) 895-1392   Fax: (202) 274-1992
Toll-free: 1-866-538-2267
Website: www.naturopathic.org